# Construction Safety, Health and Well-being in the COVID-19 Era

This edited book presents a significant and timely contribution to our understanding of a broad range of issues pertaining to COVID-19 and its relationship to occupational safety, health and well-being (OSHW) in the global construction industry.

The editors first introduce the industry and its poor OSHW history before highlighting some of the broader impacts of the pandemic on the sector. The book is then divided into two sections. Section One focuses on the management of COVID-19 transmission risk. It captures insights, practices, technologies and lessons learned in relation to what has and is being done to prevent or mitigate the risk of COVID-19 transmission among the construction workforce. *Construction Safety, Health and Well-being in the COVID-19 Era* also details case studies, lessons and best practices for managing sites and workforces when infections inevitably do occur. Section Two brings together international chapters discussing the impacts of COVID-19 on the OSHW of the construction workforce both on and off-site, as well as the management of those impacts. Furthermore, this presents implications of the pandemic (at the short-, medium- and long-term) for other performance measures of construction projects such as cost, schedule, quality and, most importantly, how the pursuit/non-pursuit of such performance measures have impacted/will impact the OSHW of construction workers and professionals in the industry.

This book addresses the gap in literature by offering global perspectives on the OSHW impacts and implications of COVID-19 in the construction industry and will help its wide readership (including construction industry organisations, professionals, researchers, government bodies/policy makers and students) to understand a broad suite of issues pertaining to COVID-19 and its relationship to OSHW in construction.

**Patrick Manu** is a professor of innovative construction and project management at the School of Architecture and Environment, University of the West of England. He is a research-active academic with an international reputation for construction safety and health research, which has underpinned exceptional contribution to knowledge transfer and external engagement in the construction industry, both in the United Kingdom and internationally. He has been involved as principal investigator (PI) and co-investigator in research projects (valued at over GBP £1.9 million) funded by several organisations. He led (as PI) an international consortium in an EPSRC-funded research to develop the first web-based application for assessing design for safety organisational capability, which won an innovation award from HS2 Ltd. He has over 120 publications.

**Clara Cheung** is a reader in the Department of Mechanical, Aerospace and Civil Engineering (MACE) at The University of Manchester (UoM). She specialises in occupational health, safety and well-being (OSHW) management in high-risk industries in the United Kingdom (UK) and internationally. Since joining UoM in 2017, Clara has secured over GBP £2.3 million external funding as PI and Co-I to improve OSHW performance in the construction industry. During the COVID period, she led a work package in the Keeping the UK Building Safely project funded by Health and Safety Executive, the UK occupational health and safety regulator, to model transmission risks of different protective measures on construction sites. Her publications, including book chapters, industry reports, conference papers and articles in leading Q1 journals, have contributed to practice and theory development in OSHW management.

**Akilu Yunusa-Kaltungo** is a reader in reliability and maintenance engineering, as well as the Head of Mechanical Engineering Education at the Department of Mechanical, Aerospace and Civil Engineering (MACE), The University of Manchester. He has a diverse range of research specialties, owing to his blend of academic and industrial experience. Some of the areas in which Akilu has developed notable international reputation include improving OSH performance across high-risk sectors, decarbonisation of high-energy industrial operations, building energy consumption prediction and optimisation, vibration-based condition monitoring of industrial machines, machine learning-based faults detection and diagnosis, construction projects risk classification, etc. Through collaborations with reputable research-focused institutions such as Health & Safety Executive (HSE-UK), Lloyd's Register Foundation (LRF), InnovateUK, EPSRC, etc. He has supported the realisation of over GBP £1.6 million external research funding, either as Principal Investigator (PI) or Co-Investigator (Co-I). He has also generated over 130 technical publications in the form of high-impact journal articles, peer-reviewed conference articles, textbooks, book chapters, government commissioned reports and professional articles.

**Fidelis Emuze** is a professor and the Head of the Department of Built Environment at the Central University of Technology, Free State (CUT), South Africa. Lean construction, health, safety and sustainability constitute the primary research interest of Professor Emuze, who is a National Research Foundation-rated researcher. He has published over 250 research outputs and received over 25 awards and recognitions. Professor Emuze is the editor of *Value and Waste in Lean Construction, Valuing People in Construction* and co-editor of *Construction Health and Safety in Developing Countries*. He authored *Construction Safety Pocketbook for South Africa* in 2020. Professor Emuze is the International Coordinator of CIB W123 – People in Construction Working Commission.

**Tarcisio Abreu Saurin** is a full professor at the Industrial Engineering Department of the Federal University of Rio Grande do Sul, Brazil. He has a PhD in industrial engineering (2002), a MS in construction management (1997) and a BS in civil engineering (1994). He was a visiting professor at Sapienza University of Rome (2022), Australian Institute of Health Innovation at Macquarie University (2018), and the University of Salford, UK (2012). His main research interests are related to resilience engineering, safety management, lean production, and complexity theory. He has carried out research and consulting projects on these topics in healthcare, construction, electricity distribution, and manufacturing. He has also supervised 70 postgraduate students (54 MS and 16 PhD) and authored a number of journal papers, book chapters, and conference papers on these topics. He is a member of the editorial board of *Safety Science* journal.

**Bonaventura Hadikusumo** is a full professor in construction management at Asian Institute of Technology, Thailand. He has been teaching and conducting research in construction project management, including construction safety management, since 1996. He has published many research articles, book chapters and books. He has been teaching and training scholars, construction professionals and government officers in construction industry in South East Asia countries. During the Covid19 pandemic, he conducted research and seminars in Covid19 management in construction projects in Singapore, China, Japan, Vietnam, Indonesia, Malaysia, Myanmar and Thailand.

# Spon Research

Publishes a stream of advanced books for built environment researchers and professionals from one of the world's leading publishers. The ISSN for the Spon Research programme is ISSN 1940–7653 and the ISSN for the Spon Research E-book programme is ISSN 1940–8005

**Improving the Performance of Construction Industries for Developing Countries**
Programmes, Initiatives, Achievements and Challenges
*Edited by Pantaleo D Rwelamila and Rashid Abdul Aziz*

**Work Stress Induced Chronic Diseases in Construction**
Discoveries Using Data Analytics
*Imriyas Kamardeen*

**Life-Cycle Greenhouse Gas Emissions of Commercial Buildings**
An Analysis for Green-Building Implementation Using A Green Star Rating System
*Cuong N. N. Tran, Vivian W. Y. Tam and Khoa N. Le*

**Data-driven BIM for Energy Efficient Building Design**
*Saeed Banihashemi, Hamed Golizadeh and Farzad Pour Rahimian*

**Successful Development of Green Building Projects**
*Tayyab Ahmad*

**BIM and Construction Health and Safety**
Uncovering, Adoption and Implementation
*Hamed Golizadeh, Saeed Banihashemi, Carol Hon and Robin Drogemuller*

**Construction Safety, Health and Well-being in the COVID-19 Era**
*Edited by Patrick Manu, Clara Cheung, Akilu Yunusa-Kaltungo, Fidelis Emuze, Tarcisio Abreu Saurin and Bonaventura Hadikusumo*

For more information about this series, please visit: www.routledge.com

# Construction Safety, Health and Well-being in the COVID-19 Era

**Edited by Patrick Manu, Clara Cheung, Akilu Yunusa-Kaltungo, Fidelis Emuze, Tarcisio Abreu Saurin and Bonaventura Hadikusumo**

Routledge
Taylor & Francis Group

LONDON AND NEW YORK

First published 2024
by Routledge
4 Park Square, Milton Park, Abingdon, Oxon OX14 4RN

and by Routledge
605 Third Avenue, New York, NY 10158

*Routledge is an imprint of the Taylor & Francis Group, an informa business*

*British Library Cataloguing-in-Publication Data*
A catalogue record for this book is available from the British Library

*Library of Congress Cataloging-in-Publication Data*
Names: Manu, Patrick, editor. | Cheung, Clara, Dr. editor. | Yunusa-
    Kaltungo, Akilu, editor. | Emuze, Fidelis, editor. | Saurin, Tarcisio, editor. |
    Hadikusumo, Bonaventura H. W., editor.
Title: Construction safety, health and well-being in the COVID-19 era /
    edited by Patrick Manu, Clara Cheung, Akilu Yunusa-Kaltungo, Fidelis
    Emuze, Tarcisio Abreu Saurin and Bonaventura Hadikusumo.
Description: Abingdon, Oxon ; New York, NY : Routledge, 2024. | Includes
    bibliographical references.
Identifiers: LCCN 2023008363 | ISBN 9781032229157 (hardback) |
    ISBN 9781032243917 (paperback) | ISBN 9781003278368 (ebook)
Classification: LCC RC965.C75 C667 2023 | DDC 363.11028/4—dc23/
    eng/20230406
LC record available at https://lccn.loc.gov/2023008363

ISBN: 978-1-032-22915-7 (hbk)
ISBN: 978-1-032-24391-7 (pbk)
ISBN: 978-1-003-27836-8 (ebk)

DOI: 10.1201/9781003278368

Typeset in Times New Roman
by Apex CoVantage, LLC

# Contents

# Contributors

**Abdullahi Muhammad** is a senior lecturer at the Department of Quantity Surveying, Ahmadu Bello University, Zaria. His research interest is in information and communications technology (ICT) in construction. He had his first degree in quantity surveying, master's in project management and PhD in quantity surveying, all from Ahmadu Bello University, Zaria. He is a member of the Nigerian Institute of Quantity Surveyors (NIQS) and a registered quantity surveyor with the Quantity Surveyors Registration Board of Nigeria (QSRBN). He has published several articles in reputable journals and has attended many conferences.

**Adetayo Onososen** is a doctoral candidate at the Department of Quantity Surveying and Construction Management, University of Johannesburg, South Africa, researching sustainable infrastructure delivery, emerging technologies in AEC, BIM, and human-robot teams in construction at the Centre of Applied Research and Innovation in the Built Environment (CARINBE). He is the sub-editor of the *Journal of Construction Innovation and Cost Management (JCICM)*. His research interests and publications cover the areas of digitalisation in construction, robotics, virtual reality and sustainable development.

**Agustina Kiky Anggraini** graduated from the Faculty of Civil Engineering, Geo and Environmental Sciences, Karlsruher Institut für Technologie, Germany, with a scholarship from the Directorate General of Higher Education, Ministry of Education and Culture, Republic of Indonesia, in 2018. After that, she joined Universitas Atma Jaya Yogyakarta. She serves as an assistant professor at the Department of Civil Engineering, Universitas Atma Jaya Yogyakarta, Indonesia. Her research interest is in water resources management and environmental engineering. Currently, she is working on a research project on the contaminant movement in groundwater.

**Albert P.C. Chan** is a chair professor of construction engineering and management, Dean of Students, Associate Director of Research Institute for Sustainable Urban Development and Able Professor in Construction Health and Safety at The Hong Kong Polytechnic University. With over 800 publications, his research has significantly impacted policy decisions in the construction industry. His team's interdisciplinary undertaking in health and safety is a multi-award-winning Anti-Heat Stress Uniform (AHSU), which decreases heat stockpiling by 28.8% and improves warm solace by 14.2%. The uniform is presently the standard clothing for all open works contracts appointed by the Hong Kong government.

**Alfredo Serpell** is a professor in the School of Engineering at the Universidad del Desarrollo, Chile. A civil engineer from the Catholic University of Chile, he obtained a M.Sc. and Ph.D. degrees in architectural and civil engineering respectively at the University of Texas at Austin, Texas, USA. During his academic life, he has worked as a researcher and consultant on the following subjects: construction and project management, conceptual cost estimation, risk management, contract management, claims analysis, productivity and quality management, and other related topics. He has more than 150 publications in journals, conferences, and in several specialized books on these topics.

**Alime Sanlı** is a Ph.D. student in the Department of Architecture and the Project and Construction Management program at Istanbul Technical University, Turkey. Her research interests are student resilience, stress management, well-being, personality, organizational resilience, and agility.

**Amir Mahdiyar** is a senior lecturer and program coordinator in the department of Construction Project Management at Universiti Sains Malaysia. He is a chartered construction manager and a chartered member of the Chartered Institute of Building. He has achieved the status of Fellow (FHEA) from HEA and served as associate editor, guest editor and reviewer of several international journals. His research areas include construction safety, risk management, green roof implementation, probabilistic cost-benefit analysis, artificial intelligence, and multi-criteria decision making.

**Andrea Yunyan Jia** is an academic at the Department of Building and Real Estate at the Hong Kong Polytechnique University (PolyU). She received her PhD from The University of Hong Kong in 2009. Before joining PolyU, she worked as a senior lecturer at the Faculty of Architecture, Building and Planning at The University of Melbourne, and in research and teaching positions at National University of Singapore, Curtin University. The University of Hong Kong, and Sichuan University. Her research is focused on institutional logics in the architecture, engineering and construction (AEC) industry and the climate.

**Anita Odame Adade-Boateng**, Ph.D., is a lecturer in construction management in the Department of Construction Technology and Management, Kwame Nkrumah University of Science and Technology (KNUST), Kumasi, Ghana. Her research interests include construction health and safety, environmental and social impact of construction, and human resources management within the construction industry. She has served as a reviewer for a number of journals and conferences, both locally and internationally. She is a member of the Ghana Institute of Surveyors (GhIS), and has over 14 years of work experience in the construction industry within quantity surveying and construction management roles.

**Aung Paing** is a planning engineer who got bachelor of engineering at West Yangon Technological University (WYTU) in Myanmar in 2019. He is also an alumni of the Asian Institute of Technology (AIT). He finished his master of engineering in construction engineering and infrastructure management at AIT in 2021. He has deep knowledge in construction planning, scheduling and monitoring. Construction management software such as Primavera P6 and Microsoft Project are his expertise.

**Babatunde Fatai Ogunbayo** obtained his Ph.D. from the University of Johannesburg in construction management, focusing on maintenance management and services. He is presently doing his post-doctoral research fellowship (PDRF) in the Department of Construction Management and Quantity Surveying, Faculty of Engineering and the Built Environment, University of Johannesburg, South Africa. As a researcher, Ogunbayo has authored, co-authored, and presented at various international conferences. He has conducted research in several areas, including maintenance management and services, construction material testing and analysis, public-private partnership, housing, building component analysis, artificial intelligence, construction health, safety, welfare, and productivity.

**Bello Mahmud Zailani** is currently a Ph.D. student at the Department of Civil Engineering, Morgan State University, USA. He has several publications in both peer-reviewed journals and conference proceedings around the world, mainly focused on health and safety management in construction. He holds a bachelor's degree in building, and a master's degree in project management, both from Ahmadu Bello University, Nigeria. He is a member of the Nigerian Institute of Building (NIOB) and the American Society of Civil Engineering (ASCE), both of which underpin and promote safety in construction practices.

**Che Khairil Izam Che Ibrahim** is an associate professor at the School of Civil Engineering, Universiti Teknologi MARA, Malaysia. He holds a PhD from the University of Auckland, New Zealand. He is currently leading a project on prevention through design in construction funded by the National Institute of Occupational Safety and Health (NIOSH), Malaysia, and has been involved in several projects funded by public and private organisations. Previously, he led a research project on multi-organisational integration funded by the Ministry of Education under the Fundamental Research Grant Scheme (FRGS) (completed in 2019), construction safety-related research funded by SOCSO (completed in 2017, 2019 and 2020) and a project evaluation framework funded by Malaysia Development Bank (completed in 2020).

**Christina M. Scott-Young** is a clinical psychologist and organizational behaviour scholar who researches in the fields of project teamwork, leadership, work readiness, resilience, wellbeing and diversity. Christina is an associate professor at RMIT University, having previously held academic positions at Pennsylvania State University, the University of South Australia and at Melbourne University, where she was awarded her PhD in management in 2008. Her research has been published in *Construction Management and Economics, Engineering*

*Construction and Architectural Management, Journal of Operations Management, International Journal of Operations and Production Management, International Journal of Project Management* and the *Project Management Journal.*

**Chunxue Liu** is a lecturer in project management at University of the West of Scotland (London Campus). She obtained her PhD in management of projects and a master's degree with distinction in management of projects from the University of Manchester. She obtained a bachelor's degree with an upper second-class honour in business and management studies from the University of Bradford. She has participated in teaching and supporting activities since 2017, and achieved Fellowship status of the AdvanceHE (FHEA) in 2021. Her research interests include leadership development, mindfulness, project management, and occupational health and safety.

**Clinton O. Aigbavboa** is a professor of sustainable human development in the Department of Construction Management and Quantity Surveying, University of Johannesburg, South Africa. He has published over 800 research papers. He is also an author of many scholarly research books published with Springer Nature and CRC Press. He has extensive knowledge in practice, research, training and teaching. He is currently the Director and Research Chair in sustainable construction management and leadership in the built environment and Director of the CIDB Centre of Excellence. Furthermore, he is the chief editor of the *Journal of Construction Project Management and Innovation* (accredited by the DHET) and a recipient of several national and international recognitions. He is an active postgraduate degree supervisor (masters and PhD) with more than 100+ masters and 45 doctoral students supervised to completion.

**David J. Edwards** is a senior professor at Birmingham City University, UK, a Distinguished Visiting Professor at University of Johannesburg and visiting professor at KNUST, Deakin University and University of South Australia. David is listed in the top 2% of global scientists and has attracted circa £15 million in funding over his career. He is reviewer for over 70 academic journals and editor for several others. David is currently working for National Highways (a UK government company) and has worked previously for various UK government bodies, the US Department of Defense and UK Ministry of Defence.

**Dayana Bastos Costa** is an associate professor in the Structural and Construction Engineering Department of the School of Engineering at the Federal University of Bahia – Brazil. She has a BSc in Civil Engineering (Federal University of Bahia) and MSc and Ph.D. in Civil Engineering – Construction Management (Federal of Rio Grande do Sul-Brazil). She was a visiting student at the University of Salford (2006–2007) in the UK and visiting professor at the Georgia Institute of Technology in the US (2014–2015). Dr. Costa's research includes construction management and technology to improve industry performance, involving aspects related to production, quality, safety and sustainability, integrating with digital technologies, such as unmanned aerial systems and building information modeling.

**Emmanuel Adinyira**, Ph.D., is an associate professor of construction project management in the Department of Construction Technology and Management, Kwame Nkrumah University of Science and Technology (KNUST) Kumasi, Ghana. His areas of specialisation include construction project management, construction safety, health and environment and construction education and training. He has served as a guest editor, editor, sectional editor, editorial board member and reviewer for several national and international journals and conferences. His global experience in construction education and training includes working as a visiting scholar at Loughborough University, UK, among others.

**Ferdinand Fassa** is the Head of Construction Engineering and Management Programme at Podomoro University. He has produced five books in Bahasa, Indonesia, namely *Pengantar Keselamatan dan Kesehatan Kerja Konstruksi/ Introduction to Construction Occupational Health and Safety* (2020), *Metode Pengadaan Jasa Konstruksi dan Proses Penawaran/Construction Procurement Methods and Bidding Process* (2020), *Manajemen Logistik Konstruksi/Construction Logistics Management* (2021), *Perencanaan Konstruksi Berkelanjutan/Sustainable Construction Planning* (2022) *and Manajemen Tim Proyek/ Project Team Management* (2022).

**Gumbert Maylda Pratama** received his master's degree from the Civil and Environmental Engineering Department, Universitas Gadjah Mada, Yogyakarta, Indonesia, in 2017. He is currently a lecturer and a junior researcher at the Civil Engineering Department of Universitas Atma Jaya. He has also been a member of the Indonesian Society for Geotechnical Engineers (ISGE) since 2017. His specialization is in geotechnical engineering, especially foundation engineering and slope stability analysis. Currently, he serves as a task force team leader of PPKM (Independent Campus Competition Program), grants from the Ministry of Education, Culture, Research and Technology Directorate General of Higher Education, Research and Technology.

**Hai Chien Pham** received a master's degree from the Asian Institute of Technology, Thailand, in 2012, and a Ph.D. from Chung-Ang University, South Korea, in 2018, both in construction management. Before pursuing his Ph.D., he had more than 15 years of solid experience in construction management. He received a PMP certification from the Project Management Institute. He is currently Head of the Department of Construction Engineering and Management, Faculty of Civil Engineering, Ton Duc Thang University, Vietnam. His research interests include BIM, VR, AR, photoreality and mobile computing, focusing on technology-enhanced applications for construction education, training, and management.

**Harijanto Setiawan** is an associate professor in the Civil Engineering Department, Universitas Atma Jaya Yogyakarta, Indonesia. He received a Ph.D. from the School of Energy, Geosciences, Infrastructure and Society, Heriot-Watt University, UK. His research interest is in the areas of construction management, project management, occupational safety and health, entrepreneurship and sustainability. He is a reviewer for academic journals, such as the *International Journal of Construction Management; Engineering, Construction and Architectural Management* and conferences, such as Euro Asia Civil Engineering Forum; Central Europe towards Sustainable Building. For several years, his research has benefited from funds from the Directorate General of Higher Education Ministry of Education and Culture, Republic of Indonesia.

**Haruna Musa Moda** is an associate professor of Occupational Health, Safety and Environment at University of Doha for Science and Technology, Qatar. He is actively engaged in research, consultancy and knowledge transfer projects in the Middle East, UK and West Africa. Dr Moda is a chartered member of the Institution of Occupational Safety and Health (IOSH) and belongs to several professional bodies that include International Commission on Occupational Health (ICOH), Workplace Health Without Borders (WHWB), Higher Education Academy.

**Henry Alinaitwe** is the Deputy Vice Chancellor in charge of Finance and Administration at Makerere University. He has served as Principal of the College of Engineering, Design, Art and Technology, Deputy Principal of the same college, Dean in the same college, and earlier as Deputy Dean of the then-Faculty of Technology. He is a professor of civil engineering and has taught at the university for more than 30 years. Henry is a Fellow of the Institution of Civil Engineers (UK) and Fellow of Uganda Institution of Professional Engineers. He is a registered engineer and has wide experience in construction.

**Innocent Musonda** holds a PhD in engineering management and qualifications in construction management and civil engineering. He is a registered civil engineer (Zambia), construction manager (South Africa), and a full member of the Chartered Institute of the Building (CIOB-UK) and the International Council for Research and Innovation in Building and Construction (CIB). He has worked for both the public and private sectors in Southern Africa. He is currently a professor in construction project management, researcher, invited speaker, founder and director of the Centre for Applied Research and Innovation in the Built Environment (CARINBE) based at the University of Johannesburg.

**Iruka Chijindu Anugwo** is a lecturer in construction project management and built environment at the Department of Construction Management and Quantity Surveying, Durban University of Technology (DUT), South Africa. Anugwo holds a Ph.D. in construction management and is an active academic. Anugwo is an emerging international researcher in areas such as construction safety and health research, construction contractors' sustainability, geopathic stress zone, and infrastructure development research, which has significantly contributed to the body of knowledge within the built environment sector and community engagement, both in South Africa and internationally. Anugwo has been involved as a principal investigator (PI) in various research projects (valued at over US $10,000) funded by several institutions. He has about 27 academic publications.

**Janet Mayowa Nwaogu** is a postdoctoral fellow at the Hong Kong Polytechnic University. She was an assistant lecturer at the Federal University of Technology, Akure, Nigeria and worked in the Nigerian construction industry, which informed her research interests. She is passionate about job satisfaction, client satisfaction, job design, and construction employees' mental health and well-being. Her research interest covers labour management, construction safety and health and other aspects of construction management.

**Jessica Borg** is a lecturer in construction management at the University of Melbourne. She is passionate about research that makes an impact on the working lives of professionals in today's complex work environments, with a particular focus on research in the context of project-based workplaces and the construction industry. Dr. Borg is best known for her research on the work readiness of built environment professionals. She continues to research in the areas of workplace transitions, early career work readiness, diversity and inclusion and professional development within project-based contexts and the construction industry.

**John Smallwood** is a professor of construction management in the Department of Construction Management, Nelson Mandela University, and the Principal of Construction Research Education and Training Enterprises (CREATE). Both his MSc and PhD (construction management) addressed construction health and safety (H&S). He has conducted extensive research and published in the areas of construction H&S, ergonomics, and occupational health (OH), but also in the areas of construction management education and training, environmental management, health and well-being, primary health promotion, quality management, risk management, and the practice of construction management.

**Junfeng Guan** is a research assistant in the Building and Real Estate Department at The Hong Kong Polytechnic University. He obtained his master's degree from the Harbin Institute of Technology in 2021. In 2018, he received a scholarship from the Jilin Provincial Government. His work focuses on the paradigm for organizational learning from accidents in view of resilient safety culture.

**Kofi Agyekum**, Ph.D., is a senior lecturer of building science, engineering and materials in the Department of Construction Technology and Management, Kwame Nkrumah University of Science and Technology (KNUST), Kumasi, Ghana. His specialisation areas include construction health and safety, building biology, circular economy in construction, building pathology, and sustainable and lean construction. He has served as a guest editor, editorial board member, and reviewer for several national and international journals and conferences. He is a professional peer reviewer and holds a recognised peer review certificate from the Web of Science Academy.

**Marcelino Danu Egardy** graduated from the construction engineering and management programme in 2022. In carrying out his bachelor's thesis, he was guided by Ir. Seng Hansen, S.T., M.Sc., Ph.D., IPM, and Mr. Ferdinand Fassa, S.T., M.T.

**Matthew Ikuabe** obtained a bachelor's of technology (B.Tech) and master's of technology (M.Tech) in quantity surveying from the Federal University of Technology, Akure, Nigeria. He was awarded his doctorate in philosophy (Ph.D.) in construction management from the University of Johannesburg, South Africa, in 2022. He is currently a post-doctoral research fellow at the CIDB Centre of Excellence, Faculty of Engineering and Built Environment, University of Johannesburg, South Africa. To his credit, he has published research works in accredited journals, book chapters, and peer-reviewed conferences. He is a corporate member of the Nigerian Institute of Quantity Surveyors.

**Mírian Caroline Farias Santos** graduated with a degree in civil engineering from the Federal University of Bahia (2016) and a master's in civil engineering (construction management and material science) from the Federal University of Bahia (2018) and specialisation in work safety engineering from Cruzeiro do Sul University (2017). Santos has experience in construction management using building information modelling. Currently, she is a PhD Student at the Federal University of Bahia, studying artificial intelligence applied to safety management.

**Mohd Amizan Mohamed @ Arifin** has his PhD in civil engineering from the Queensland University of Technology (QUT), Brisbane, Australia. He received his diploma in civil engineering, bachelor's in civil engineering with honours and master's in civil engineering (construction) from the MARA University of Technology, Malaysia. He is currently a senior lecturer and the Head of the Division for Construction Business and Project Management (CBPM) at the School of Civil Engineering, College of Engineering, UiTM Shah Alam, Malaysia. Since 2020, he has conducted much research on how COVID-19 impacted the Malaysian construction industry. He currently focuses his research on the international construction business and artificial intelligence (AI) for construction and disaster management.

**Mojtaba Ashour** is a doctoral student and a graduate assistant in the Department of Interior Architecture and Environmental Design at Bilkent University. His research is primarily concerned with decision making for the realization of sustainable development goals, and well-being of stakeholders and occupants.

**Motheo Meta Tjebane** is a lecturer at the renowned Mangosuthu University of Technology (MUT) in South Africa, where she imparts her knowledge and expertise to aspiring scholars. Concurrently, she is pursuing her doctoral studies at the prestigious Centre of Applied Research and Innovation in the Built Environment (CARINBE) at the University of Johannesburg, South Africa. She has carved a distinct niche for herself, focusing her research efforts on the fascinating domains of artificial intelligence, building information modelling (BIM), and sustainability within the built environment. Her studies and publications delve into the intersection of these disciplines, exploring innovative ways to integrate AI, BIM and sustainability principles to optimize the construction and design processes. She plays a pivotal role in guiding and supporting aspiring researchers, fostering their academic growth and nurturing their potential.

**Mu'awiya Abubakar** is a senior lecturer in the Department of Building, Ahmadu Bello University, Zaria-Nigeria. His research interest is in construction safety management. He holds a B.Sc. in Building and M.Sc. and Ph.D. in construction management from Ahmadu Bello University. He is a member of the Nigerian Institute of Building (NIOB) and registered with the Council of Registered Builders of Nigeria (CORBON). He was at the M.E. Rinker Sr. School of Construction Management, University of Florida, as a visiting Ph.D. scholar. He has over 30 publications in reputable journals and has refereed conference proceedings.

**Nader Naderpajouh** is the Senior Lecturer, Director of Research Education, and Post-Graduate Coordinator, and leads the Organizing for Resilience in the Built Environment (ORIBE) research group. His main area of research focuses on collective actions and organizing across social, technical and ecological systems. He serves as Associate Editor for the *Journal of Management in Engineering* published by the American Society of Civil Engineers (ASCE), as a member of the editorial board of the *International Journal of Project Management* (IJPM), and serves as a referee for over 30 academic journals. He is actively engaged with research communities, industry partners and government agencies across Australia, New Zealand, Europe, USA, UK, the Middle East and Asia.

**Naomi Borg** is a casual tutor at the University of Melbourne and at RMIT University, as well as a project manager in the construction industry, having delivered multiple projects across sectors. Naomi is also a research assistant at RMIT and Melbourne University with a passion for combining industry knowledge and research. She is a Certified Practicing Project Practitioner (CPPP) with the Australian Institute of Project Management (AIPM) and a Project Management Industry (PMI) member. She has presented on resilience at various national and international conferences.

**Nazirah Mohd Apandi** is a senior lecturer in the School of Civil Engineering, University Technology MARA (UiTM), Shah Alam. Throughout her career, she has been involved in concrete repair and strengthening works, structure design and disaster issues. She is active in publishing articles related to her research interests. She focused on research related to building damage assessment based on pre-disaster and post-disaster events.

**Nghia Hoai Nguyen** received his doctorate degree in management technology from SIIT, Thammasat University, Thailand in 2018. He has over 10 years of experience in the Vietnamese construction industry, especially in construction management and real estate development. He joined the academic area in 2011. He is currently working as a Dean of School of Civil Engineering and Construction

Management, International University, Ho Chi Minh City, Viet Nam – Vietnam National University, Ho Chi Minh City, Vietnam. Nghia has published his research in various domestic and international journals and conferences.

**Nikdokht Ghadiminia** is a Senior Lecturer in Built Environment at the School of Engineering, Technology and Design, Canterbury Christchurch University. She is a researcher and co-author at the IoT Security Foundation (IoTSF) and also part of the leading team in cybersecurity in the built environment working group. She received her Ph.D. in security minded digital transformation in the built environment from Birmingham City University, and achieved her BEng and MSc (Hons.) degree in civil engineering from the University of Birmingham (UK). As a Chartered Member of the CIOB (MCIOB), Future Leader's CIOB Board Member and a fellow of the Higher Education Academy (FHEA), she is actively involved in research in digital construction, digital twins, BIM and cybersecurity in the built environment.

**Nur Izzati Sofia Shuhaimi** holds a First Class with Honours bachelor's degree in civil engineering from Universiti Teknologi Mara. She has extensive experience in working with various people in the construction sector with a focus on quality control and quality assurance as well as civil and structure. Currently, she is a civil and structural engineer at Perunding Rekacekap Sdn. Bhd., a company that provides high standard personalized consultancy services that create cost-effective and sound engineering solutions for the specific needs of individuals. As a civil and structural engineer, she is responsible for the project designs of residential developments that focus on the safety and capability in withholding external elements.

**Obuks A. Ejohwomu** is currently an associate professor (senior lecturer) in project management at the University of Manchester. He is an award-winning research-active academic with a world-leading profile for delivering impact-driven research in construction engineering and management, particularly in the areas of digitalisation, productivity, health and safety and the future sustainable built environment. In this capacity, he has co-authored over 82 publications spanning journals and conferences, book and book chapters, technical reports and government documents. He has supported governmental organisations in the UK, as well as across the world in countries like South Africa, Ghana and Nigeria.

**Pinar Irlayici Cakmak** is an associate professor in the Department of Architecture and Project and Construction Management Graduate Program at Istanbul Technical University, Turkey. She has a Ph.D. degree and an MSc in project and construction management. Her research interests are in the areas of project and construction management, contract management, dispute resolution and cost management.

**Qingyao Qiao** is a post-doctoral research fellow at the University of Hong Kong. Prior to this, he completed his PhD degree at the University of Manchester, where he also worked as a research associate. He obtained his B.E. degree in civil engineering from Nanjing Tech University, China, in 2015. He received a M.Sc. in civil engineering from Shenzhen University in 2018. His research interests include building energy consumption prediction, machine learning application, feature engineering and data mining, agent-based modelling, project safety control measure and occupational health and safety.

**Raja Muhamad Amir Hamzah Raja Mohd Azlan** holds an honors bachelor's degree in civil engineering from Universiti Teknologi Mara Shah Alam. He has experience working with construction workers during the Covid-19 pandemic. Now he is a civil and structural engineer at OMK Jurutera Perunding Sdn. Bhd., a company that provides C&S design and consultancy services to clients. He would like to be a professional engineer who can accept challenges as an opportunity to grow.

**Richard Irumba** is the Director of Physical Planning at Kampala Capital City Authority. He previously served as a lecturer in the College of Engineering, Design, Art and Technology, Makerere University. His research interests include construction safety and health, housing, land management, system dynamics and spatial econometric applications in real estate and construction. He is a registered and practicing surveyor, a Fellow of the Institution of Surveyors of Uganda, and a member of both the African Real Estate Society and the Commonwealth Association of Surveyors and Land Economists. He holds a Ph.D. from KTH Royal Institute of Technology, Sweden.

**Rose Matete** is a PhD candidate as a professional construction health and safety (H&S) agent (Pr. CHSA) and is a member of the South African Council of Projects and Construction Management Professions (SACPCMP) and a consultant with over 16 years of experience in construction H&S. Rose is also a part-time lecturer in the Department of Built Environment at the Central University of Technology, Free State, South Africa. She is an upcoming researcher who is passionate about research in construction (H&S), and she holds an MSc in built environment in construction H&S.

**Ruifeng Cao** received a B.E. degree in mechanical engineering from Taiyuan University of Science and Technology, China, in 2015. He participated in a joint master's programme with Taiyuan University of Technology, China, and the University of Manchester, UK, and received the M.Sc. degree in mechanical engineering design from the University of Manchester in 2019. He is currently pursuing a Ph.D. degree with the Department of Mechanical, Aerospace and Civil Engineering, the University of Manchester, UK. His research interests include mechanical fault diagnosis, condition monitoring, occupational health and safety and machine learning.

**Saeed Reza Mohandes** is a postdoctoral research associate at the University of Manchester (UoM), undertaking research on the area of construction project management (CPM) using artificial intelligence (AI)-based techniques. Prior to joining the UoM, he worked as a postdoctoral fellow at Hong Kong Polytechnic

University, focusing on the application of AI-based techniques in infrastructure management. Furthermore, he has been appointed associate editor, guest editor and reviewer for the leading journals in the area of CPM. His research areas include the application of leading AI-based techniques and technologies to construction safety, green construction, energy building analysis, infrastructure management and facility management.

**Salman Saeidlou** is a senior lecturer in mechanical/material engineering and the Course Director of Manufacturing Engineering Degree Apprenticeship at the School of Engineering Technology and Design, Canterbury Christ Church University (CCCU), UK. Salman is a Chartered Mechanical Engineer (CEng, MIMechE). He is also a Senior Fellow of the Higher Education Academy (SFHEA) and has broad-ranging teaching and supervision experience in undergraduate and postgraduate engineering courses at UK higher education institutions. His research interests include intelligent manufacturing systems, distributed systems, agent-based modelling, big data analytics in manufacturing, data mining and machine learning. Salman has been implementing the CDIO methodology into various engineering modules at CCCU.

**Samuel A. Adekunle** obtained his bachelor's of science and master's of science in quantity surveying from the University of Lagos, Nigeria and PhD in construction management from the University of Johannesburg. He has several publications in accredited peer-reviewed journals, book chapters and conferences, which have earned him recognition and awards and a growing international reputation. Samuel has been involved in several research projects in different capacities. In addition, he has served as a panel member on several platforms and seminars discussing and presenting BIM adoption strategies in developing economies. Samuel has been involved in several construction projects as a quantity surveyor and project manager.

**Seng Hansen** is a senior lecturer in the construction engineering and management programme at Podomoro University, Jakarta. In addition to being active in two professional associations, he has produced several books, including *Manajemen Kontrak Konstruksi/Construction Contract Management* (2015), *Quantity Surveying* (2017), *Construction Contract Management Body of Knowledge* (2021), *100 Tanya-Jawab Permasalahan Kontrak Konstruksi Indonesia/100 Questions and Answers on Indonesian Construction Contractual Issues* (2021) and *Gambar Konstruksi/Construction Drawings* (2022).

**Siti Rashidah Mohd Nasir** is an associate professor at the School of Civil Engineering, Universiti Teknologi MARA, Malaysia. She obtained her PhD in civil engineering from Universiti Teknologi Malaysia. She is currently leading a research project on industrial building systems funded by the Ministry of Education under the Fundamental Research Grant Scheme (FRGS), and another research project on COVID-19 under university research grants (MyRA and Professor Grant). In addition, she has led collaborative industry research funded by LLM (completed in 2017) and TNB (completed in 2018).

**Syahirah Intan Mohd Sheffie** holds a master's of science in Teaching English to Speakers of Other Languages (MSc TESOL) from the University of Edinburgh, United Kingdom, and a bachelor's of education with honours in Teaching English as a Second Language (TESL) from the University of Exeter, United Kingdom. As a practising educator for over a decade, her expertise includes English language curriculum reforms in Malaysia since 2010. Her professional working experiences as the Assistant Director at the Ministry of Education Malaysia involved multilateral and bilateral diplomatic relations, including as an editor and speechwriter for the ministers, director generals and directors of several ministries and divisions. She has written, published and co-authored journal articles. She is also a proofreader and an editor of journal articles, conference papers, and proceedings, successfully submitted and presented in countries such as Malaysia, Australia, South Korea and Thailand. She presented at international conferences, won several international education design innovation awards and is a co-member of a higher education team with ongoing research securing funds from the UN SDG40 and the Ministry of Higher Education Malaysia. Her current interest in the sophistication of education has seen her taking up responsibility as a mentor transverse from young learners' education to postgraduate research.

**Thanwadee Chinda** is an associate professor at the School of Management Technology, Sirindhorn International Institute of Technology, Thammasat University, Thailand. She received her Ph.D. in engineering management from Griffith University, Australia. Her research areas are in construction management, forecasting model, structural equation modelling, and system dynamics modelling. Her publications have appeared in *Journal of Construction Engineering and Management, Civil Engineering and Environmental Systems, Engineering Management Journal, International Journal of Occupational Safety and Ergonomics, International Journal of Construction Management, and Engineering, Construction,* and *Architectural Management.*

**Thembani Moyo** is a post-doctoral fellow at the Centre for Applied Research + Innovation in the Built Environment (CARINBE), University of Johannesburg. His research interests leverage a combination of experimental and empirical approaches to continue making a significant contribution in the pursuit of merging the Fourth Industrial Revolution (4IR) and urban planning. Driven by a relentless pursuit of knowledge, Thembani has made remarkable contributions to the academic community. His expertise is evidenced by a series of highly regarded academic publications, wherein he has shared groundbreaking insights and novel perspectives. His research outputs have been influential in shaping the discourse surrounding the integration of 4IR and urban planning. In addition to his publications, Thembani is recognized as a distinguished resource person for research seminars. Through his engaging presentations and thought-provoking discussions, he enriches the scholarly community by sharing his wealth of knowledge and expertise.

**Thi-Thanh-Mai Pham** is currently a lecturer of the faculty of International Trade, College of Foreign Economic Relation, Ho Chi Minh City, Vietnam. Her research interests focus on solutions for improving education, training, and business management.

**Victor Nnannaya Okorie** is an associate professor and currently serving as the Assistant Dean of Faculty of Environmental Sciences, University of Benin. He holds a doctor of philosophy degree in construction management from the Nelson Mandela Metropolitan University, Port Elizabeth, South Africa in 2014. He is an Incorporate Member of the Chartered Institute of Building (ICIOB), United Kingdom, Professional Member of the Nigerian Institute of Quantity Surveyors (MNIQS) and Registered Quantity Surveyor (RQS). His research interest is on construction health and safety (H&S) with focus on culture, behaviour and leadership in relation to construction health and safety performance.

**Victoria Maame Afriyie Kumah,** BSc (First Class Honours) is currently a research and teaching assistant at the Department of Construction Technology and Management, Kwame Nkrumah University of Science and Technology (KNUST), Kumasi, Ghana. Her areas of specialization include green and sustainable construction, and construction health and safety.

**Wen Yi** is an assistant professor at the Hong Kong Polytechnic University. Dr. Wen Yi was a senior lecturer at Massey University, New Zealand. She has over 50 publications and is part of the team that undertook the research, which led to the multi-award-winning Anti-Heat Stress Uniform (AHSU). Her research interest covers optimization in construction management, construction safety and health and construction engineering and management.

**Yahaya Makarfi Ibrahim** is a professor of quantity surveying in the Department of Quantity Surveying, Ahmadu Bello University, Nigeria. He holds a B.Sc. in quantity surveying from Ahmadu Bello University, Nigeria, an M.Sc. and PhD in construction project management from Heriot-Watt University, Edinburgh, UK. He has over 50 publications in reputable journals and conference proceedings around the world. He has been involved as a co-investigator and principal investigator in research projects funded by many organisations. He led (as PI) the TETFund funded research project that developed the first web-based e-tendering portal for public procurement in Nigeria.

**Yang Yang** is a research assistant professor of urban sustainability policy at the Hong Kong Polytechnic University (PolyU). Dr. Yang (also known as Dr. Jackie Y. Yang) was a senior officer at the Construction Industry Council in Hong Kong. In 2014, Dr. Yang's health and safety research received the OSH Student Research Scholarship from the Hong Kong Occupational Safety and Health Council. With over 20 publications, she has made a tremendous impact in the construction industry. She is part of the team that undertook the research that led to the multi-award-winning Anti-Heat Stress Uniform (AHSU). Her research interest covers occupational safety and health and industry policy.

# Foreword

The COVID-19 pandemic changed the world, and the built environment sector was no exception. The global construction sector was forced to consider worker health, safety, and well-being and placed these human rights at the forefront at their business. Unfortunately, across the globe, construction remains one of the most dangerous and fatal occupations. The sector struggles with higher-than-average divorce and suicide rates. Mental health must remain a central focus and emerge as a deep-rooted value within the construction sector in the post-COVID era.

This book places the pandemic in context along with the key safety, health, and well-being challenges facing the global construction sector. What will we learn from this book? Well, certainly it is hoped another pandemic does not occur for this book to be directly utilised. But the pandemic forced change and was something new to manage. The construction sector became more adaptable, nimble, and innovative. The authors of these excellent chapters also bring out that adaptability and innovation through coping with the pandemic. The global perspectives included in this book provide the reader with a diverse understanding of best practices that emerged during the pandemic. The same adaptability shown throughout the pandemic and evidenced by this book should be viewed as parallel to the ever-evolving and changing technologies in the construction sector such as wearables, artificial intelligence, monitoring devices, and other rapid changes in equipment and technology. This book highlights case studies and best practices to understand and better manage change; the pandemic simply happened to be that change agent. The key learning points contained within are generalisable to future technological change, and thus I have no doubt this textbook will be impactful far into the future.

The International Council for Research and Innovation in Building and Construction (CIB) has active Working Commissions on Health, Safety and Well-being in Construction (W099) and People in Construction (W123). W099 and W123 remained quite active during the pandemic, hosting two very well-attended and interactive online international conferences. The group and its leadership were adaptive to change and disruption, setting an example for other Working Commissions within CIB. This book also sets a wonderful example of forward thinking, innovation, and creativity while sharing case studies, research, and best practices from across the globe.

I am very keen to support this publication and hope that it makes an important contribution to improving the lives of construction workers and their families across the world.

Michael Behm, PhD CSP
Professor, Occupational Safety, East Carolina University
Past CIB Programme Director (2019–2022)
Past Coordinator, CIB W099 (2012–2019)

# 1 Construction safety, health and well-being in the COVID-19 era

## An introduction

*Patrick Manu, Clara Cheung, Akilu Yunusa-Kaltungo, Fidelis Emuze, Tarcisio Abreu Saurin, Bonaventura Hadikusumo and Saeed Reza Mohandes*

## Introduction

Globally, the construction sector accounts for a high and disproportionate number of occupational fatalities, injuries, and illnesses (International Labour Organisation, 2015; Health and Safety Executive, 2021; Eurostats, 2022). Workers in the construction industry are three to six times more likely than other workers to die from work-related accidents (International Labour Organisation, 2015). Furthermore, construction workers are more likely to suffer from an occupational illness than other workers (Health and Safety Executive, 2021). The industry is also notorious for poor workforce well-being, as evidenced by the prevalence of anxiety, stress, depression, and fatigue (Rees-Evans, 2020; RSM UK Consulting LLP, 2021). The nature of work at construction sites is physically more demanding than most other industries. The existence of a large number of workers on the work site coupled with the prevalence of hazards causes the likelihood of incident occurrence to surge. The incidents and work conditions in construction (e.g. time pressure, high level of subcontracting, job insecurity, long hours of work, long commutes, and dynamic work environment) commonly result in injuries, illnesses, deaths, and poor well-being outcomes for the workforce (Haslam, 2005; Manu et al., 2014; Rees-Evans, 2020; Tijani et al., 2021). Poor occupational safety, health, and well-being (OSHW) is a concerning issue for the workers, their families, companies, and government bodies since it has adverse impacts on the overall economic and social status of these stakeholders. Moreover, these impacts dampen the morale of the worker, which results in performing tasks inefficiently (De Prins et al., 2020). Between 2020 and 2030, globally, the construction sector's output is forecasted to increase by about USD $4.5 trillion to reach circa USD $15 trillion (Oxford Economics, 2021). This growth could adversely affect the OSHW of construction workers if adequate safeguards are not implemented. The gloomy outlook for construction OSHW has recently been exacerbated by the global COVID-19 pandemic.

The construction sector is highly labour-intensive and works are much more difficult to control due to the rapidly changing nature of construction sites, the multiplicity of site hazards, activities, and trades, and the transience of construction projects. Moreover, construction site operations are often undertaken by teams

DOI: 10.1201/9781003278368-1

of tradespeople/workers who work in close proximity to each other. There is also less mechanisation of construction activities in some countries, which implies a greater physical presence of workers on construction sites and by extension implies greater exposure of the workforce to occupational health and safety hazards. The construction workforce is thus highly susceptible to COVID-19 transmission, infection, and related deaths. For instance, in England and Wales, construction occupations were reported to be among the occupations with the highest rates of death involving COVID-19 (Office for National Statistics, 2021a). Aside from the COVID-19-related deaths associated with the construction industry, the pandemic seriously impacted the industry in several ways. For instance, the number of employment opportunities dropped seriously, which was partially because of the work interruptions induced by the limitations imposed to prevent the spread of the coronavirus. In addition, there was a lack of personal protective equipment because healthcare employees placed high demand on such equipment. The interruption of supply chains and lack of employees/workers because of quarantines caused numerous construction projects to be stopped or suspended (Rouhanizadeh et al., 2019). The Associated General Contractors of America reported that 28% of their members had to stop or postpone construction projects due to the spread of COVID-19 (Pamidimukkala and Kermanshachi, 2021). Therefore, construction is highly impacted by COVID-19 (Koh, 2020).

Despite the significant toll of the COVID-19 pandemic, there is generally a dearth of published studies relating to the OSHW impacts and implications arising from the pandemic within construction. However, there is a growing interest in this area, as shown by calls for journal special issues on COVID-19 in the construction industry. Given that the COVID-19 pandemic has impacted nations on all continents in both similar and different manners/scales, a compendium of studies that offers comprehensive global coverage of the OSHW situation induced by the pandemic in the construction industry would be very useful to multiple stakeholders. This book addresses this gap by offering global perspectives on the OSHW implications of COVID-19 in the construction industry. In this introductory chapter, the status of OSHW in the construction industry is first highlighted. Following this, the impacts of COVID-19 are elaborated on. This is followed by a discussion regarding the OSHW opportunities and challenges induced by the pandemic in the construction industry. Finally, a summary of the chapters presented in the book is provided.

## COVID-19 impacts on industry

COVID-19 can be transmitted among people, causing symptoms such as fever, fatigue, dry cough, and breath shortness (Shi et al., 2020). As of January 2023, it had spread to more than 200 countries and territories, with over 750 million cases and resulting in over six million COVID-19-related deaths (World Health Organisation, 2023).

The COVID-19 pandemic seriously affected not only the people's health status but also the global economy (International Monetary Fund, 2021). For instance, a period of recession started in the United States in February 2020, which was termed the 'Recession of COVID-19' (Chodorow-Reich and Coglianese, 2021). In April 2020, a high unemployment rate of 14.7% was recorded in the United States because of the economic downturn, which was much worse than the 3.8% rate of February 2020 (Pamidimukkala and Kermanshachi, 2021).

Like other industrial sectors, the COVID-19 pandemic significantly affected the construction industry (Alsharef et al., 2021). Apart from the risks induced by the nature of construction work, construction workers and professionals are at high risk of being infected by aerosol and droplet contamination (Zheng et al., 2021). The restrictions imposed on construction projects as a result of the pandemic negatively affected economic growth, augmented the unemployment rate, interrupted supply chains of construction materials, and interrupted many investments (Bsisu, 2020; Ogunnusi et al., 2020). For instance, in the UK the value of new construction work in 2020 recorded an over-15% drop from £119.087 billion in 2019 (Office for National Statistics, 2021b). Several stakeholders of the construction sector were impacted by the crisis of COVID-19 at a global level (Ogunnusi et al., 2020).

**Opportunities and challenges for OSHW in construction**

Apart from the economic concerns induced by the COVID-19 pandemic, the OSHW of construction workers was also affected (Bourne et al., 2022). A number of reasons resulted in this situation, including the occurrence of health hazards to workers on remote construction sites while commuting because of overcrowding on transport and the nonexistence of risk control measures, and adverse impacts on workers' mental health because of the augmented anxiety amongst them (Iqbal et al., 2021). The emergence of COVID-19 offers a number of both opportunities and challenges regarding the OSHW of construction workers. As regards the opportunities, the pandemic has brought about the following upsides (Dobrucali et al., 2022; Bourne et al., 2022).

(1) The respective firms have been tilted towards the adoption of the latest technologies (e.g., sensors) to be brought into practice. The use of said technologies can benefit the concerned decision-makers by providing them with constant monitoring of the OSHW status of the ongoing projects, such as checking whether the workers have worn the required personal protective equipment (PPE) or when the respective workers come into contact with dangers, to name but a few.

(2) The respective firms have been adopting more flexible working conditions (e.g., working from home) for the workers compared to the pre-pandemic era, thereby improving the OSHW of all the groups involved in the projects.

(3) The respective companies have introduced more health practices for cleaning up and improving the related conditions of sites, which has made the work environment safer for the workers.

(4) Another point is related to the new communication channels among the stakeholders involved in a project, which has been accelerated by the increased adoption of information and communication technologies during the pandemic.

Challenges to the OSHW of construction personnel arising from the pandemic include the following (Amoah and Simpeh, 2020; Sierra, 2021; Stiles et al., 2021; Yang et al., 2021):

(1)  The supply of appropriate and sufficient PPEs by contractors is one of the major impediments to achieving a safe working environment for the involved workers.
(2)  There is always a threat of adherence to compliance from the side of the concerned regulators and policymakers; during the pandemic, it was observed that some construction projects did not implement a social distancing strategy on the respective sites, thereby posing dangers to the health of all the involved crew members. This was more apparent at the beginning of the pandemic when very few rules and regulations existed, if any.
(3)  Another challenge is related to the proper sanitisation of the materials used on construction sites; if a frequent and appropriate sanitation strategy is in place, there are fewer infections spreading across the sites.
(4)  Last but not least, superstition is another stumbling block to improving the OSHW of construction projects during the pandemic. Some crew members were of the opinion that COVID-19 was for a particular group of people, and that they could not contract it if they boosted their immune systems.

Further information regarding the challenges and opportunities is covered in the subsequent chapters of this book.

## Overview of chapters

There are 25 chapters in the book, which have been grouped into three thematic sections. Collectively, the chapters provide insights from over 10 countries across six world regions – Africa, Asia, Australia, Europe, North America, and South America. A brief description of the chapters is presented here.

Chapter 1 is 'Construction safety, health and well-being in the COVID-19 era: an introduction.' In this introductory chapter, Manu et al. highlight the gap in the literature regarding the lack of a comprehensive compendium of studies about the OSHW impacts and implications arising from the COVID-19 pandemic within the construction domain. The chapter gives a high-level view of the OSHW status of the construction industry, the impacts of COVID-19 on industries, and the OSHW opportunities and challenges arising from the pandemic within the construction industry.

### Section 1: management of COVID-19 transmission risk

Chapter 2 is 'The transmission of COVID-19 in construction: a systematic review of findings from statistical and modelling techniques.' In this chapter, Cao et al. used the PRISMA way of compiling a systematic literature review to beam the searchlight on modelling techniques related to the need to limit exposure to COVID-19. The chapter outlined and explained five modelling techniques with their corresponding features. Knowing the characteristics and strength of each technique is vital to making informed decisions that will save lives on construction sites.

Chapter 3 is 'Health and safety measures for managing the COVID-19 pandemic in the construction industry: a comparison study.' This chapter by Chan et al. used semi-structured interviews conducted with the management staff of construction projects from Nigeria and China. The study outcomes revealed that both countries had construction site health and safety control measures, including body temperature monitoring, face mask-wearing, disinfection of offices, and sanitisation of employees. However, unlike Nigeria, China complemented the aforementioned measures with sophisticated technology-based approaches like big data analysis, onsite tracer apps, and health QR codes, which aided real-time management of COVID-19 transmission on construction sites.

Chapter 4 is 'Towards improving health management of construction projects during the COVID-19 pandemic.' In this chapter, Mahdiyar et al. frame the need to limit exposure to COVID-19 on construction sites. The chapter examined COVID-19 in Hong Kong to highlight how the effects of preventative measures were handled on-site. The chapter reinforced the benefits of health measures and ranked the importance of identified measures. The implication of the shared results is that decision- or policymakers should brainstorm about the effects of preventive measures before deployment.

Chapter 5 is 'An overview on the measures taken to tackle COVID-19 impacts on Nigerian construction sites: a case study of South-South Geo-Political Zone.' In this chapter, Okorie and Anugwo investigate the measures taken to mitigate the spread of COVID-19 among construction companies in Nigeria. They conducted interviews with 24 small, medium, and large companies. While they found the implementation of measures such as wearing face masks, social distancing, and temperature reading, they also reported that workers' attitude towards the measures as well as the implementation of the measures is relatively better among the large companies than the small and medium-sized companies. This echoes the challenges faced by small and medium-sized companies in effectively managing the safety, health, and well-being of workers.

Chapter 6 is 'COVID-19 pandemic: challenges in practising new norms for construction workers.' In this chapter, Mohamed @ Arifin et al. identify the new norms and practices for construction workers in the COVID-19 pandemic, examine the challenges of using those new norms and practices, and depict ways to practise them in the Klang Valley area in Malaysia. This study concludes that following the MOH (Ministry of Health) Malaysia's SOP (Standard Operating Procedure) at construction sites enabled construction employees to normalise new norms and practices more effectively during the pandemic.

Chapter 7 is 'Health and safety in the construction industry during the COVID-19 pandemic: case study of Vietnam.' In this chapter, Pham et al. investigate measures to prevent COVID-19 infection at construction sites in Vietnam, highlighting twelve solutions such as the reduction of the number of workers during safety training and the elimination of night work shifts. Three high-level lessons learned are also discussed: strict compliance with government policies, flexible approach in policy implementation, and strong commitments of project stakeholders. Finally, based on an industry-wide survey, the authors found that government regulations were perceived as effective in curbing the spread of COVID-19 in construction sites.

Chapter 8 is 'Construction safety culture management during the COVID-19 pandemic.' This chapter addresses the role of safety culture in construction sites in order to reduce infection rates. Based on interviews with experts from small, medium, and large construction sites, Chinda proposed recommendations for the management of safety culture in a pandemic context. The recommendations account for five types of safety culture enablers: leadership, policy and strategy, people, resources, and processes. Several examples related to each enabler are discussed in the chapter.

Chapter 9 is 'Policy assessment framework to measure the efficacy of mask-wearing arrangements during the COVID-19 outbreak: case studies from Jakarta, Indonesia.' In this chapter, Hansen et al. explore the effectiveness of mask-wearing policy implementation on two construction projects in Jakarta, Indonesia. To do so, a qualitative approach together with semi-structured interviews are adopted. From the results obtained, differences in policy implementation between the two observed case studies are noted. It is also observed that the enforcement control and strategies undertaken by contractors have an unavoidable impact on workers' perception about the effectiveness of mask-wearing policy implementation. The findings also reveal the need to update the mask-wearing policy in both projects for future improvements.

Chapter 10 is 'Construction sector in Indonesia: occupational health and safety during the outbreak of COVID-19.' Setiawan et al. investigate the OHS of construction projects during the outbreak of COVID-19 in Indonesia using a qualitative approach. To this end, the existing regulations related to OHS during the pandemic are explored, followed by an exploration of the health protocols implemented in construction projects. It is seen that Indonesian contractors commit to implementing the guidance that regulates the implementation of health protocols in every workplace; thus, they established a procedure enabling the organisation of all the activities on construction project sites.

### Section 2: impact of COVID-19 on occupational safety, health and well-being (OSHW)

Chapter 11 is 'Individual and organisational support mechanisms to foster career resilience during the COVID-19 pandemic.' In this chapter, Borg et al. explore the impacts of the pandemic on the well-being of project managers in the construction industry. Based on a survey with 148 project managers, the authors concluded that 61% of them reported high levels of personal resilience during the pandemic. Many attributed their personal resilience to organisational support mechanisms, such as an intensified focus on health and well-being, maintaining connections with work teams, training and development opportunities, and job security. The chapter also presents recommendations to foster personal and career resilience in construction companies.

Chapter 12 is 'Assessing how pandemic lockdown upended construction work creed in Free State and Limpopo, South Africa.' In this chapter, Matete and Emuze report on a qualitative inquiry into the impact of the COVID-19 pandemic lockdowns on workplace rules about the health, safety, and well-being of construction workers in South Africa. Based on interviews with 25 participants, they discuss several impacts, including: the impact on hazard identification and risk assessment; the impact on the implementation of the safety and health plan; the impact on the bi-weekly toolbox talks; the impact on safety and health induction of workers; impact on the provision and use of PPE; and impact on the provision and use of welfare facilities on site.

Chapter 13 is 'COVID-19 pandemic: a case study of mental health of migrant construction workers at Ttdi Sentralis, Selangor, Malaysia.' Migrant construction workers can be more prone to adverse safety, health, and well-being outcomes. Against this backdrop, in this chapter, Mohamed @ Arifin et al. investigate the effect of the COVID-19 pandemic on the mental health of migrant construction workers in Malaysia. They also investigated ways to mitigate this effect. Among the top factors that affected the mental health of migrant workers are: worrying about their financial difficulties; fear of losing job; and feeling helpless about the inability to help family during the lockdown. Suggestions to mitigate the effects of the pandemic on the mental health of migrant workers include: a good work environment that boosts work morale; provision of leaves of absence for sickness; recognition/praise by the work boss.

Chapter 14 is 'COVID-19 and the Ghanaian construction industry: current state of impact and mitigation measures.' In this chapter, Agyekum et al. examine the impact of the COVID-19 pandemic on Ghanaian construction with specific attention to control measures. A major impact identified in the chapter is anxiety, which underscores the importance of psychological safety in construction. The control measures deployed in Ghanaian construction helped limit the disease's spread. Some of the measures include mandatory screening and strict hygiene protocol on site.

Chapter 15 is 'Developing resilient construction professionals in the COVID-19 era: examining architecture students' personality perspective.' In this chapter, Sanh and Cakmak investigate the relationship between the personality types and resilience skills, stress factors experienced by architecture students during the pandemic, and provide recommendations on how to cope with stress and develop resilience. They found there are significant relationships between Enneagram personality types and resilience skills and stress factors experienced during the pandemic. The study also suggests the Enneagram as a practical guide to enhance and build resilience at the university level and beyond.

Chapter 16 is 'Safety, health and wellbeing of construction workers in Nigeria – opportunities and challenges associated with the COVID-19 pandemic.' In this chapter, Moda et al. show that the pandemic negatively affected project delivery on multiple fronts. The chapter turns readers' attention to coping mechanisms used in Nigerian construction during the pandemic. Some of the mechanisms are useful in similar context in developing countries.

Chapter 17 is 'Construction site management during COVID-19 in Myanmar.' In this chapter, Paing and Hadikusumo examine the effect of COVID-19 and its regulations imposed by Myanmar government on construction project management. Based on the four case studies, they identified the different and common construction safety management approaches that could be useful for construction projects to implement in the pandemic period and beyond.

### Section 3: implications of the COVID-19 pandemic for construction project performance

Chapter 18 is 'Intricacies and lifeline for the construction industry amidst the Coronavirus pandemic.' In this chapter, Adekunle et al. conduct an investigation into the impact of the COVID-19 pandemic on the construction industry in the developing country. Based on a bibliometric analysis undertaken, four cardinal perspectives are obtained, including economic, safety, labour availability, and legal impacts. Moreover, an outlook for the construction industry in developing countries post-COVID-19 is provided via data from two African countries. The essence of information management for improving the OHSW of construction projects during the pandemic is also discussed.

Chapter 19 is 'Assessment of COVID-19 control and prevention measures: lessons learned at construction sites.' In this chapter, Costa and Santos develop the lessons learned at construction sites through the evaluation of COVID-19 control and prevention measures in Brazil. Based the analysis of the seven categories of COVID-19 control measures, they highlight the organisation and hygiene category as having the highest degree of implementation. Meanwhile, personal care responsibilities, creating awareness, and changing the work regime were partially implemented.

Chapter 20 is 'COVID-19 and shock events in the AEC Sector: perspectives on mitigating measures.' In this chapter, Musonda et al. initially examine the impacts of shock-wave events such as COVID-19 on construction projects, as well as generate lessons that could improve the resilience of construction projects against future shock-wave events. Following consultations with experts in built environment within the sub-Saharan Africa region via focus group discussions, it was identified that measures such as digital transformation, policy, standards/contract guidelines, capacity development, improved information management/awareness, health and safety, training/upskilling, employee-worker relationship, and risk identification are immensely critical.

Chapter 21 is 'Implication of COVID-19 SOP compliance to project-based construction workers in Malaysia.' In this chapter, Nasir and Che Ibrahim study the impact of construction workers' compliance with health and safety (H&S) standard operating procedures (SOP) on project performance. Following conducting 25 semi-structured interviews with construction professionals from Peninsular Malaysia, Sabah, and Sarawak, it was revealed that factors such as shortage of workers, workers' utilities and test kits, poor management, working hours restrictions at sites, vaccination and quarantine, safety awareness, and SOP compliance were the dominant factors responsible for heightened H&S incidents during COVID-19 pandemic.

Chapter 22 is 'Facing the impacts of COVID-19 in construction: the case of Chile.' This chapter describes how the Chilean construction industry coped with the pandemic, both at the institutional level and at each company's level. Based on the lessons learned, Serpell recommends the following key measures of control: industrialisation in construction to reduce the exposition of workers at the site; use of technology to supervise workers and help protect them; dissemination of good practices for handling the pandemic and application of new business models to maintain the operation; teleworking; collaboration with suppliers; and contracts with clarity regarding the consequences from a pandemic like COVID-19.

Chapter 23 is 'Factors that led to an increase of building collapses during the COVID-19 lockdown period in the Greater Kampala Metropolitan Area, Uganda.' In this chapter, Alinaitwe and Irumba sought to understand the influence of a 16-month COVID-19 related lockdown on increased cases of building collapses in the Greater Kampala Metropolitan Area of Uganda. The examination of five case studies revealed a multi-causal relationship whereby the majority of causes were inherent, but exacerbated by the lockdown. The most dominant factors identified include poor supervision of building works, poor monitoring of works by local authorities, lack of approved building plans, poor construction methods, and failure to conduct site investigations.

Chapter 24 is 'A digital approach to health and safety management on-site: a silver lining of the COVID-19 pandemic.' In this chapter, Ghadiminia and Saeidlou pursued the following three main objectives via semi-structured interviews with construction professionals in the United Kingdom: (1) investigate the limitations brought by the COVID-19 pandemic to construction site; (2) explore the digital technologies introduced to overcome the limitations; and (3) investigate the feasibility of the digital technologies in tackling health and safety on-site. While presenting findings addressing these objectives, Ghadiminia also recommended further research to identify missing links between the anticipated potentials of the technologies and the real benefits derived from a mature digitalisation of health and safety management on site.

Chapter 25 is 'Digitalisation differently: an inclusive digital twin model for climate risk management in major projects in the post-COVID era.' Local weather conditions such as heat can make construction workers susceptible to heat stress during work on site. Construction projects in locations with a high risk of heat stress thus need to have systems for managing heat-related weather information. In this chapter, Jia et al. draw on pre-COVID-19 site observations and literature pertaining to industry 4 technologies to propose a digital twin model for managing weather information in major projects in the post-COVID-19 era. They suggest that the model can assist contractors and frontline workers to prepare for health risks resulting from extreme or changing weather conditions.

## References

Alsharef, A., Banerjee, S., Uddin, S.M.J., Albert, A., & Jaselskis, E. (2021). Early impacts of the COVID-19 pandemic on the United States construction industry. *International Journal of Environmental Research and Public Health*, 18, 1559.

Amoah, C., & Simpeh, F. (2020). Implementation challenges of COVID-19 safety measures at construction sites in South Africa. *Journal of Facilities Management*, 19(1), 111–128.

Bourne, N., Cao, R., Cheung, C., Clarke, S., Collinge, W., Hartwig, A., Howells, A., Johnson, S., Kirkham, R., Ling, D., Mann, C., Manu, P., Qiao, Q., Saba, S., van Tongeren, M., & Yunusa-Kaltungo, A. (2022). Keeping the UK building safely phase 2. *PROTECT COVID-19 National Core Study: Buxton*. Available at https://sites.manchester.ac.uk/covid19-national-project/2023/01/17/3726/ (Accessed 24 January 2023).

Bsisu, K.A.D. (2020). The impact of COVID-19 pandemic on Jordanian civil engineers and construction industry. *International Journal of Engineering Research and Technology*, 13(5), 828–830.

Chodorow-Reich, G., & Coglianese, J. (2021). Projecting unemployment durations: A factor-flows simulation approach with application to the COVID-19 recession. *Journal of Public Economics*, 197, 104398.

De Prins, P., Stuer, D., & Gielens, T. (2020). Revitalizing social dialogue in the workplace: The impact of a cooperative industrial relations climate and sustainable HR practices on reducing employee harm. *The International Journal of Human Resource Management*, 31, 1684–1704.

Dobrucali, E., Sadikoglu, E., Demirkesen, S., Zhang, C., & Tezel, A. (2022). Exploring the impact of COVID-19 on the United States construction industry: Challenges and opportunities. IEEE Transactions on Engineering Management.

Eurostats. (2022). Accidents at work: Statistics by economic activity. *Eurostats*. Available at https://ec.europa.eu/eurostat/statistics-explained/index.php?title=Accidents_at_work_-_statistics_by_economic_activity (Accessed 9 August 2022).

Haslam, R.A., Hide, S.A., Gibb, A.G.F., Gyi, D.E., Pavitt, T., Atkinson, S., & Duff, A.R. (2005). Contributing factors in construction accidents. *Applied Ergonomics*, 36(4), 401–415.

Health and Safety Executive. (2021). Construction statistics in Great Britain, 2021. *Health and Safety Executive*. Available at www.hse.gov.uk/statistics/industry/construction.pdf (Accessed 9 August 2022).

International Labour Organisation. (2015). *Construction: A hazardous work*. Available at www.ilo.org/safework/areasofwork/hazardous-work/WCMS_356576/lang-en/index.htm (Accessed 22 July 2020).

International Monetary Fund. (2021). *World economic outlook*. Available at www.imf.org/en/Publications/WEO/Issues/2021/10/12/world-economic-outlook-october-2021 (Accessed 24 January 2023).

Iqbal, M., Ahmad, N., Waqas, M., & Abrar, M. (2021). COVID-19 pandemic and construction industry: Impacts, emerging construction safety practices, and proposed crisis management. *Brazilian Journal of Operations & Production Management*, 18, 1–17.

Koh, D. (2020). Migrant workers and COVID-19. *Occupational and Environmental Medicine*, 77, 634–636.

Manu, P., Ankrah, N., Proverbs, D., & Suresh, S. (2014). The health and safety impact of construction project features. *Engineering Construction and Architectural Management*, 21(1), 65–93.

Office for National Statistics. (2021a). *Coronavirus (COVID-19) related deaths by occupation, England and Wales: Deaths registered between 9 March and 28 December 2020*. Available at www.ons.gov.uk/peoplepopulationandcommunity/healthandsocialcare/causesofdeath/bulletins/coronaviruscovid19relateddeathsbyoccupationenglandandwales/deathsregisteredbetween9marchand28december2020 (Accessed 23 January 2023).

Office for National Statistics. (2021b). *Construction statistics, Great Britain: 2020*. Available at www.ons.gov.uk/businessindustryandtrade/constructionindustry/articles/constructionstatistics/2020/pdf (Accessed 24 January 2023).

Ogunnusi, M., Hamma-Adama, M., Salman, H., & Kouider, T. (2020). COVID-19 pandemic: The effects and prospects in the construction industry. *International Journal of Real Estate Studies*, 14.

Oxford Economics. (2021). Future of construction. *Oxford Economics*. Available at www.oxfordeconomics.com/resource/future-of-construction/#:~:text=Global%20construction%20output%20in%202020,growth%20and%20recovery%20from%20COVID (Accessed 9 August 2022).

Pamidimukkala, A., & Kermanshachi, S. (2021). Impact of Covid-19 on field and office workforce in construction industry. *Project Leadership and Society*, 2, 100018.

Rees-Evans. (2020). Understanding mental health in the built environment. *CIOB*. Available at www.ciob.org/industry/research/Understanding-Mental-Health-Built-Environment?gclid=CjwKCAjwi8iXBhBeEiwAKbUofQX6exbnl9vfDzkkfgltgQQGhQTBoMERU4jPJfTmVRz1AjRYwEku6RoCbn8QAvD_BwE (Accessed 9 August 2022).

Rouhanizadeh, B., Kermanshachi, S., & Nipa, T.J. (2019). Identification, categorization, and weighting of barriers to timely post-disaster recovery process. In *Computing in civil engineering 2019: Smart cities, sustainability, and resilience* (pp. 41–49). Reston, VA: American Society of Civil Engineers.

RSM UK Consulting LLP. (2021). Mental health and wellbeing research: Final report. *CITB*. Available at www.citb.co.uk/media/ffwjadqn/citb_mental_health_and_wellbeing_research_report.pdf (Accessed 9 August 2022).

Shi, Y., Wang, G., Cai, X.P., Deng, J.W., Zheng, L., Zhu, H.H., Zheng, M., Yang, B., & Chen, Z. (2020). An overview of COVID-19. *Journal of Zhejiang University-SCIENCE B*, 21(5), 343–360.

Sierra, F. (2021). COVID-19: Main challenges during construction stage. *Engineering, Construction and Architectural Management*, 29, 1817–1834.

Stiles, S., Golightly, D., & Ryan, B. (2021). Impact of COVID-19 on health and safety in the construction sector. *Human Factors and Ergonomics in Manufacturing & Service Industries*, 31, 425–437.

Tijani, B., Nwaeze, J.F., Jin, X., & Osei-Kyei, R. (2021). Suicide in the construction industry: Literature review. *International Journal of Construction Management*. doi: 10.1080/15623599.2021.2005897.

World Health Organisation. (2023). *WHO coronavirus (COVID-19) dashboard*. Available at https://covid19.who.int/ (Accessed 30 January 2023).

Yang, Y., Chan, A.P.C., Shan, M., Gao, R., Bao, F., Lyu, S., Zhang, Q., & Guan, J. (2021). Opportunities and challenges for construction health and safety technologies under the COVID-19 pandemic in Chinese construction projects. *International Journal of Environmental Research and Public Health*, 18, 13038.

Zheng, L., Chen, K., & Ma, L. (2021). Knowledge, attitudes, and practices toward COVID-19 among construction industry practitioners in China. *Frontiers in Public Health*, 8, 599769.

# Section One

# Management of COVID-19 transmission risk

# 2 The transmission of COVID-19 in construction

## A systematic review of findings from statistical and modelling techniques

*Ruifeng Cao, Clara Cheung, Akilu Yunusa-Kaltungo, Patrick Manu, Chunxue Liu and Qingyao Qiao*

## Introduction

According to the World Health Organization (WHO), the COVID-19 pandemic has caused a huge loss of human life and posed unprecedented challenges to public health. The outbreak of COVID-19 forced governments worldwide to impose various restrictions, including mobility restrictions, socio-economic restrictions, and social distancing regulations, to reduce the spread of the disease (de Bruin et al., 2020). Although these restrictions have positively impacted the spread of COVID-19, they have caused significant losses to the construction industry (Jones et al., 2020). As social distancing was the main way to curtail the spread of the pandemic, the construction sector was severely affected because of the labour-intensiveness of the execution of construction projects. Despite the implementation of strict restrictions, previous studies have revealed that the construction industry has the highest COVID-19 infection rate among other industries such as medical care, manufacturing and transportation, with a hospitalisation rate that was five times the average level of other industries (Allan-Blitz et al., 2020; Pasco et al., 2020).

Recent studies, particularly in epidemiology, have shown how different statistical and modelling techniques such as linear programming, dynamic programming, structural equation modelling, and agent-based modelling (ABM) can predict the spread of COVID-19 (Saldaña and Velasco-Hernández, 2022; Afzal et al., 2022). However, there is limited research reviewing which modelling techniques could be used to understand how construction workers interact, resulting in predicting the transmission rate on site. In addition, the approach for selecting the most appropriate modelling method is still unclear. This study conducts a systematic literature review of modelling applications in the spread of COVID-19 in construction, with specific interest in the modelling purposes and limitations to guide researchers in selecting appropriate modelling techniques.

## Methodology

The Preferred Reporting Items for Systematic Reviews and Meta-Analyses (PRISMA) protocol (Liberati et al., 2009; Moher et al., 2010) was used to define

DOI: 10.1201/9781003278368-3

the literature search methodology, which helped to identify, select, and evaluate the literature that is relevant to modelling techniques used by the construction industry against COVID-19. The review questions guiding this study are as follows:

1. What modelling techniques have been commonly used by the construction industry to manage workers' health and safety conditions during the COVID-19 pandemic?
2. What are the characteristics and functions of these modelling techniques?
3. What are the main purposes of those modelling applications?

Considering the interdisciplinary nature of this study, Scopus was selected as the database for this systematic literature review due to its high reputation as the largest abstract and citation database of peer-reviewed literature (Vieira and Gomes, 2009; Adriaanse and Rensleigh, 2011; Aghaei Chadegani et al., 2013). Based on the outlined research questions, the preliminary search string for the identification stage was generated as TITLE-ABS-KEY ("model*" AND "COVID" AND ("construction*" OR "building*")). There were 2027 outputs in total identified through the advanced search in Scopus. After a rough review, it was found that a large number of documents were about DNA construction or the construction of organisations, rather than the construction industry. Therefore, the number of the search outputs was further narrowed down based on the screening criteria such as year of publication, document type, publication stage, and language, as well as the stricter search string to focus on the construction industry and workers' health and safety. Only the journal articles or review papers that were published from January 2020 to the present (10th June 2022) and written in English were included. The refined search

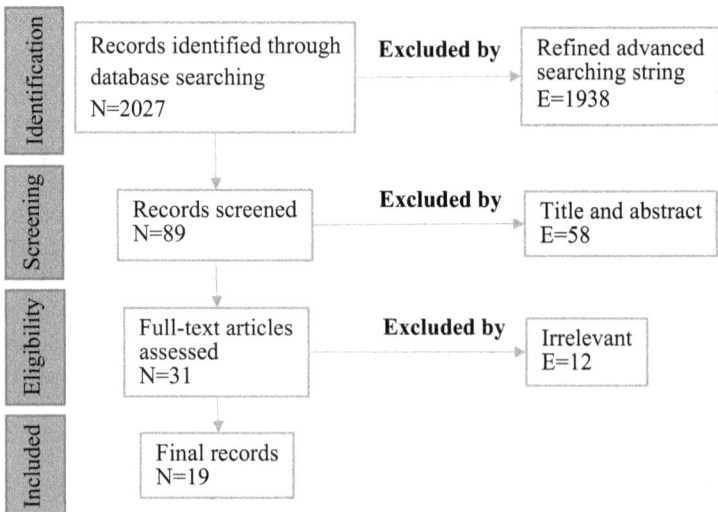

*Figure 2.1* PRISMA based systematic literature review flowchart.

string with screening criteria was then determined as TITLE-ABS-KEY ("model*" AND "COVID" AND ("construction site*" OR "construction work" OR "construction workers" OR "construction industry" OR "construction sector" OR "building construction" OR "building site*" OR "building sector")) AND (LIMIT-TO (LANGUAGE, "English")) AND (LIMIT-TO (DOCTYPE, "ar") OR LIMIT-TO (DOCTYPE, "re")). There were 89 records left with the refined search string. Then, the title and abstract analysis was implemented to exclude the out-of-scope articles. The full text of the remaining 31 articles were further assessed for relevance. Finally, 19 journal articles were determined to fully meet the scope of the review and were thus included in this study. Figure 2.1 shows the PRISMA flowchart with the number of documents and the inclusion and exclusion criteria applied in each phase.

## Results and discussion

Based on the review, it was found that the five commonly used simulation and modelling techniques in the construction industry against COVID-19 are: 1) SIR/SEIR modelling (Susceptible – Infectious – Recovered modelling or Susceptible – Exposed – Infectious – Recovered modelling), 2) Agent-based modelling (ABM), 3) Statistical modelling, 4) Building information modelling (BIM), and 5) Artificial Intelligence (AI) approach. Figure 2.2 illustrates the annual distribution of articles using the five modelling techniques included into this systematic literature review. At first glance, the number of articles related to statistical modelling and ABM are the largest in the past few years, closely followed by the number of articles related to the AI approach. The number of applications of the other modelling techniques are the same. The applications of ABM, statistical modelling, and AI approach are

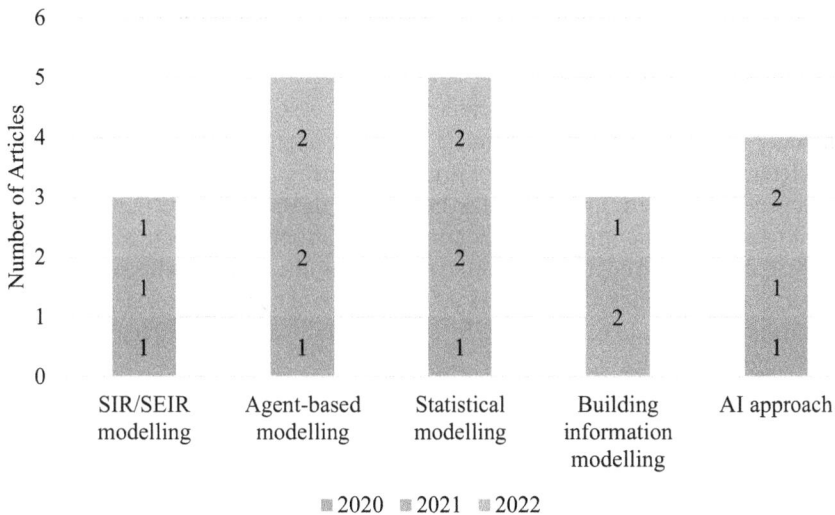

*Figure 2.2* Yearly distribution of articles related to the different modelling techniques.

growing from one article per method in 2020 to two articles per method in 2022. One of the articles selected in this review study discussed both BIM and AI approaches for construction health and safety under the COVID-19 pandemic (Yang et al., 2021).

### *SIR/SEIR modelling*

SIR (Susceptible – Infectious – Recovered) and SEIR (Susceptible – Exposed – Infectious – Recovered) modelling are mathematical modelling techniques in which the population is assigned to compartments with labels in order. The flow patterns of people progressing between the compartments are indicated in the order of labels; for instance, SEIR means people are first at the stage of being susceptible, followed by being exposed, infectious, and finally recovered. The modelling purpose is to estimate the reproductive number, understand the pattern of epidemic spread, and predict the number of infected people and duration of a pandemic. SIR/SEIR models' core required data is the line list for individual confirmed cases (e.g., confirmed cases, severity status and date of recovery, discharge, or death). This modelling technique is particularly useful for predicting transmission at a meta-population level and has been widely used by epidemiologists for over 100 years (Adiga et al., 2020b). The main drawback of this technique is that it requires large population data to make the prediction, and it cannot simulate the impact of complex interventions (e.g., voluntary home isolation, school closures, etc.) on disease spread across different social and spatial scales (Adiga et al., 2020b).

Afkhamiaghda and Elwakil (2020) developed a preliminary model using the SIR modelling technique and indicator of coronavirus (COVID-19) spread in the construction industry in order to provide a guide for construction workers. The developed model has also considered construction spending, the number of workers, and the density of the regions. Research results identified the factors related to the construction industry that affect the speed of the spread of the virus, including the quantity of the work that needs to be performed, the area of the jobsite, and the daily output of the work crew.

Chen et al. (2021) combined a detailed SEIR disease model of COVID-19 with a model of the US economy to estimate the direct impact of labour supply shock to different sectors including the construction industry. Results indicated a trade-off between economic losses and the number of deaths and infections avoided. When more epidemic prevention measures were strictly implemented, including longer lockdown and compliance with interventions, the economic losses would be greater, and the number of deaths and infections would be lower. Besides, a shorter lockdown period could be overcome by a higher compliance to nonpharmaceutical interventions, and vice versa.

Yuan et al. (2022) developed a dual-community model including the susceptible – exposed – infectious/asymptomatic – hospitalised – recovered – pathogen (SEI/AHR-P) model for construction workers and the susceptible – exposed – infectious/asymptomatic – hospitalised – recovered (SEI/AHR) model for their close contacts. It further discussed effectiveness of nonpharmaceutical interventions implemented in the construction industry, as well as the effectiveness of vaccination.

*Agent-based modelling (ABM)*

ABM is a class of computational models that simulate the simultaneous operations and interactions of multiple agents (e.g., human and its environment) to recreate and predict the appearance of complex phenomena. It is a kind of a microscale model, and the simulating process is one of emergence, which can be expressed as "the whole is greater than the sum of its parts." ABM was used to predict the spread of disease in time series and evaluate the impact of different interventions on epidemic outcomes. Consequently, it can help find the most effective intervention from a suite of interventions. ABM has been widely used in the research on the construction industry to simulate construction activities (Lu et al., 2016; Ji et al., 2019). A few studies have recently adopted ABM to simulate the spread of COVID-19 in the industry (Cuevas, 2020; Araya, 2021a), which outlined the potential of using ABM to evaluate the impact of different epidemic prevention measures in construction sites on health risk and worker performance. The key advantages of ABMs are that they can stimulate complex social interactions, individual and collective behavioural adaptation, and different intervention measures (Adiga et al., 2020a), and the agents' interactions can be visualised on the open-source modelling platform such as NetLogo. The main drawback is that it relies on the quality of assumptions put in the model.

Ronchi and Lovreglio (2020) proposed a microscopic crowd model that allows the representation of each person's location and interactions with the physical space/other people. Although this study does not provide a complete disease transmission model, it shows the ability of this model to investigate the occupant exposure in buildings based on the microscopic people movement. Araya (2021a) proposed an ABM framework to simulate the spread of COVID-19 among construction workers and found the spread may reduce the workforce of a project by approximately between 30% and 90%. Araya (2021b) then presented an ABM approach to quantifying the benefits of using multiple working shifts to reduce the spread of COVID-19 among construction workers. Araya (2022) also simulated the influence of multiskilled construction workers in the deficit of workers during COVID-19 pandemic using an ABM approach. In order to enhance the performance of ABM by introducing randomness, Gerami Seresht (2022) introduced a stochastic multi-agent framework to predict the spread of COVID-19 in construction projects using ABM and Monte Carlo simulation. The proposed framework was applied to simulate the spread of COVID-19 in a residential building project case study, and to assess the effectiveness of face-covering for preventing disease transmission.

*Statistical modelling*

Statistical modelling includes techniques such as regression and structural equation modelling. It is a mathematical model that embodies statistical assumptions that idealise the data-generating process (Cox, 2006). It usually specifies a mathematical relationship between many variables, both random and non-random. This type of model is purely phenomenological. The key associations of essential factors are examined to estimate epidemiological parameters or predict disease risk, but mechanisms of transmission processes are not considered (Becker et al., 2021). The advantages of statistical models are the effectiveness and efficiency in short-term forecasting projections (Adiga et al., 2020a), and they are easy and fast to build up. The main limitation is that it overly simplifies the relationships among the variables in the model.

Pasco et al. (2020) developed a decision analytical model based on a mathematical model of COVID-19 transmission with stratification of age and risk group of construction workers to assess the association between construction work during the COVID-19 pandemic and hospitalisation rates for construction workers and the surrounding community. Onubi et al. (2021) utilised the partial least squares structural equation modelling technique to analyse a sample of 312 construction site workers to obtain the determinants of COVID-19-related safety behaviour on construction sites in Nigeria. Olanrewaju et al. (2021) developed a questionnaire instrument that included 24 Covid-preventive measures on construction sites and then applied Principal Component Analysis to structure the 24 measures into four components. The results indicated that project cost increased by more than 20% due to the cost of health and safety regulations against COVID-19, site productivity decreased by up to 50% and personnel shortages increased by 40%. Aslan and Türkakın (2022) used multi-objective genetic algorithm, resource-constrained project scheduling techniques, and modelling of COVID-19 infection rate to obtain an optimal solution considering project duration, total cost, and pandemic risk. Radzi et al. (2022) applied partial least squares structural equation modelling to identify the causal relationships between COVID-19 impacts and response strategies in the construction industry.

### *Building information modelling (BIM)*

BIM is a virtual multidimensional model of construction engineering that provides a complete and consistent construction engineering information database (Fargnoli and Lombardi, 2020). The information database includes geometric information, professional properties, state information of building components, and state information of non-component objects (such as space and motion behaviour). With the help of such model and information database, the information integration of construction engineering is significantly improved, thus providing a platform for engineering information exchange, and sharing for stakeholders of construction projects within the overall project life cycle. Although BIM cannot be directly used to predict the spread of COVID on construction sites, its visualisation ability can better help the project team understand the current health and safety status (Rice, 2021), as well as the effectiveness and level of compliance to various nonpharmaceutical interventions (Yang et al., 2021).

Rice (2021) identified the feasibility of integrating the application of BIM with the measurement of various building health indicators. Meanwhile, Yang et al. (2021) pointed out that the appliance of BIM platform enhanced the communication and coordination of the project team when implementing social distance measures. Previous literature and market reviews have shown that BIM technology has been developed and applied to epidemic prevention measures at the construction site. However, this technology was seldom used in the projects studied by this research. Afterwards, Hosny et al. (2022) created a 4D BIM combined with Monte Carlo simulation for modelling uncertainties of productivity and workspace sizes occurring onsite to check the compliance to social distancing and other required safety buffering.

### Artificial intelligence (AI) approach

Artificial intelligence (AI) technologies help build models to make predictions or decisions by using computer algorithms that improve automatically through experience based on sample data, known as "training data," instead of being explicitly programmed to do so (Mitchell, 1997). The model aims to predict transmission growth rate in time-series and analyse interventions as well as contact tracing. AI-based models are particularly useful in forecasting and short-term projections (Adiga et al., 2020a). Techniques such as artificial neural networks (ANN) have the ability of self-learning without prior knowledge, and thus their application in the prediction of infectious diseases has become increasingly prominent (Adiga et al., 2020b). These models have used a wide variety of data for conducting prediction, including (i) social media data, (ii) weather data, (iii) incidence curves and (iv) demographic data (Adiga et al., 2020b). The main challenge of using AI is that it highly relies on a considerable amount of data.

Neisani Samani et al. (2020) developed a modelling strategy using location-based social network and artificial neural network technologies to identify the risk zone of transmission diseases temporally. Yang et al. (2021) evaluated AI-powered fever monitoring and AI-based safety monitoring technologies for health and safety management in the construction sector during the COVID-19 pandemic. Sadeh et al. (2022) developed a supervised machine learning linear regression model and applied a probabilistic risk-based cost estimate Monte Carlo simulation to evaluate the data collected from Occupational Safety and Health Administration of the US government, Centers for Disease Control, and the World Health Organization. Cédric Cabral et al. (2022) proposed a concept of intelligent building sites management using AI to organise several construction sites in real-time to fulfil multiple requirements including sustainable development goals and COVID-19.

### Comprehensive comparison

In order to discuss the applicability of different modelling techniques, three of the stages of pandemic response were considered in this research, including early stage, acceleration stage, and mitigation stage (Adiga et al., 2020a). Due to the high dependence on the assumptions of building the models, and the difficulty of obtaining corresponding information for assumptions at the early stage, ABM cannot be used at the early stage of pandemic. Similarly, due to the lack of sufficient data at the beginning of the epidemic, AI approaches are difficult to apply on the modelling of epidemic for analysis and prediction at the early stage. The other three modelling techniques can be applied in all three stages.

In terms of modelling purpose, SIR/SEIR modelling, statistical modelling, and AI approaches were applied to estimate epidemiological parameters (Adiga et al., 2020a; Adiga et al., 2020b). Four modelling techniques except BIM were used for growth rate and time-series forecasting. There are applications of ABM and BIM for intervention analyses (Ronchi and Lovreglio, 2020; Gerami Seresht, 2022; Hosny et al., 2022). Only ABM can meet the requirements to model the spatial spread of the disease at different scales: state, county, and community levels (Adiga et al., 2020a). BIM and AI approaches can be utilised for contact tracing (Yang et al., 2021).

Regarding the data needs for modelling, all five modelling techniques request line lists for individual confirmed cases and time-series data on disease outcomes. In addition, ABM and BIM need spatial representation as well as activity data and representation behaviours in order to consider individual differences and complex interactions (Gerami Seresht, 2022; Hosny et al., 2022). While the modelling purpose is for contact tracing, BIM and AI approaches require GPS traces data (Adiga et al., 2020a; Yang et al., 2021). Overall, SIR/SEIR modelling techniques require relatively fewer data types and smaller total amount, while AI approaches require the most and the largest.

Traditional SIR/SEIR modelling can only be applied to the large population scale, while the population scales of BIM applications are normally small. Due to the complexity of AI approaches, the operating speed of AI-based models is the slowest among the five technologies. The running speed and consumption of computing resources are much faster and lower for using SIR/SEIR modelling and statistical modelling.

The visualisation ability of ABM and BIM would be highly appreciated by the construction industry during application, which also assist in understanding the effects of interventions. Another feature that would be valued by industry, easiness of implementation, exists in SIR/SEIR modelling, ABM and BIM. Four modelling techniques except BIM contain the ability for short-term projections, while only SIR/SEIR modelling and ABM are competent to do long-term projections.

Based on this review, a comprehensive comparison of the five modelling techniques was created as shown as Table 2.1.

**Implications for practice and/or research**

Considering the insights from the literature review results, this study proposes the hybrid simulation/modelling of the risk of transmission of COVID-19 on construction site using the ABM and SIR/SEIR technique. ABM is selected because of its ability to simulate how humans interact with others and the environment over time (Adiga et al., 2020b), which aligns well with the complexity of construction site activities that are often labour-intensive and time- and space-constrained in nature. The combination with SIR/SEIR can make up for the deficiency of the assumption

*Table 2.1* Comparison of the five commonly used modelling techniques.

| Evaluation criteria | | SIR/SEIR modelling | ABM | Statistical modelling | BIM | AI approach |
|---|---|---|---|---|---|---|
| Pandemic Stages | Early stage | Yes | No | Yes | Yes | No |
| | Acceleration stage | Yes | Yes | Yes | Yes | Yes |
| | Mitigation stage | Yes | Yes | Yes | Yes | Yes |
| Modelling Purpose | Epidemiological parameter estimation | Yes | No | Yes | No | Yes |
| | Spatial spread across scales | No | Yes | No | No | No |
| | Growth rate and time-series forecasting | Yes | Yes | Yes | Yes | Yes |
| | Intervention analyses | No | Yes | No | Yes | No |
| | Contact tracing | No | No | No | Yes | Yes |
| Data Needs | Line lists for individual confirmed cases | Yes | Yes | Yes | Yes | Yes |
| | Spatial representation | No | Yes | No | Yes | No |
| | Activity data and representation behaviours | No | Yes | No | Yes | No |
| | Time-series data on disease outcomes | Yes | Yes | Yes | Yes | Yes |
| | GPS traces | No | No | No | Yes | Yes |
| Characteristics | Data amount requirement | Small | Medium | Medium | Medium | Large |
| | Population scales | Large | Large and small | Large and small | Small | Large and small |
| | Consider individual differences and complex interactions | No | Yes | No | Yes | No |
| | Rely on the quality of assumptions | No | Yes | No | No | No |
| | Operating speed | Fast | Medium | Fast | Medium | Slow |
| | Consider spatial information | No | Yes | No | Yes | Yes |
| Abilities | Visualisation | No | Yes | No | Yes | No |
| | Easy to use | Yes | Yes | Yes | Yes | No |
| | Short-term projections | Yes | Yes | Yes | No | Yes |
| | Long-term projections | Yes | Yes | No | No | No |
| | Understanding the effects of interventions | No | Yes | No | Yes | No |

*Table 2.2* Proposed data framework for hybrid ABM-SEIR models of COVID-19 transmission on construction site.

| Environment data | Agent (i.e., workers on site) properties | Agent (i.e., workers on site) behaviours |
|---|---|---|
| For example:<br>• Site layout<br>• Construction type<br>• Scale of the site<br>• Number of workers<br>• Transmission rate<br>• Location of work (i.e., indoor/outdoor/underground) | For example:<br>• Workload distribution of the construction site<br>• Schedule of the construction workers<br>• Work type of construction workers<br>• Location and proximity<br>• Vaccination rate<br>• Positive cases<br>• Mode of transportation to work | For example:<br>• Response to the different on-site epidemic prevention measures<br>• Risk perception of getting infected<br>• Safety leadership/culture<br>• Interaction frequency and duration<br>• On-site epidemic prevention measures (e.g., wear masks, washing hands, keep social distances) |
| *Possible Data Sources:*<br>Building Information Modelling (BIM); Construction Management Plan | *Possible Data Sources:*<br>Construction Management Plan; Questionnaire | *Possible Data Sources:*<br>Wearable Devices; Questionnaire |

for transmission dynamics of infectious diseases in ABM. In addition, ABM can be a highly visualised and easy-to-use tool once the verification, calibration, and validation models are constructed.

It is also proposed to simulate the transmission of COVID-19 and construction projects' working progress using the hybrid ABM-SEIR models from an on-site individual workers' perspective. The agent-based approach explicitly models the individual contact patterns in the modelling so that the epidemic prevention measures can be analysed at a micro-level. An agent-based model consists of three components: 1) agents' properties, behaviours, and environment; 2) agents' interactions with environments; and 3) agents' relationship and interactions with other agents (Macal and North, 2005). The model can be developed based on the standard procedure recommended by Wilensky and Rang (2015). Using the agents' properties, behaviours, and environment as the foundation, a data framework has been proposed and showed in Table 2.2 to build and test the hybrid models in future.

## Conclusions

The aim of this study is to develop an awareness of the simulation and modelling techniques used by the construction industry to manage the COVID-19 transmission risk on construction sites. A systematic literature review was conducted to identify the most commonly used simulation and modelling techniques in construction, and 19 journal articles were selected to review in detail based on PRISMA guideline.

As a result, five modelling techniques were compared comprehensively, including 1) SIR/SEIR modelling, 2) Agent-based modelling (ABM), 3) Statistical modelling, 4) Building information modelling (BIM), and 5) AI approach. The comparison covers several criteria including suitability for stages of pandemic; modelling purpose; data requirements; characteristics; and capabilities. The review reveals that each of these techniques have their unique strengths that make them useful for modelling COVID-19 transmission risk in construction under various scenarios/conditions or stages of COVID-19 pandemic. Finally, a data framework is proposed for future activities, to build and test the hybrid ABM-SEIR models, which are to simulate the transmission of COVID-19 and construction projects' working progress from the individual workers' perspective. The conclusions of this chapter are also applicable to other infectious diseases that are transmitted between close contacts, providing ideas for the construction industry to deal with possible future pandemics.

## References

Adiga, A., Chen, J., Marathe, M., Mortveit, H., Venkatramanan, S., & Vullikanti, A. (2020a). Data-driven modeling for different stages of pandemic response. *Journal of the Indian Institute of Science*, 100, 901–915.

Adiga, A., Dubhashi, D., Lewis, B., Marathe, M., Venkatramanan, S., & Vullikanti, A. (2020b). Mathematical models for COVID-19 pandemic: A comparative analysis. *Journal of the Indian Institute of Science*, 100, 793–807.

Adriaanse, L.S., & Rensleigh, C. (2011). Comparing web of science, scopus and Google scholar from an environmental sciences perspective. *South African Journal of Libraries and Information Science*, 77, 169–178.

Afkhamiaghda, M., & Elwakil, E. (2020). Preliminary modeling of Coronavirus (COVID-19) spread in construction industry. *Journal of Emergency Management*, 18, 9–17.

Afzal, A., Saleel, C.A., Bhattacharyya, S., Satish, N., Samuel, O.D., & Badruddin, I.A. (2022). Merits and limitations of mathematical modeling and computational simulations in mitigation of COVID-19 pandemic: A comprehensive review. *Archives of Computational Methods in Engineering*, 29, 1311–1337.

Aghaei Chadegani, A., Salehi, H., Yunus, M., Farhadi, H., Fooladi, M., Farhadi, M., & Ale Ebrahim, N. (2013). A comparison between two main academic literature collections: Web of science and scopus databases. *Asian Social Science*, 9, 18–26.

Allan-Blitz, L.-T., Turner, I., Hertlein, F., & Klausner, J.D. (2020). High frequency and prevalence of community-based asymptomatic SARS-CoV-2 infection. *MedRxiv*.

Araya, F. (2021a). Modeling the spread of COVID-19 on construction workers: An agent-based approach. *Safety Science*, 133.

Araya, F. (2021b). Modeling working shifts in construction projects using an agent-based approach to minimize the spread of COVID-19. *Journal of Building Engineering*, 41.

Araya, F. (2022). Modeling the influence of multiskilled construction workers in the context of the covid-19 pandemic using an agent-based approach. *Revista de la Construccion*, 21, 105–117.

Aslan, S., & Türkakın, O.H. (2022). A construction project scheduling methodology considering COVID-19 pandemic measures. *Journal of Safety Research*, 80, 54–66.

Becker, A.D., Grantz, K.H., Hegde, S.T., Bérubé, S., Cummings, D.A.T., & Wesolowski, A. (2021). Development and dissemination of infectious disease dynamic transmission models during the COVID-19 pandemic: What can we learn from other pathogens and how can we move forward? *The Lancet Digital Health*, 3, e41–e50.

Cédric Cabral, F.Y., Patrick Joël, M.M., Ursula Joyce Merveilles, P.N., Marcelline Blanche, M., Georges Edouard, K., & Chrispin, P. (2022). Using AI as a support tool for bridging construction informal sector mechanisms to sustainable development requirements. *Journal of Decision Systems*, 31(S1), 226–240.

Chen, J., Vullikanti, A., Santos, J., Venkatramanan, S., Hoops, S., Mortveit, H., Lewis, B., You, W., Eubank, S., Marathe, M., Barrett, C., & Marathe, A. (2021). Epidemiological and economic impact of COVID-19 in the US. *Scientific Reports*, 11.

Cox, D.R. (2006). *Principles of statistical inference*. Cambridge: Cambridge University Press.

Cuevas, E. (2020). An agent-based model to evaluate the COVID-19 transmission risks in facilities. *Computers in Biology and Medicine*, 121, 103827.

De Bruin, Y.B., Lequarre, A.-S., Mccourt, J., Clevestig, P., Pigazzani, F., Jeddi, M.Z., Colosio, C., & Goulart, M. (2020). Initial impacts of global risk mitigation measures taken during the combatting of the COVID-19 pandemic. *Safety Science*, 128, 104773.

Fargnoli, M., & Lombardi, M. (2020). Building Information Modelling (BIM) to enhance occupational safety in construction activities: Research trends emerging from one decade of studies. *Buildings*, 10, 98.

Gerami Seresht, N. (2022). Enhancing resilience in construction against infectious diseases using stochastic multi-agent approach. *Automation in Construction*, 140.

Hosny, A., Nik-Bakht, M., & Moselhi, O. (2022). Physical distancing analytics for construction planning using 4D BIM. *Journal of Computing in Civil Engineering*, 36.

Ji, T., Wei, H.-H., & Chen, J. (2019). Understanding the effect of co-worker support on construction safety performance from the perspective of risk theory: An agent-based modeling approach. *Journal of Civil Engineering and Management*, 25, 132–144.

Jones, W., Chow, V., & Gibb, A. (2020). COVID-19 and construction: Early lessons for a new normal. *Loughborough University*, (August), 1–18.

Liberati, A., Altman, D.G., Tetzlaff, J., Mulrow, C., Gøtzsche, P.C., Ioannidis, J.P., Clarke, M., Devereaux, P.J., Kleijnen, J., & Moher, D. (2009). The PRISMA statement for reporting systematic reviews and meta-analyses of studies that evaluate health care interventions: Explanation and elaboration. *Journal of Clinical Epidemiology*, 62, e1–e34.

Lu, M., Cheung, C.M., Li, H., & Hsu, S.-C. (2016). Understanding the relationship between safety investment and safety performance of construction projects through agent-based modeling. *Accident Analysis & Prevention*, 94, 8–17.

Macal, C.M., & North, M.J. (2005). Tutorial on agent-based modeling and simulation. Proceedings of the Winter Simulation Conference, p. 14.

Mitchell, T.M. (1997). *Machine learning*. New Delhi: McGraw Hill Education India.

Moher, D., Liberati, A., Tetzlaff, J., & Altman, D.G. (2010). Preferred reporting items for systematic reviews and meta-analyses: The PRISMA statement. *International Journal of Surgery*, 8, 336–341.

Neisani Samani, Z., Karimi, M., & Alesheikh, A. (2020). Environmental and infrastructural effects on respiratory disease exacerbation: A LBSN and ANN-based spatio-temporal modelling. *Environmental Monitoring and Assessment*, 192.

Olanrewaju, A., Abdulaziz, A., Preece, C.N., & Shobowale, K. (2021). Evaluation of measures to prevent the spread of COVID-19 on the construction sites. *Cleaner Engineering and Technology*, 5.

Onubi, H.O., Yusof, N.A., & Hassan, A.S. (2021). Perceived COVID-19 safety risk and safety behavior on construction sites: Role of safety climate and firm size. *Journal of Construction Engineering and Management*, 147, 04021153.

Pasco, R.F., Fox, S.J., Johnston, S.C., Pignone, M., & Meyers, L.A. (2020). Estimated association of construction work with risks of COVID-19 infection and hospitalization in Texas. *JAMA Network Open*, 3.

Radzi, A.R., Rahman, R.A., & Almutairi, S. (2022). Modeling COVID-19 impacts and response strategies in the construction industry: PLS-SEM approach. *International Journal of Environmental Research and Public Health*, 19.

Rice, L. (2021). Healthy BIM: The feasibility of integrating architecture health indicators using a Building Information Model (BIM) computer system. *Archnet-IJAR*, 15, 252–265.

Ronchi, E., & Lovreglio, R. (2020). EXPOSED: An occupant exposure model for confined spaces to retrofit crowd models during a pandemic. *Safety Science*, 130.

Sadeh, H., Mirarchi, C., Shahbodaghlou, F., & Pavan, A. (2022). Predicting the trends and cost impact of COVID-19 OSHA citations on US construction contractors using machine learning and simulation. Engineering, Construction and Architectural Management.

Saldaña, F., & Velasco-Hernández, J.X. (2022). Modeling the COVID-19 pandemic: A primer and overview of mathematical epidemiology. *SeMA Journal*, 79, 225–251.

Vieira, E., & Gomes, J. (2009). A comparison of Scopus and Web of Science for a typical university. *Scientometrics*, 81, 587–600.

Wilensky, U., & Rand, W. (2015). *An introduction to agent-based modeling: Modeling natural, social, and engineered complex systems with NetLogo*. Cambridge, MA: MIT Press.

Yang, Y., Chan, A.P.C., Shan, M., Gao, R., Bao, F., Lyu, S., Zhang, Q., & Guan, J. (2021). Opportunities and challenges for construction health and safety technologies under the COVID-19 pandemic in Chinese construction projects. *International Journal of Environmental Research and Public Health*, 18.

Yuan, Z., Hsu, S.C., Cheung, C.M., & Asghari, V. (2022). Effectiveness of interventions for controlling COVID-19 transmission between construction workers and their close contacts. *Journal of Management in Engineering*, 38.

# 3 Health and safety measures for managing the COVID-19 pandemic in the construction industry

## A comparison study

*Albert P.C. Chan, Yang Yang, Janet Mayowa Nwaogu, Wen Yi and Junfeng Guan*

### Introduction

The construction sector is a major part of an economy in terms of revenue provision, unemployment reduction, and poverty alleviation (Agyekum et al., 2022; Nwaogu and Chan, 2021; Omatule Onubi et al., 2021). However, construction employees, especially site workers, work in unhygienic conditions and are susceptible to the spread of infectious diseases on sites; they are exposed to harsh weather, which causes them to sweat profusely (Olanrewaju et al., 2021). Thus, COVID-19 presents a health and safety challenge to the construction sector. The COVID-19 pandemic led to the loss of lives, economic recession, struggling businesses, high unemployment rates, and ways of gathering (Yang et al., 2021). To effectively continue construction projects during the COVID-19 period, some industry-friendly health and safety anti-epidemic measures must be sought (Ebekozien and Aigbavboa, 2021; Olanrewaju et al., 2021). Such measures include workforce education, hand washing, wearing face masks, regular temperature checks, staggered shifts, remote working, 6-foot physical distance between workers, and engaging a COVID-19 supervisor to ensure compliance (Ebekozien and Aigbavboa, 2021; Agyekum et al., 2022).

Studies have been conducted regarding COVID-19 and its impact on the construction industry (Sami Ur Rehman et al., 2022; Agyekum et al., 2022; Olanrewaju et al., 2021; Yang et al., 2021; Simpeh and Amoah, 2021; Ebekozien and Aigbavboa, 2021; Alsharef et al., 2021). The studies have been conducted in Nigeria (Ebekozien and Aigbavboa, 2021), China (Yang et al., 2021), the United Arab Emirates (Sami Ur Rehman et al., 2022), Ghana (Agyekum et al., 2022), South Africa (Simpeh and Amoah, 2021), the United States of America (Alsharef et al., 2021), and the United Kingdom. (Jallow et al., 2021). The studies focused only on the impact of COVID-19 on the construction industry and/or general health and safety measures employed to manage the spread of COVID on construction sites. In contrast, Ebekozien and Aigbavboa (2021) examined the role of how digital technologies such as cyber-physical systems, big data, blockchain, digital twin, augmented reality, robots, and 3D printing curtailed the spread of the COVID-19 pandemic on construction sites in Nigeria. Yang et al. (2021) detailed the role of health and safety technologies in managing COVID-19 on construction sites and

DOI: 10.1201/9781003278368-4

the issues associated with technology adoption in Chinese construction projects. However, comparative investigations into health and safety measures taken to curb the spread of the COVID-19 disease on construction projects while the industry is trying to deliver on its economic goals are lacking.

This study moves the conversation forward by evaluating the health and safety measures employed for managing construction projects in Nigeria and China under the COVID-19 pandemic. A comparative study between Nigeria (a Lower Middle-Income Country) and China (an Upper Middle-Income Country) is deemed necessary because several Chinese companies are engaged in infrastructure projects in Nigeria. Confronted with significant infrastructure needs, Nigeria sought so much help from China that Chinese investments in Nigeria between 2009 and 2010 increased from US$6 billion to US$8 billion (Babatunde and Low, 2013). Information from this study can help investors learn what is expected of them and technologies to adopt to enhance the safety of their workers and continuity of their projects during the COVID-19 era.

This study aims to examine the health and safety measures deployed in the construction industry of China and Nigeria in the COVID-19 era to facilitate effective pandemic planning. The specific objectives were: (i) to determine the health and safety measures used to respond to the COVID-19 pandemic unique to each country; (ii) to determine strategies used to manage or engage the construction projects during the COVID-19 pandemic. This study will inform policies that can help the construction industry ensure good health among its employees in order to meet its development and economic goals. The findings of this study will be helpful to governments of various economic statuses and their construction industries as they implement safety policies to prevent the spread of the COVID-19 disease and other epidemics to ensure the well-being of construction workers.

## Perspectives and concepts

### *Measures recommended for the fight against COVID-19*

The construction site has been described as an epicentre for spreading infectious diseases (Olanrewaju et al., 2021). This implies that working on construction sites during a pandemic such as COVID-19 is risky for employees and challenging for employers. Therefore, actions that are vital to curbing the spread of the disease must be implemented. In 2020, during the wake of the pandemic, measures recommended by the World Health Organization (WHO) to control the pandemic on construction sites were classified into general guidelines, screening process before entering sites, preventive measures related to the use of transportation, and procedure to follow in case of contagion (Agyekum et al., 2022). The general guidelines recommend that contractors restrict visitors' entry, assign a central point for implementing and monitoring COVID-19 prevention measures, ensure that employees who fall ill stay home, and hold health-related pep talks each day to discuss COVID-19. It also stipulates taking of body temperature, ensuring that employees practice hand-washing before entering the site or project office, ensuring social distancing on construction sites, observing all safety protocols, and following further instructions given by their local authorities (Agyekum et al., 2022).

Yang et al. (2021) classified the anti-epidemic measures employed on Chinese construction projects into three categories: personal, managerial, and technological. Personal control measures included mask-wearing, daily disinfection of work sites and offices, vaccinations, quarantine, health screening for temperature checkups, setting up isolation rooms, and conducting regular nucleic acid tests (Yang et al., 2021). Managerial controls included developing an emergency plan, online meetings, rescheduling jobs, and purchasing hygiene items. Health and safety technologies measures include using an onsite tracer app, health QR code, and COVID-19 big data analysis. The COVID-19 big data analysis in China identifies high-risk and low-risk COVID-19 areas. Big data technology is deployed through a health code system to prevent and control COVID-19 in China (Wu et al., 2020). The big data health code system is divided into three colour levels: red, yellow, and green. People with red or yellow codes will be quarantined. At the same time, green indicates that the person did not go to a virus-infected area and can carry out regional activities and movement. If someone with green codes has been to high-risk areas or is in contact with high-risk people, their code will turn red and they will have to be quarantined (Wu et al., 2020). In essence, the colour-coded health QR codes are used as electronic certificates to differentiate the COVID-19 status of individuals, and the QR codes are presented when using public services or before being allowed into the workplace (Sharara and Radia, 2022).

Simpeh and Amoah (2021) noted that government measures recommended for health and safety with regards to COVID-19 in the workplace in South Africa comprise four key aspects: plan for reopening workplaces following the lockdown, administrative actions, social distancing measures, and health and safety measures (Simpeh and Amoah, 2021). Administrative measures are instituted to minimise the number of workers at the workplace to ensure social (physical) distancing and raise awareness about COVID-19 among their workers (Simpeh and Amoah, 2021). Simpeh and Amoah (2021) further pointed out that the recommended health and safety measures include symptom screening, sanitisation (hygiene), ventilation, and PPE (e.g., use of mask, face shield, sanitisers, disinfectants, and hand gloves).

Agyekum et al. (2022) mentioned that health and safety measures outlined by the Government of Ghana are those put in place by construction firms in Ghana to fight COVID-19. They include sanitising of workers, use of PPEs, shift working times, regular COVID-19 testing and checks, use of screening questionnaires, and isolation of workers who show symptoms of sickness. In Nigeria, governmental recommendations for businesses changed rapidly. By August 2020, the recommendations for the manufacturing industry (which includes the construction sector) were four, namely: ensure the provision of sanitisers and appropriate PPEs to all workers, limit the number of workers to 75% to allow physical distancing, mandatory use of non-medical face masks and conducting of temperature checks (NCDC, 2020).

**Methodological approach**

This study adopted the qualitative methodology to probe in-depth the views and experiences of participants on the subject. With qualitative methodology, a particular phenomenon can be understood from the perspective of those experiencing it (Vaismoradi et al., 2013). A semi-structured interview, a qualitative data collection method, was used to collect data from 34 purposively selected respondents. This semi-structured interview approach was adopted because it could facilitate an interactive discussion. The interview was carried out using an interview guide adapted from Yang et al. (2021) via Zoom for 30 minutes (see Appendix I).

The interviewees were selected by purposive sampling to ensure the reliability of the interview and data collected. The interviewees were from varying professional backgrounds, firm sizes, and different positions. They included project managers, product managers, project general managers, directors, health and safety officers, and site supervisors. Following Yang et al. (2021), interviewees with work experience of at least three years were invited to the survey. Twenty-four interview invitations were emailed to potential respondents in China and Nigeria, of which 23 were received from China and 11 from Nigeria. Since similar qualitative studies (Agyekum et al., 2022; Ebekozien and Aigbavboa, 2021) interviewed nine to 12 professionals, the sample size of the interview survey is considered adequate.

**Data analysis**

The audio recordings were transcribed and analysed in the MAXQDA Plus software version 2022. The interviews with the practitioners in Nigeria were conducted in English, while others conducted with practitioners in the People's Republic of China were conducted in Chinese. The researchers translated Chinese scripts into English (Yang et al., 2021). Content analysis through deductive and inductive reasoning was used to determine the themes, and it followed the procedure described in Yang et al. (2021). Themes and categories were first drawn from the context of the data and later refined using themes in existing literature (Nwaogu et al., 2021).

**Results and discussion**

The interviewees provided relevant information on the response of their construction firms to COVID-19. When asked, "Can you describe how you respond to the COVID-19 pandemic and how you manage or engage in construction projects under the Covid-19 era?" the interviewees indicated that in the COVID-19 era, health and safety measures employed on the construction sites included checking body temperature before accessing the workplace, using PPEs (wearing face masks), disinfection of the site and offices, and sensitisation of employees (see Figure 3.1). As shown in Figure 3.1, the interviewees further revealed that the projects were managed using various strategies (approaches), such as online meetings, rediscussing the project cost and time with clients, using mechanised equipment, and planning for anti-epidemic items at the tender stage.

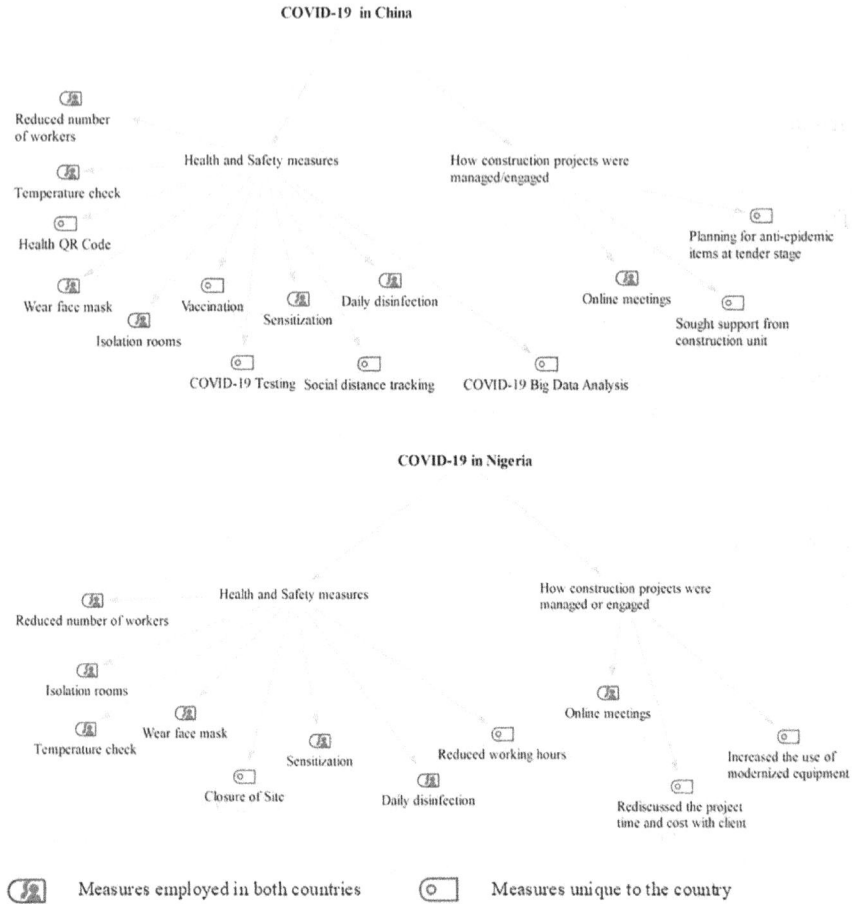

*Figure 3.1* COVID-19 response in the construction industry of China and Nigeria.

### Health and safety measures

Following the classification of health and safety measures detailed in Simpeh and Amoah (2021) and Yang et al. (2021), the measures can be further categorised into anti-epidemic public health measures, lockdown, administrative controls, and health and safety technology. Figure 3.2 and Figure 3.3 illustrate transcripts on health and safety measures employed by construction firms in Nigeria and China, respectively.

#### Administrative actions

The administrative actions taken included sensitising workers, reducing the work hours, and minimising the number of site workers at the workplace to allow for social distancing. These findings align with the recommended administrative

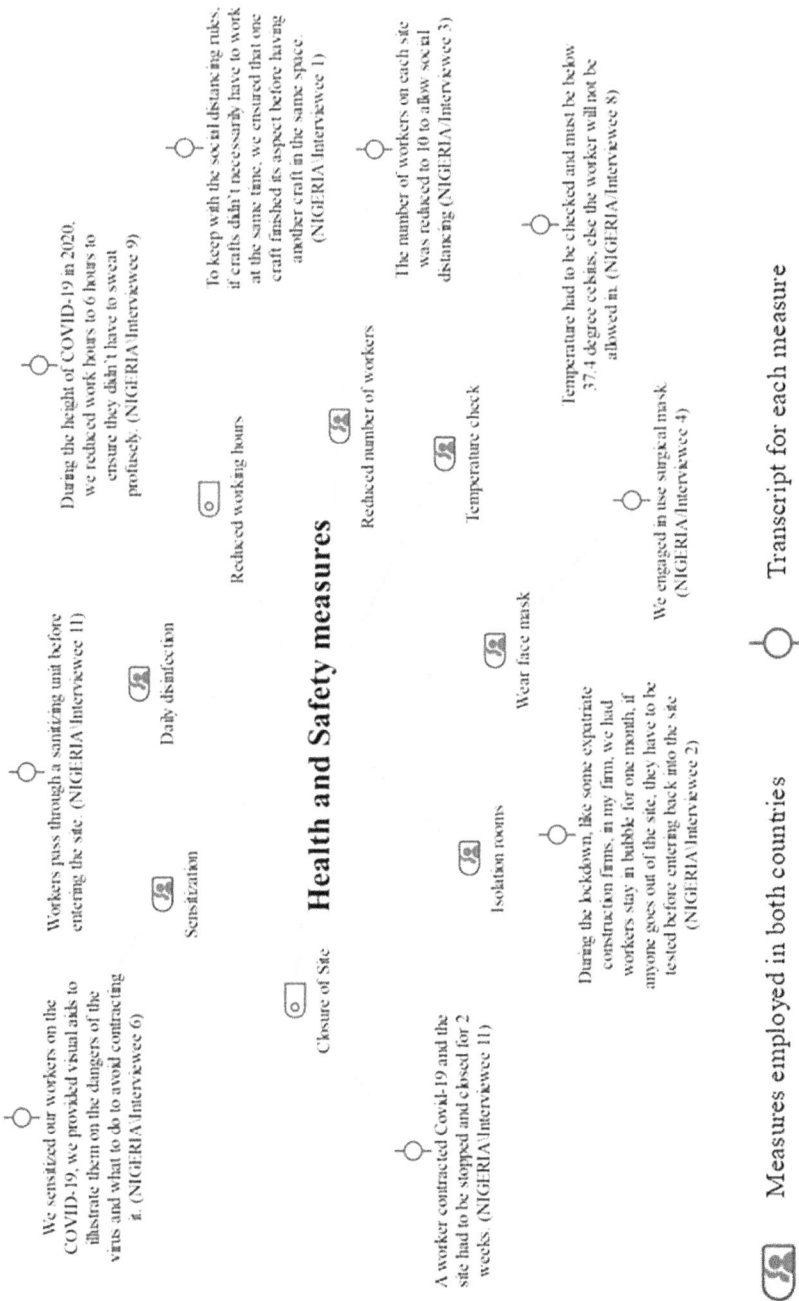

We sensitised our workers on the COVID-19, we provided visual aids to illustrate them on the dangers of the virus and what to do to avoid contracting it. (NIGERIA/Interviewee 6)

Workers pass through a sanitising unit before entering the site. (NIGERIA/Interviewee 11)

During the height of COVID-19 in 2020, we reduced work hours to 6 hours to ensure they didn't have to sweat profusely. (NIGERIA/Interviewee 9)

To keep with the social distancing rules, if crafts didn't necessarily have to work at the same time, we ensured that one craft finished its aspect before having another craft in the same space. (NIGERIA/Interviewee 1)

The number of workers on each site was reduced to 10 to allow social distancing (NIGERIA/Interviewee 3)

Temperature had to be checked and must be below 37.4 degree celsius, else the worker will not be allowed in. (NIGERIA/Interviewee 8)

**Health and Safety measures**

Sensitization

Daily disinfection

Reduced working hours

Reduced number of workers

Temperature check

Closure of Site

Isolation rooms

Wear face mask

We engaged in use surgical mask (NIGERIA/Interviewee 4)

A worker contracted Covid-19 and the site had to be stopped and closed for 2 weeks (NIGERIA/Interviewee 11)

During the lockdown, like some expatriate construction firms, in my firm, we had workers stay in bubble for one month, if anyone goes out of the site, they have to be tested before entering back into the site (NIGERIA/Interviewee 2)

Measures employed in both countries

Transcript for each measure

*Figure 3.2* Some health and safety measures employed in the Nigerian construction industry.

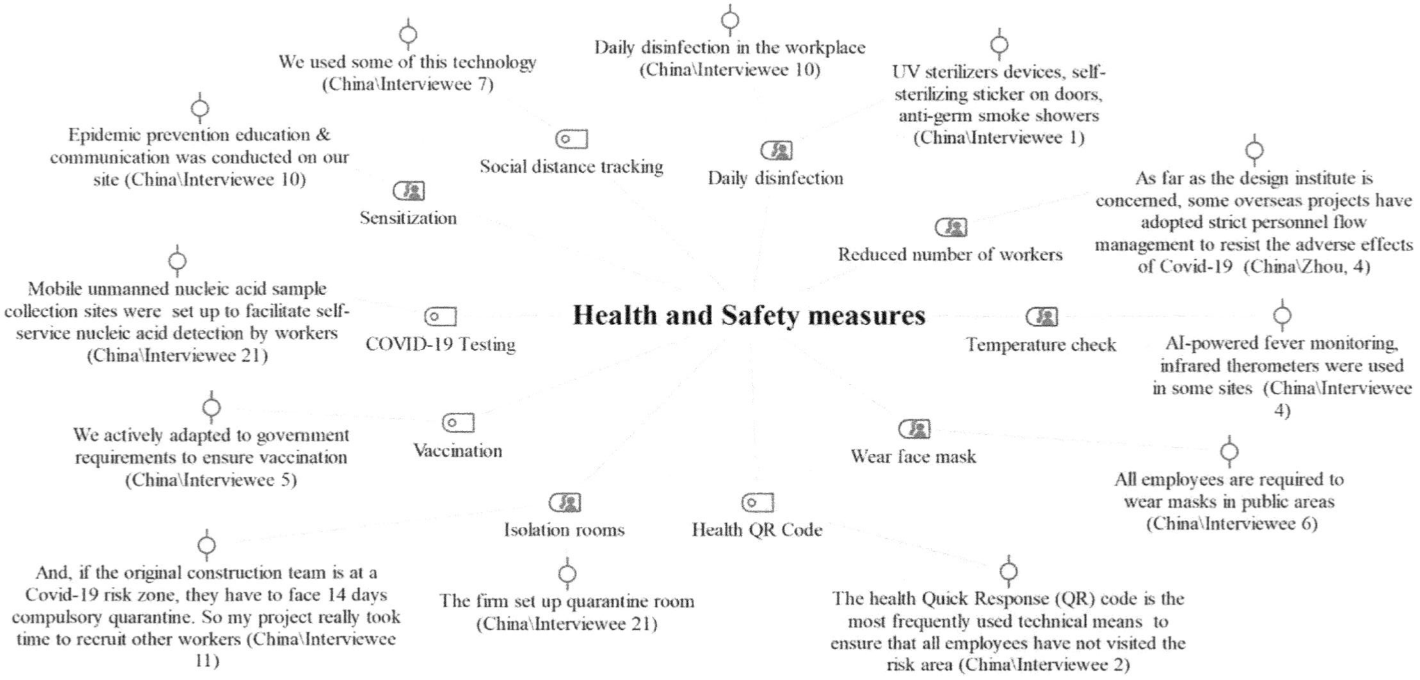

*Figure 3.3* Some health and safety measures employed in the Chinese construction industry.

actions mentioned in Simpeh and Amoah (2021). It was deduced that work hours were reduced on some sites in Nigeria, unlike in China. Like Nigeria/Interviewee 9 stated, "Since they said that COVID-19 can spread through sweat, in April 2020 during that lockdown, in my place of work, we reduced work hours to 4 hours to 6 hours to ensure they didn't have to sweat profusely".

Based on the interviews, it was deduced that in Nigeria, the number of craftsmen and administrative staff was reduced, while in China, the interviewees indicated that only the number of administrative staff was reduced. As detailed in Figure 3.2, the number of craftsmen on a particular site in Nigeria was reduced to 10 to allow social distancing (Nigeria/Interviewee 3). Also, Interviewee 1 mentioned that "to keep to the social distancing rules, if crafts didn't necessarily have to work at the same time, we ensured that one craft finished its aspect before having another craft in the same space".

*Anti-epidemic public health measures*

The anti-epidemic public health measures taken by construction firms in both countries included checking body temperature (using infrared thermometers or AI-powered fever monitoring devices) before accessing the workplace, wearing face masks, and daily disinfection of the workplace. These measures are part of those recommended by WHO for contractors (Agyekum et al., 2022). While workers on construction sites in Nigeria mainly had to pass through a sanitising unit before entering the site" (see Figure 3.2), it was deduced that various kinds of sterilising units were adopted in China (see Figure 3.3).

> ultraviolet (UV) sterilisers devices, self-sterilising sticker on doors, anti-germ smoke showers are used to disinfect the workplace.
>
> (China\Interviewee 1)

Although wearing face masks by employees was compulsory in both countries, construction firms in China made provisions for masks, as boxes of 50 pieces were periodically distributed to employees. "We regularly distribute masks and disinfectants to frontline workers" (China\Interviewee 20). This corroborates Simpeh and Amoah (2021), who reported that some construction companies in South Africa supplied PPEs to their workers.

On some sites in Nigeria and China, periodic safety meetings/daily toolbox meetings were also used to educate and reeducate the workers about the COVID-19 pandemic. This finding agrees with Simpeh and Amoah (2021), who suggested that most companies in South Africa revise their induction, toolbox talk, and training sessions to include COVID-19.

> Every Monday, we always had a safety meeting to remind the workers about the intensity of the COVID-19 virus. We reminded them not to throw handkerchiefs, tissues anywhere to ensure cleanliness and reduce the spread of diseases.
>
> (Nigeria/Interviewee 8)

*Health and safety technologies*

It was deduced that aside from public health measures, health and safety technologies such as health QR code systems, COVID-19 testing, social distance tracking, and COVID-19 big data analysis were employed in China, but not in Nigeria (see Figure 3.2 and Figure 3.3). This finding is similar to Yang et al. (2021), where the health QR code system was reported in Mainland China but not in Hong Kong or Dubai. Nevertheless, the technologies appeared not to be used on all sites in China, as revealed by China\Interviewee 4 and China\Interviewee 7.

> AI-powered fever monitoring, social distance tracking, health QR code, nucleic acid detection technologies. Some of the above techniques are used.
>
> (China\Interviewee 7)

> technologies such as online collaboration platforms, AI-powered fever monitoring, social distance tracking can be used. But they are not used.
>
> (China\Interviewee 4)

Some transcripts from the interviewees on the health and safety technologies not included in Figure 3.3 are detailed here:

> At present, we require all personnel entering the workplace to undergo temperature testing and keep records, show the Health QR Code, and wear masks. We regularly organise nucleic acid tests for all employees and encourage them to get vaccinated.
>
> (China\Interviewee 9)

> We adopted the "Covid-19 big data analysis map" to avoid entering medium- and high-risk areas to reduce the probability of personnel being infected. Employees' health QR code has been maintained as normal. Using mobile signalling data to track the movement of internal personnel helps to track social distance.
>
> (China\Interviewee 3)

The use of the health and safety technologies such as health quick response (QR) code systems, COVID-19 testing, social distance tracking, and COVID-19 big data analysis in the Chinese construction industry may have been influenced by governmental requirements instituted for businesses. According to Yang et al. (2021), "the COVID-19 big data analysis enables the management to identify medium- and high-risk areas within China and formulate corresponding coping strategies for workers from those risk areas". While some of these measures are unique to China's construction industry, they can be implemented and tested in other countries. For instance, the digital approach of using QR codes with big data analytics has been reported successful in containing and tackling the COVID-19 pandemic in China (Sharara and Radia, 2022).

*Lockdown*

The measures in this theme category include the closure of site and creation of isolation rooms on site. For some construction companies in China and Nigeria, isolation rooms had to be set up. While in China, the isolation rooms appeared to be a place where workers would stay temporarily for some hours, as inferred from China/Interviewee 20, in Nigeria, the workers had to be isolated together on some construction sites for one month so that construction activities could continue (Nigeria\Interviewee 2):

> We set AI-powered fever monitoring devices at the construction site entrance. If we find employees with abnormal body temperature, we will immediately take them to the quarantine room for observation.
>
> (China\Interviewee 20)

> During the lockdown, like some expatriate construction firms, in my firm, we had workers stay in a bubble for one month; if anyone goes out of the site, they have to be tested before entering back into the site.
>
> (Nigeria\Interviewee 2)

Likewise, it was deduced that in 2020, some sites had to be closed for 14 days in Nigeria. "A worker contracted Covid-19, and the site had to be stopped and closed for two weeks" (Nigeria\Interviewee 11). This could affect such firms' ability to meet the contract conditions as the contract duration may have to be extended due to the closure, as pointed out in Agyekum et al. (2022).

### Strategies used to manage or engage construction projects during the COVID-19 pandemic

When asked how construction projects were managed or engaged during the COVID-19 pandemic, it was deduced that a variety of strategies (i.e., approaches) were taken to manage the project. The most recurring strategy among 80% of interviewees in China and all the interviewees in Nigeria was conducting administrative and site meetings online. However, the potential of online meetings could not be entirely tapped in some cases because of confidentiality concerns (China/ Interviewee 3). The issue of confidentiality draws attention to some factors affecting effective information sharing and the adoption of digital assets in various supply chains. This is why information confidentiality preservation with regard to the use of information technology and digital assets is receiving increased attention (Ghondaghsaz et al., 2022).

> Because our company has high-level confidentiality measures, raw data is not allowed to be uploaded to the Internet. Therefore, we cannot use remote collaboration to continue the project's development. We can only handle schedule adjustments and design changes through online meetings, but work

involving big data governance and analysis cannot be performed. In the late period of Covid-19, the government adjusted anti-epidemic policy, and we gradually resumed the operation of the project by health QR codes and nucleic acid testing.

(China/Interviewee 3)

Among the 20% in China that indicated that online meetings were not conducted, it was due to the nature of their job (China/Interviewee 22). This further suggests that flexible work schedules (e.g., teleworking) would not fit all professions in the construction industry, as noted by Nwaogu and Chan (2021).

For teams specialising in software, jobs can be easily converted to online mode, and remote meetings have become the norm. My team's biggest challenge is the inability to communicate face-to-face, which inevitably damages communication efficiency.

(China/Interviewee 22)

Interviewees in Nigeria indicated that since the number of craftsmen had to be reduced, the firms resorted to using mechanised equipment to replace labour. According to an interviewee:

we employed the concrete placement equipment to reduce the number of artisans needed for concrete placement. You know, for a medium firm like ours, we do more manual placement, but now we have to engage the services of the concrete pump even for small jobs. The construction workers were reduced to meet social distancing rules.

(Nigeria/Interviewee 9)

Aside from the strategies discussed here, it was deduced that some companies in Nigeria addressed issues relating to the project cost and time with clients. For instance, Nigeria/Interviewee 3 stated:

we had to meet with the client to rediscuss project time frame and cost. We also discussed cost because craftsmen were reduced to 10 people on a site to meet social distancing rules. So, we had to discuss the impact of the Covid-19 regulations on project delivery time and cost.

Additionally, interviewees from China revealed that they managed their construction project by seeking financial support from the construction unit in their province. Some interviewees hinted that they have started including the cost of anti-epidemic items at the tender stage so they can include it in the bid (see China/Interviewee 6). This may be unique to China since the COVID-19 rules are still strictly enforced, unlike in Nigeria.

At the contract level, the builder needs to increase the stock of anti-epidemic items and arrange anti-epidemic measures (such as infrared thermometers, masks, medicines, monitoring stations, personnel deployment). At the tender stage, anti-epidemic costs in the contract are regarded as measure cost (or start-up cost).

(China/Interviewee 6)

These findings support previous studies that have suggested that health and safety concerns should be costed for during the tendering process (Sumner and Farrell, 2003; Boadu et al., 2021). While globally every construction project is deemed to have a health and safety manual and/or plan (Nwaogu and Chan, 2021), in developing countries, they are given low priority, and health and safety objectives are not clearly spelt out (Boadu et al., 2021). They mostly focus on accident prevention, while other health-related issues are not catered for or properly planned for (Nwaogu and Chan, 2021). With the COVID-19 experience, anti-epidemic measures should be catered for in such a document.

**Implications**

The construction industry in China and Nigeria followed laid-down government measures/protocols for curbing COVID-19 unique to each country. Some of the measures/protocols are part of those recommended by WHO. These form the shared similarities between the health and safety measures adopted in Chinese and Nigerian construction industries to curb the spread of COVID-19. The difference between the health and safety measures adopted in both industries emanates from:

(i) The difference in government recommended measures and regulations for businesses and the country – the local authority regulations and recommendations in China appeared to be more rigorous than the protocols by WHO and those recommended by the Nigerian government.
(ii)     Infrastructural development: China is at the forefront of the Fourth Industrial Revolution (Ito, 2019). Therefore, it is more convenient for the construction industry in China to adopt health and safety technologies leveraging information technology because of heightened infrastructural development in China.

The findings offer some implications for the diffusion of health and safety technologies in the construction industry. Regularly distributing masks to workers would help with compliance and ensure that they do not repeat used face masks the next day. Therefore, it is recommended that some epidemic or pandemic support be provided for businesses. Construction firms in China leveraged sophisticated technologies to curb the spread of COVID-19. Therefore, some of these measures can be implemented and tested in Nigeria and other countries. The government should provide financial support or subsidies to construction firms interested in technology transformation to relieve the financial burden on such firms. This would boost technological and infrastructural development in the country.

## Conclusions

The COVID-19 pandemic has impacted businesses directly or indirectly and brought a new reality to how everyone carries out their daily jobs. This study determined health and safety measures that Chinese and Nigerian construction firms instituted to curb their employees' exposure to the COVID-19 disease. Semi-structured interview was conducted among 34 purposively selected construction practitioners. The data collected were content analysed. The respondents' views were sought around two specific areas: how they responded to the COVID-19 pandemic with reference to health and safety measures and strategies used to manage or engage the construction project.

The responses indicate that most of WHO's health and safety measures and local authority measures for each country were implemented on construction sites. Health and safety measures employed on construction sites in China and Nigeria are checking body temperature before accessing the workplace, wearing face masks, disinfection of the site and offices, sensitisation of employees, minimising the number of workers, and setting up isolation rooms. It was gathered that construction firms managed their projects and the impact of the pandemic using various approaches, such as conducting online meetings, rediscussing the project cost and time with clients, use of mechanised equipment, and planning for anti-epidemic items at the tender stage.

It was deduced that the potential of online meetings could not be entirely tapped because of confidentiality concerns. Hence, this study recommends that further study should probe trust and confidentiality concerns with respect to the use of health and safety technology and remote working engaged in curbing COVID-19. Additionally, it is recommended that further research should be conducted to determine the impact of COVID-19 on the construction bidding process and health and safety plans for construction projects.

## Acknowledgement

The study forms part of the research project funded by the National Natural Science Foundation of China (No. 71971186). The authors are grateful to the funding body and all the interviewees for their contribution.

## References

Agyekum, K., Kukah, A.S., & Amudjie, J. (2022). The impact of COVID-19 on the construction industry in Ghana: The case of some selected firms. *Journal of Engineering, Design and Technology*, 20, 222–244. doi: 10.1108/JEDT-11-2020-0476.
Alsharef, A., Banerjee, S., Uddin, S.M., Albert, A., & Jaselskis, E. (2021). Early impacts of the COVID-19 pandemic on the United States construction industry. *International Journal of Environmental Research and Public Health*, 18. doi: 10.3390/ijerph18041559.

Babatunde, O.K., & Low, S.P. (2013). Chinese construction firms in the Nigerian construction industry. *Habitat International*, 40, 18–24. https://doi.org/10.1016/j.habitatint.2013.01.002.

Boadu, E.F., Sunindijo, R.Y., & Wang, C.C. (2021). Health and safety consideration in the procurement of public construction projects in Ghana. *Buildings*, 11, 128.

Ebekozien, A., & Aigbavboa, C. (2021). COVID-19 recovery for the Nigerian construction sites: The role of the fourth industrial revolution technologies. *Sustainable Cities and Society*, 69, 102803. https://doi.org/10.1016/j.scs.2021.102803.

Ghondaghsaz, N., Chokparova, Z., Engesser, S., & Urbas, L. (2022). Managing the tension between trust and confidentiality in mobile supply chains. *Sustainability*, 14, 2347.

Ito, A. (2019). Digital China: A fourth industrial revolution with Chinese characteristics? *Asia-Pacific Review*, 26, 50–75. doi: 10.1080/13439006.2019.1691836.

Jallow, H., Renukappa, S., & Suresh, S. (2021). The impact of COVID-19 outbreak on United Kingdom infrastructure sector. *Smart and Sustainable Built Environment*, 10, 581–593. doi: 10.1108/SASBE-05-2020-0068.

NCDC. (2020). *Guidelines for employers and businesses in Nigeria*. Available at https://covid19.ncdc.gov.ng/media/files/COVID19GuideforBusinessesAugust2020_V3.pdf (Accessed 21 June 2022).

Nwaogu, J.M., & Chan, A.P.C. (2021). Evaluation of multi-level intervention strategies for a psychologically healthy construction workplace in Nigeria. *Journal of Engineering, Design and Technology*, 19, 509–536. doi: 10.1108/JEDT-05-2020-0159.

Nwaogu, J.M., Chan, A.P.C., Naslund, J.A., Hon, C.K., Belonwu, C., & Yang, J. (2021). Exploring the barriers to and motivators for using digital mental health interventions among construction personnel in Nigeria: Qualitative study. *JMIR Formative Research*, 5, e18969.

Olanrewaju, A., Abdulaziz, A., Preece, C.N., & Shobowale, K. (2021). Evaluation of measures to prevent the spread of COVID-19 on the construction sites. *Clean Eng Technol*, 5, 100277. doi: 10.1016/j.clet.2021.100277.

Omatule Onubi, H., Yusof, N.A., & Sanusi Hassan, A. (2021). Perceived COVID-19 safety risk and safety behavior on construction sites: Role of safety climate and firm size. *Journal of Construction Engineering and Management*, 147, 04021153. doi: 10.1061/(ASCE)CO.1943-7862.0002201.

Sami Ur Rehman, M., Shafiq, M.T., & Afzal, M. (2022). Impact of COVID-19 on project performance in the UAE construction industry. *Journal of Engineering, Design and Technology*, 20, 245–266. doi: 10.1108/JEDT-12-2020-0481.

Sharara, S., & Radia, S. (2022). Quick Response (QR) codes for patient information delivery: A digital innovation during the coronavirus pandemic. *Journal of Orthodontics*, 49, 89–97.

Simpeh, F., & Amoah, C. (2021). Assessment of measures instituted to curb the spread of COVID-19 on construction site. *International Journal of Construction Management*, 1–19. doi: 10.1080/15623599.2021.1874678.

Sumner, S., & Farrell, P. (2003). The influence of clients on health and safety standards in construction. Proceedings of the 19th Annual Association of Researchers in Construction Management (ARCOM) Conference, University of Brighton, pp. 193–202.

Vaismoradi, M., Turunen, H., & Bondas, T. (2013). Content analysis and thematic analysis: Implications for conducting a qualitative descriptive study. *Nursing & Health Sciences*, 15, 398–405.

Wu, J., Wang, J., Nicholas, S., Maitland, E., & Fan, Q. (2020). Application of big data technology for COVID-19 prevention and control in China: Lessons and recommendations. *Journal of Medical Internet Research*, 22, e21980–e21980. doi: 10.2196/21980.

Yang, Y., Chan, A.P., Shan, M., Gao, R., Bao, F., Lyu, S., Zhang, Q., & Guan, J. (2021). Opportunities and challenges for construction health and safety technologies under the COVID-19 pandemic in Chinese construction projects. *International Journal of Environmental Research and Public Health*, 18, 13038.

# Appendix I

**Title of project:** Health and safety measures for managing the COVID-19 pandemic in the construction industry: a comparison study

You are invited to participate in a study led by Professor Albert P.C. Chan and Dr. Jackie Yang, staff members of the Department of Building and Real Estate in The Hong Kong Polytechnic University (PolyU). The study forms part of the research project funded by the National Natural Science Foundation of China (No. 71971186).

This study aims to examine the implementation of construction Health and Safety (H&S) measures in China and Nigeria in the COVID-19 era to facilitate effective pandemic planning for the effective deployment of H&S measures. Your response is valuable to us because we can help the construction industry meet its development and poverty alleviation goals with it.

If you choose to participate in the study, we would like to meet and talk with you over Zoom. This will take about 25–30 minutes. We would ask you a short series of questions about the impact of COVID-19 oil construction activities and steps taken by your organisation to ensure that projects are delivered within time without jeopardising the health of workers. We will make the questions available to you before the interview. You can also see the questions overleaf.

The talk is a structured interview that will take 25 to 30 minutes, and the audio will be recorded so that it can be transcribed and analysed later. Audio recordings and transcriptions will be stored in password-protected cloud servers. All information related to you will remain confidential and identifiable by codes only known to the researchers, and your details will not be stored or reported in any research outputs. Also, none of the activities will cause any physical discomfort.

You have the right to withdraw from the study at any phase without penalty of any kind. If you want to obtain more information about this study, don't hesitate to contact Dr. Janet Mayowa Nwaogu (email: janet.nwaogu@connect.polyu.hk).

Thank you for being so interested in participating in this study.

Yours faithfully,
Dr. Jackie Yang, Principal Investigator.

**The interview questions**

1. Please, for record purposes, what service does your company render, what is your position, how many years of work experience in the industry?
2. Can you describe how you respond to Covid-19 pandemic and how you manage/engage in construction projects under Covid-19 pandemic?

# 4 Towards improving health management of construction projects during the COVID-19 pandemic

*Amir Mahdiyar, Mojtaba Ashour,
David J. Edwards and Saeed Reza Mohandes*

## 1 Introduction

The construction industry is responsible for a considerable number of worker injuries and fatalities around the globe (Mohandes et al., 2022c). The outbreak of COVID-19 has also introduced significant concerns within the construction industry. Apart from contracting the virus itself, some of these consequences are monetary in nature, such as operational delays, suspension of projects, and the increase in costs (Agyekum et al., 2022). There are, however, other aspects that directly affect the well-being of workers, such as unexpected workforce reduction, working hours and salary reductions, as well as unpaid leaves (Ahmed et al., 2022). Given the unpredictable effects of the COVID-19 pandemic and the inherent complexity of construction projects, the construction risks threatening the workers' occupational health and safety (OHS) should be managed through innovative approaches. The existence of various COVID-19-related uncertainties to which the construction workers could be exposed has made the process of safety risk management a challenge for construction managers. This is due to the responsibilities of construction managers for the safety, health, and well-being of workers (Bavafa et al., 2018), while construction activities are not to be stopped for a long period. Consequently, construction managers have implemented various types of health strategies and measures to cope with the OHS risks COVID-19 has brought to construction sites (Alsharef et al., 2021).

Research conducted on construction safety risk management using novel approaches is myriad (please see (Mohandes et al., 2022a) for more examples and additional information), albeit those approaches might not be efficient considering the effects of COVID-19. Moreover, several studies have investigated the impacts of COVID-19 on health-related issues (e.g., (Agyekum et al., 2022; Ahmed et al., 2022; Olanrewaju et al., 2021)); however, there is a notable lack of studies focusing on preventative measures to be implemented for curbing those adverse impacts. Hence, this book chapter aims to identify and prioritize the health strategies and measures in curbing the effect of COVID-19 on construction workers' OHS-related issues. To this end, a pool of health measures was retried from reviewing recently published research and presented to Hong Kong experts to check their applicability in the Hong Kong construction industry. In a round of structured interviews,

DOI: 10.1201/9781003278368-5

the experts were also given the opportunity to provide their opinion regarding any additional health measures that must be added to the list. Then, the final list of health strategies and measures was ranked according to their importance in reducing the impact of COVID-19 on construction workers' safety and health using the Best Worst method.

The remainder of this chapter is as follows. Section 2 provides a background on the health measures implemented to prevent the spread of COVID-19. Section 3 defines the research methodology and the methods used to achieve the objectives of the research. Section 4 shows the results of the research and discusses the findings. Also, the implications of the findings are discussed in this section. Finally, the conclusions and recommendations are presented in Section 5.

## 2   Preventive strategies

While the construction industry has accrued an infamous reputation for its health and safety risks and accident rates (Mohandes and Zhang, 2021), the dire consequences of the COVID-19 outbreak on the workforce have presented new challenges (Alsharef et al., 2021; Araya, 2021; del Rio-Chanona et al., 2020). Among these challenges is the lower well-being level of construction workers who are working under immense pressure in a high-risk environment (Stiles et al., 2021). Recent studies suggested that the spread of COVID-19 among workers could potentially reduce up to 90% of the workforce involved in a construction project (i.e., being sick and not able to work) by implementing sagacious safety and health measures (Araya, 2021). Considering the significant share of the construction industry in the economy, as well as the labor-intensive nature of it (Aslan and Türkakın, 2022), various measures have been put forward to prevent the spread of COVID-19 and to mitigate its ensuing consequences (Assaad and El-adaway, 2021; Nnaji et al., 2022; Olanrewaju et al., 2021). In the wake of the third year post the initial COVID-19 outbreak, most measures adopted concentrate mainly on prevention. This section provides a brief background on some of the effective preventive strategies within the construction industry that were identified via a comprehensive literature review of the existing body of knowledge.

There are several industry guidelines and best practices provided by construction-related organizations from around the globe (i.e., see (CCOHS, 2021; Construction Industry Council, 2021; OSHA, 2021; Safe Work Australia, 2022)). These strategies are often concerned with a few common major aspects, such as social distancing, monitoring, disinfection, and hygiene, as well as more recently focused measures which rely heavily on governmental and managerial decisions (i.e., incentives, remote work, etc.). Apart from the aforementioned, recent research has also discussed some of the best practices. For instance, Olanrewaju et al. (2021) found that providing hygienic workplaces, adequate personal protective equipment (PPE), and education for workers about the risks of COVID-19, as well as managerial components relating to monitoring, policies, and incentives are among the most successful preventive measures. Nnaji et al. (2022) reported that respondents from the construction industry perceive that social distancing measures and use of technologies (i.e., video conferencing (Burton et al., 2021)) are considerably more effective than screening and controlling measures. This echoes the earlier findings of Pamidimukkala and Kermanshachi (2021) suggesting that exploiting communication technologies and virtual solutions, coupled with more flexible working schedules may not only reduce COVID-19-related risks, but also increase workers' productivity and mental well-being. In addition, Gan and Koh (2021) suggest that isolation of positive (or symptomatic), quarantine requirements for close contacts, and enforced social distancing on site are the best-combined strategy for preventing large-scale outbreaks.

Briggs et al. (2022) reported a comprehensive best practices guideline that was adopted in practice and resulted in significantly decreasing the number of COVID-19 cases among workers. The authors discuss strategies and measures such as PPE, personal hygiene, social distancing, screening, quarantining, and tracking, as well as the responsibilities of safety teams in an industrial construction environment. Stiles et al. (2021) stressed the important role of management in a pandemic situation and reported on observations within the UK construction industry. They (*ibid*) posited that while there may be awareness about numerous guidelines that are provided (especially by governmental or industry-related organizations), there may still be confusion about their correct implementation (i.e., how often should disinfection be carried out in certain spaces and for certain objects/surfaces). Additionally, they posited that some of the necessary safety steps are not conducted due to the very existence of COVID-19 preventive measures. For instance, routine safety on-site meetings are no longer conducted face-to-face so as to reduce contact. Nevertheless, they are being conducted in other forms (i.e., over the phone, in online meetings, in open spaces, etc. as pointed out by Briggs et al., (2022)). Thus, for many of the existing practices, it is merely the medium of instruction that has changed, but the content either remains the same or has improved.

The reported strategies within the existing literature encompass numerous specific measures that are further categorized based on the opinion of experts within the industry and with consideration to the context of the present research, the details of which are thoroughly discussed in the succeeding sections. Additionally, a summary of the discussed strategies and specific measures – both from the existing literature as well as those added by experts participating in this research – are presented in Table 4.1 (please refer to Section 4).

## 3   Methodology

To achieve the objectives specified in this study, a hybrid methodological approach is employed. First, a systematic review for identifying the beneficial measures and strategies in dealing with the detrimental impact of COVID-19 menacing construction projects was undertaken. Afterward, with a view to achieving a detailed list of relative measures and strategies, as well as validating the findings from literature, further interviews with qualified concessioners (experts) were carried out. Furthermore, in order to rank the importance of the identified measures and strategies and determine the critical ones, the Best Worst Method (BWM) was utilized. There are two major reasons for employing BWM in this research (Mohandes et al., 2022b; Tetteh et al., 2022). First, the experts invited to fill out the questionnaires do not need to conduct laborious and time-consuming pairwise comparisons among the measures identified in this study (as compared to the other similar techniques such as analytical hierarchy process, analytical network process, etc.), and second, fewer pairwise comparisons to be undertaken by the experts bring about an improved consistency related to the calculated measures' weights, obtaining more precise and accurate responses. The following are elaborations on the aforementioned stages straddled within the methodological approach employed in this research.

### 3.1 Data collection

Since the collection of reliable and prudent data from experts having rich experience in Hong Kong was a must for achieving the specified objectives, two strict criteria were considered: the obtainment of at least an undergraduate degree in the area of construction engineering and management, and the involvement in at least one project (either ongoing or completed) during the pandemic. Based on these criteria, twenty-six qualified experts were shortlisted who contributed to the study (see Figure 4.1).

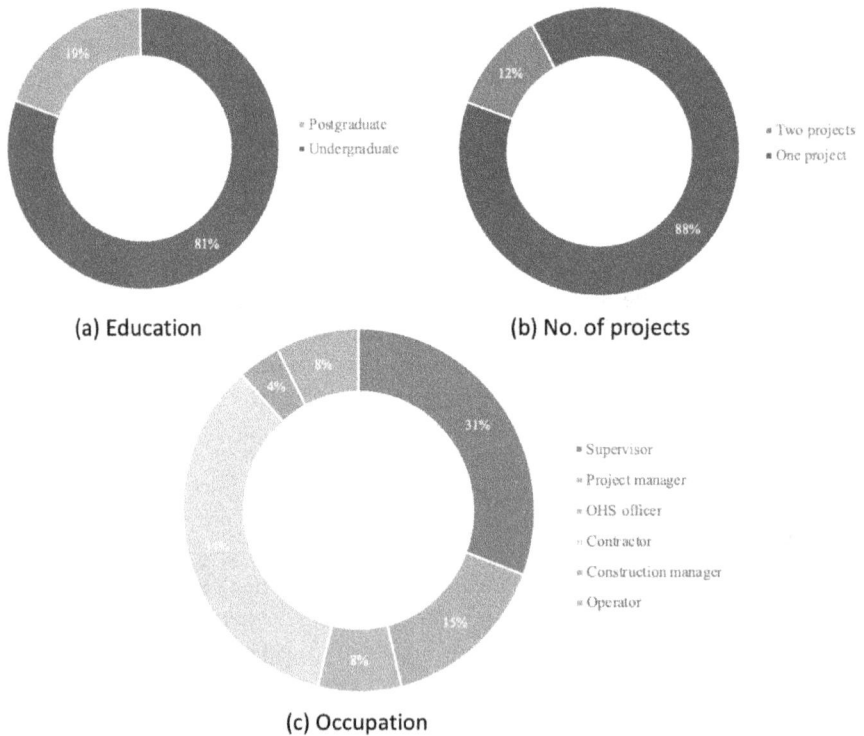

(a) Education

(b) No. of projects

(c) Occupation

*Figure 4.1* Experts' profiles based on their: (a) level of education, (b) NO. of projects being undertaken during the pandemic, and (c) professional occupation held.

### 3.2   Systematic review and experts' interviews

As the first objective of the study, there was a dire need to identify the relative strategies and measures playing a role in curbing the negative impacts associated with COVID-19 on construction projects. In doing so, a systematic review of the studies published on the concerned topic was carried out (please see (Salihu et al., 2022) for more details on the review approach). First, combinations of relevant keywords in the Scopus search engine were used during the bibliometric review. Following this, a number of filters for the exclusion of irrelevant papers were considered. Then, to increase the number of relevant papers, the snowballing technique was employed (Owolabi et al., 2022). In the final stage, each paper for identifying the relative strategies and measures was scrutinized. Once a detailed list was garnered, then further interviews with three experts, who were willing to participate in open-ended sessions, were carried out. In the interviews held, each expert was asked to provide their points of view on the prepared list, by either adding any missing items or removing irrelevant ones. In this way, a comprehensive list of strategies, measures, and their respective definitions was provided.

### 3.3   Best Worst Method utilization

The Best Worst Method (BWM), which works based on pairwise comparison, was originally proposed for the solution of the Multi-Criteria Decision-Making (MCDM) problems (Salimi and Rezaei, 2018). In comparison with other MCDM methods, BWM offers two key advantages: 1) it requires less pairwise comparison data in comparison with a full-pairwise comparison matrix; and 2) the results obtained by BWM show higher consistency compared to those of other MCDM methods that utilize a full-pairwise comparison matrix (Durdyev et al., 2022); this was the key reason justifying the application of BWM to the present research. The method has been already applied to solve different complex decision-making problems in construction management science (cf. Mahdiyar et al., 2020; Tabatabaei et al., 2020; Zhang and Mohandes, 2020). Due to these advantages, this study employs the BWM for calculating the importance weights of identified strategies and measures. The following are the elaborations of the steps taken to utilize the BWM:

Step 1. Determining a set of decision criteria. This step involves identifying the decision criteria, which could be presented at different levels. In this study, there were 32 specific measures under six corresponding strategies.

Step 2. Identifying the best (i.e., the most significant/important measures or strategies) and the worst (i.e., the least significant/important measures or strategies), considering the opinions offered by the expert(s).

Step 3. Determining the preference of the best decision criterion over all the other decision criteria with the help of a nine-point scale. The scales used in this study were adapted from the study carried out by Gupta (2018).

Step 4. Determining the preference of all the decision criteria over the worst criterion (W), with the use of a nine-point scale; the outcome will be the others-to-worst vector.

Step 5. Exploring the optimum weights using the following equation.

$$\text{Min } \zeta$$

s.t.

$$\left| \frac{a_B}{a_j} - c_{Bj} \right| \le \zeta, \text{ for all } j$$

$$\left| \frac{a_j}{a_W} - c_{jW} \right| \le \zeta, \text{ for all } j \tag{1}$$

$$\sum_j a_j = 1$$

$$a_j \ge 0, \text{ for all } j$$

where $a_B$, $a_j$, $a_W$, $c_{Bj}$, and $c_{jW}$ are respectively: the most significant measure/strategy chosen by an expert; the other significant measure/strategy against which the comparison is made; the least significant measure/strategy chosen by an expert; the extent of comparison to which the chosen most significant measure/strategy is more important than the other one; and the extent of comparison to which the other measure/strategy is more important than the least important one.

Step 6. Check the consistency of the responses provided by each expert, according to a study carried out by Ahmadi et al. (2017).

Step 7. Aggregation of the weights that have been calculated for all the experts involved in the study.

Step 8. Determining the critical measures and strategies using the proposed threshold values. Once the aggregated weights for all the measures and strategies were calculated, then two threshold values (viz. one for the group of strategies and the one for the measure group).

## 4   Results and discussion

Based on the systematic review and experts' interviews, an exhaustive list of fecund strategies and specific measures was garnered (see Table 4.1). Five strategies and twenty-eight measures were gathered from reviewing the literature while one strategy and nine measures were identified through structured interviews. Cumulatively, six strategies and thirty-seven specific measures were identified for further investigation.

The results produced from the BWM employment are illustrated in Figures 4.2 and 4.3. Figure 4.2 reveals that SG5, SG2, and SG3 are the most critical strategies for dealing with the impacts of COVID-19 on the OHS of construction workers. By examining Figure 4.3, one can observe that M5, E6, and E2 are the most important preventive measures, while S3, S4, S5, S6, T1, T2, T3, T5, and M6 are the least critical ones. The weights provided in Figure 4.3 are the global weights of the measures which are based on the importance of the measures as well as their respective strategies. Notably, the consistency of the responses provided by all the experts who participated in BWM was below 0.1.

*Table 4.1* List of preventative strategies and measures.

| Strategy | ID | Specific measures | References | | | | | | | |
|---|---|---|---|---|---|---|---|---|---|---|
| | | | 1 | 2 | 3 | 4 | 5 | 6 | 7 | 8 |
| Monitoring and Screening **(SG1)** | S1 | Ensuring frequent wash/ disinfection of hands | ✓ | ✓ | | | | | | |
| | S2 | Ensuring the use of special/ suitable PPE when the job requires close physical distance, such as facemask, gloves, face shields, etc. (less than 1.5 m) | ✓ | ✓ | ✓ | | | | | |
| | S3 | Avoiding handshake, hugging, and close contact | | ✓ | | | | | | |
| | S4 | Preventing sharing of foods or drinks among employees/ workers | | | ✓ | | | | | |
| | S5 | Routine examination of symptoms (i.e., daily temperature checks) | ✓ | ✓ | | ✓ | ✓ | | | |
| | S6 | Pre-assignment health survey for workers (may include travel history) | ✓ | | | | | ✓ | | |
| | S7 | Conducting regular COVID-19 tests | | | | ✓ | ✓ | | | |
| | S8 | Enforcing self-isolation/ quarantine for positive cases | ✓ | ✓ | | ✓ | | | | |
| Contact Control and Social Distancing **(SG2)** | C1 | Scheduling works in separate spaces/offices to minimize contact and crowd | | ✓ | ✓ | ✓ | ✓ | ✓ | | |
| | C2 | Limiting the interactions among working teams (i.e., varying entrance/break/lunch times) | ✓ | ✓ | ✓ | ✓ | ✓ | ✓ | | |
| | C3 | Working remotely where and when possible and suspending non-critical face-to-face works | | ✓ | ✓ | | ✓ | | | ✓ |
| | C4 | Providing food/drink on sites to limit workers' commute during working hours | | ✓ | | | | | | |
| | C5 | Providing separate accommodation facilities for workers assigned to varying teams/jobs | | ✓ | | ✓ | | | | |
| | C6 | Limiting the number of workers in small areas (i.e., lift, car, trailers, etc.) | | | | | | | | ✓ |
| | C7 | Opting for off-site/remote fabrication | | | | | ✓ | | | |

*(Continued)*

*Table 4.1* (Continued)

| Strategy | ID | Specific measures | References | | | | | | | |
|---|---|---|---|---|---|---|---|---|---|---|
| | | | 1 | 2 | 3 | 4 | 5 | 6 | 7 | 8 |
| Equipment, Hygiene, and Disinfection **(SG3)** | E1 | The regular supply of appropriate masks, sanitizers, and other necessary PPEs (i.e., face shields) | | ✓ | | | ✓ | ✓ | | |
| | E2 | Regular disinfection of objects and surfaces (i.e., door handles, lift buttons, etc.) | | ✓ | | | ✓ | ✓ | | |
| | E3 | Sites to be regularly fumigated (i.e., at the end of shifts) | | ✓ | | | | | | |
| | E4 | Providing larger washing facilities/areas | | | | | ✓ | | | |
| | E5 | Employing third-party cleaning teams | | | | | ✓ | | | |
| | E6 | Employing ultraviolet sanitation techniques | | | | | ✓ | | | |
| Technology, Training, and Awareness **(SG4)** | T1 | Providing intuitive health advisory information (i.e., posters, infographics, etc.) to increase employees' awareness about COVID-19 | | ✓ | | | | | | |
| | T2 | Informing workers about regulations set by government and health authorities (i.e., acceptable social distance, hygiene practices, etc.) | | ✓ | | | | ✓ | | ✓ |
| | T3 | Providing training on the use of online tools for those working from home | | | | | | | ✓ | ✓ |
| | T4 | Providing/using BIM and AR/VR-based technologies for virtual inspection and sharing information | | | | | | | | ✓ |
| | T5 | Using wearable technologies (i.e., wristbands or other smart PPEs) for tracking and checking the workers | | | | ✓ | ✓ | | | |
| Managerial **(SG5)** | M1 | Providing healthcare incentives for workers (increasing the likelihood of self-report) | | ✓ | | | | | | |
| | M2 | Prolonging project/work duration/lowering working hours (where possible) to facilitate effective implementation of preventive measures by employees | | | | | | | | ✓ |

| Strategy | ID | Specific measures | References | | | | | | | |
|---|---|---|---|---|---|---|---|---|---|---|
| | | | *1* | *2* | *3* | *4* | *5* | *6* | *7* | *8* |
| | M3 | Conducting constant supervision on-site by qualified personnel to ensure the COVID-19-related measures (which includes checking the number of workers, the flow and interactions of workers, hygiene of the workplace, etc.) | AEI | | | | | | | |
| | M4 | Making payments and exchange of any documentation online (e.g., electronic signature, etc.) | AEI | | | | | | | |
| | M5 | Boosting the mental health of workers by adding more flexibilities to the working hours | AEI | | | | | | | |
| | M6 | Build up dispatch areas for the items delivered to the sites (to reduce the contact among the workers) | AEI | | | | | | | |
| Governmental **(SG6)** | G1 | Providing subsidies for workers' absenteeism (those who contracted the virus) | AEI | | | | | | | |
| | G2 | Introducing a point-based system for the contractors (e.g., bonus points for the firms adhered to the recent government's regulations concerning the development of the virus, and negative points for those who breached) | AEI | | | | | | | |
| | G3 | Providing the workers with a series of free consultation during the pandemic (to boost their mental health) | AEI | | | | | | | |
| | G4 | Conducting ad-hoc inspection of the sites | AEI | | | | | | | |
| | G5 | Involving the workers in interactive social activities and gaming through online platforms on weekends | AEI | | | | | | | |

*Note:* AEI indicates the items added by the experts in the held interview.

1: (Briggs et al., 2022), 2: (Olanrewaju et al., 2021), 3: (Aslan and Türkakın, 2022), 4: (Gan and Koh, 2021), 5: (Nnaji et al., 2022), 6: (Alsharef et al., 2021), 7: (Stiles et al., 2021), 8: (Pamidimukkala and Kermanshachi, 2021).

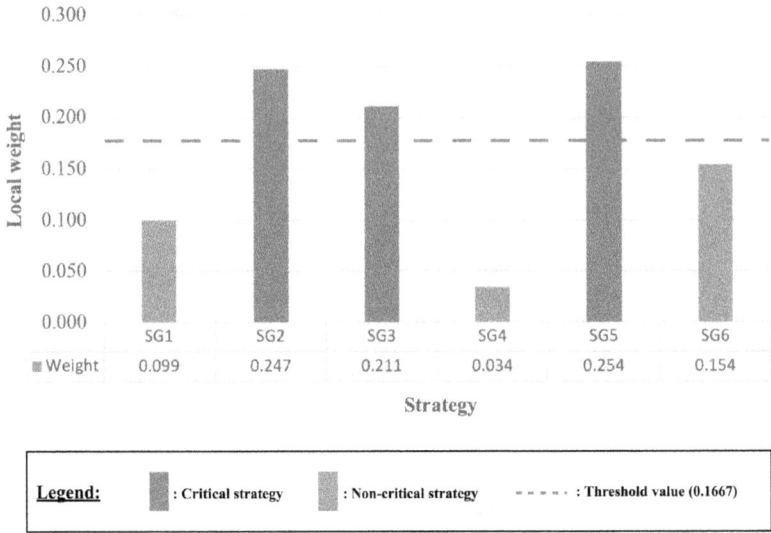

*Figure 4.2* Calculated weights of strategies and illustration of critical ones with regard to the threshold value.

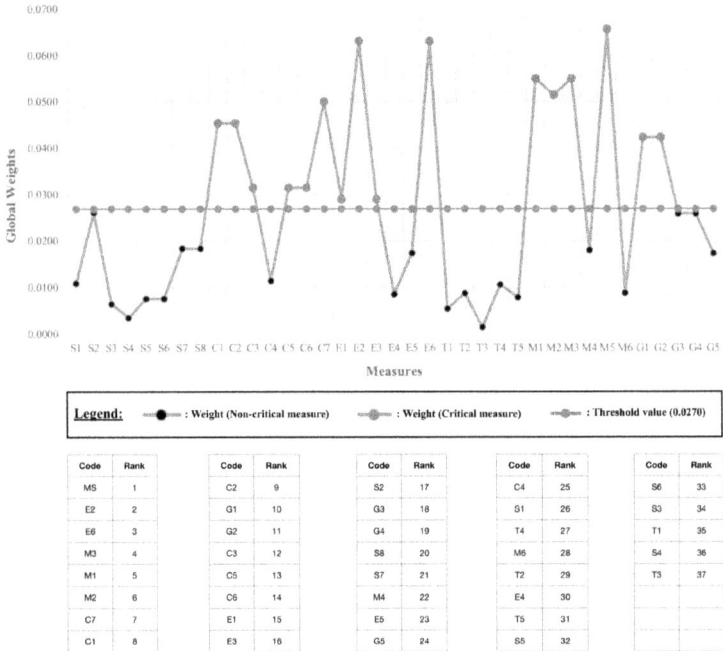

*Figure 4.3* Calculated global weights of measures and illustration of critical ones with respect to the threshold value.

The results have shown the significance of managerial measures (i.e., flexible working hours, healthcare incentives, etc.) in both curbing the COVID-19 effects and improving the well-being of workers. This is particularly of interest considering the psychological burden of working during the pandemic and the consequential loss of productivity. When appropriate and well-planned health measures are put into place in a company, the involved workers feel relaxed, improving their psychological modes, which in turn leads to increasing workers' productivity working within the respective firm. In light of this, finding a managerial measure as the most influential one (M5) indicates the value of adaptation in extreme or unknown situations and displays ways in which the construction sector can demonstrate resilience in the face of an outbreak. In line with existing literature, the current findings presented also point to the importance of strictly following social distancing and disinfection practices (SG2, SG3). A finding that concurs with the earlier research of Law et al. (2021). Nevertheless, it is found that the focus should primarily be on appropriate enforcement through constant supervision by qualified personnel (M3), indicating yet again the crucial role of management in the effective implementation of common measures (e.g., E2). The research findings provide academic and practical implications. As regards the theoretical implication, researchers may use the identified measures for developing their theoretical frameworks. Moreover, this study provides the researchers with the most critical health measures to be undertaken. In this way, they can build up their models by only focusing on the crucial ones. In this way, they are given hindsight in developing their models for unraveling the inherent relationships that may exist among the measures identified in this research. Concerning the managerial implications, the newly identified measures through structured interviews can be adopted by managers in real-life cases to improve the safety of construction workers on construction sites. In addition, in case of the occurrence of another pandemic due to COVID-19, or another contagious disease in a post-COVID-19 pandemic, adopting such strategies and measures will help alleviate their negative effects on OHS of construction workers.

## 5  Conclusion and recommendations

This research identified and prioritized the beneficial health measures for dealing with the detrimental impact of COVID-19 concerning construction projects. The former was achieved using structured interviews and the findings showed that six strategies – including "monitoring and screening," "contact control and social distancing," "equipment, hygiene, and disinfection," "technology, training and awareness," "managerial," and "governmental" – and thirty-seven measures contribute towards improving constructing safety management. The latter was carried out using an MCDM approach (i.e., Best Worst method) and findings revealed that "managerial," "contact control and social distancing," and "equipment, hygiene and disinfection" are the most critical health strategies in curbing COVID-19 effects on OHS issues of construction workers, in that order. In addition, the most influential measures are "Boosting the mental health of workers by adding more flexibilities to the working hours," "Regular disinfection of objects and surfaces (i.e., door handles, lift buttons, etc.)," and "Employing ultraviolet sanitation techniques." The research findings are limited to Hong Kong as all data were collected from Hong Kong experts, so future research with a similar scope could be carried out and their findings can be discussed in tandem with the findings of this present study. Moreover, the outcomes of this research provide a snapshot of influential preventive strategies and measures, while future research may focus on the investigation of inner dependencies among the impact of the identified measures.

## Acknowledgment

The authors express their sincere appreciation to all the experts contributing to this study.

## References

Agyekum, K., Kukah, A.S., & Amudjie, J. (2022). The impact of COVID-19 on the construction industry in Ghana: The case of some selected firms. *Journal of Engineering, Design and Technology*, 20, 222–244.

Ahmadi, H.B., Kusi-Sarpong, S., & Rezaei, J. (2017). Assessing the social sustainability of supply chains using Best Worst Method. *Resources, Conservation and Recycling*, 126, 99–106.

Ahmed, S., Haq, I., & Anam, S.M.A. (2022). Impacts of COVID-19 on the construction sector in the least developed countries. *International Journal of Building Pathology and Adaptation*, ahead-of-print. https://doi.org/10.1108/IJBPA-04-2022-0059.

Alsharef, A., Banerjee, S., Uddin, S.M.J., Albert, A., & Jaselskis, E. (2021). Early impacts of the COVID-19 pandemic on the United States construction industry. *International Journal of Environmental Research and Public Health*, 18, 1559.

Araya, F. (2021). Modeling the spread of COVID-19 on construction workers: An agent-based approach. *Safety Science*, 133, 105022.

Aslan, S., & Türkakın, O.H. (2022). A construction project scheduling methodology considering COVID-19 pandemic measures. *Journal of Safety Research*, 80, 54–66.

Assaad, R., & El-adaway, I.H. (2021). Guidelines for responding to COVID-19 pandemic: Best practices, impacts, and future research directions. *Journal of Management in Engineering*, 37, 06021001.

Bavafa, A., Mahdiyar, A., & Marsono, A.K. (2018). Identifying and assessing the critical factors for effective implementation of safety programs in construction projects. *Safety Science*, 106, 47–56.

Briggs, B., Friedland, C.J., Nahmens, I., Berryman, C., & Zhu, Y. (2022). Industrial construction safety policies and practices with cost impacts in a COVID-19 pandemic environment: A Louisiana DOW case study. *Journal of Loss Prevention in the Process Industries*, 76, 104723.

Burton, E., Edwards, D.J., Roberts, C., Chileshe, N., & Lai, J.H.K. (2021). Delineating the implications of dispersing teams and teleworking in an Agile UK construction sector. *Sustainability*, 13, 9981.

CCOHS. (2021). *Coronavirus (COVID-19)-tips: Construction sector* [WWW Document]. Available at www.ccohs.ca. www.ccohs.ca/covid19/construction/ (Accessed 17 April 2022).

Construction Industry Council. (2021, January). *Good practice on preventive measures against COVID-19 for construction site* (English Version) [WWW Document]. Available at www.cic.hk/eng/main/safety-corner/referencematerials/. www.cic.hk/files/page/51/20210121_Good%20Practice%20on%20Preventive%20Measures%20Against%20COVID-19%20for%20Construction%20Sites.pdf (Accessed 17 April 2022).

del Rio-Chanona, R.M., Mealy, P., Pichler, A., Lafond, F., & Farmer, J.D. (2020). Supply and demand shocks in the COVID-19 pandemic: An industry and occupation perspective. *Oxford Review of Economic Policy*, 36, S94–S137.

Durdyev, S., Mohandes, S.R., Tokbolat, S., Sadeghi, H., & Zayed, T. (2022). Examining the OHS of green building construction projects: A hybrid fuzzy-based approach. *Journal of Cleaner Production*, 130590.

Gan, W.H., & Koh, D. (2021). COVID-19 and return-to-work for the construction sector: Lessons from Singapore. *Safety and Health at Work*, 12, 277–281.

Gupta, H. (2018). Evaluating service quality of airline industry using hybrid best worst method and VIKOR. *Journal of Air Transport Management*, 68, 35–47.

Law, R.C.K., Lai, J.H.K., Edwards, D.J., & Hou, H. (2021). COVID-19: Research directions for non-clinical aerosol-generating facilities in the built environment. *Buildings*, 11, 282.

Mahdiyar, A., Mohandes, S.R., Durdyev, S., Tabatabaee, S., & Ismail, S. (2020). Barriers to green roof installation: An integrated fuzzy-based MCDM approach. *Journal of Cleaner Production*, 122365.

Mohandes, S.R., Durdyev, S., Sadeghi, H., Mahdiyar, A., Hosseini, M.R., Banihashemi, S., & Martek, I. (2022a). Towards enhancement in reliability and safety of construction projects: Developing a hybrid multi-dimensional fuzzy-based approach. *Engineering, Construction and Architectural Management*, ahead-of-print.

Mohandes, S.R., Karasan, A., Erdoğan, M., Ghasemi Poor Sabet, P., Mahdiyar, A., & Zayed, T. (2022b). A comprehensive analysis of the causal factors in repair, maintenance, alteration, and addition works: A novel hybrid fuzzy-based approach. *Expert Systems with Applications*, 208, 118112.

Mohandes, S.R., Sadeghi, H., Fazeli, A., Mahdiyar, A., Hosseini, M.R., Arashpour, M., & Zayed, T. (2022c). Causal analysis of accidents on construction sites: A hybrid fuzzy Delphi and DEMATEL approach. *Safety Science*, 151, 105730.

Mohandes, S.R., & Zhang, X. (2021). Developing a holistic occupational health and safety risk assessment model: An application to a case of sustainable construction project. *Journal of Cleaner Production*, 291, 125934.

Nnaji, C., Jin, Z., & Karakhan, A. (2022). Safety and health management response to COVID-19 in the construction industry: A perspective of fieldworkers. *Process Safety and Environmental Protection*, 159, 477–488.

Olanrewaju, A., AbdulAziz, A., Preece, C.N., & Shobowale, K. (2021). Evaluation of measures to prevent the spread of COVID-19 on the construction sites. *Cleaner Engineering and Technology*, 5, 100277.

OSHA. (2021). *Protecting workers: Guidance on mitigating and preventing the spread of COVID-19 in the workplace* [WWW Document]. Available at www.osha.gov. www.osha.gov/coronavirus/safework (Accessed 17 April 2022).

Owolabi, T.A., Mohandes, S.R., & Zayed, T. (2022). Investigating the impact of sewer overflow on the environment: A comprehensive literature review paper. *Journal of Environmental Management*, 301, 113810.

Pamidimukkala, A., & Kermanshachi, S. (2021). Impact of Covid-19 on field and office workforce in construction industry. *Project Leadership and Society*, 2, 100018.

Safe Work Australia. (2022). *COVID-19 for workplaces pack* [WWW Document]. Available at covid19.swa.gov.au. https://covid19.swa.gov.au/covid-19-print-pack/737/733 (Accessed 17 April 2022).

Salihu, C., Hussein, M., Mohandes, S.R., & Zayed, T. (2022). Towards a comprehensive review of the deterioration factors and modeling for sewer pipelines: A hybrid of bibliometric, scientometric, and meta-analysis approach. *Journal of Cleaner Production*, 351, 131460.

Salimi, N., & Rezaei, J. (2018). Evaluating firms' R&D performance using best worst method. *Evaluation and Program Planning*, 66, 147–155.

Stiles, S., Golightly, D., & Ryan, B. (2021). Impact of COVID-19 on health and safety in the construction sector. *Human Factors and Ergonomics in Manufacturing & Service Industries*, 31, 425–437.

Tabatabaei, M.H., Amiri, M., Ghahremanloo, M., Keshavarz-Ghorabaee, M., Zavadskas, E.K., & Antucheviciene, J. (2020). Hierarchical decision-making using a new mathematical model based on the best-worst method. *International Journal of Computers Communications & Control*, 14, 710–725.

Tetteh, M.O., Chan, A.P.C., Mohandes, S.R., & Agyemang, D.Y. (2022). Diagnosing critical barriers to international construction joint ventures success in the developing country of Ghana. *Construction Innovation*, ahead-of-print.

Zhang, X., & Mohandes, S.R. (2020). Occupational health and safety in green building construction projects: A holistic Z-numbers-based risk management framework. *Journal of Cleaner Production*, 275, 122788.

# 5 An overview on the measures taken to tackle COVID-19 impacts on Nigerian construction sites

## A case study of the South-South geo-political zone

*Victor Nnannaya Okorie and*
*Iruka Chijindu Anugwo*

## Introduction

COVID-19 was first recognized by the world in 2019 and started in the region of Wuhan, China (Alozie et al., 2020; WHO, 2020a). The rate at which COVID-19 spread across the world prompted the World Health Organization (WHO) to declare it a pandemic on 11th March 2020 (WHO, 2020b). The rate of transmissions and infections continued to rise globally, as the total number of infected persons worldwide stood at 10 million as of 30th June 2020 (WHO, 2020a; Alozie et al., 2020). As noted by WHO (2020a), on 21st January 2021, about 95,612,831 infections and 2,066,176 deaths due to the COVID-19 pandemic were reported globally. According to the International Labour Organisation (ILO) (2020), before the COVID-19 pandemic, the construction sector in many countries accounted for about 7.7% of global employment, with the projection of 12% in 2030 indicating that the construction industry would contribute to 17.4% of global gross domestic product (GDP). This implies that the construction industry is a major contributor to the economic and social development of any nation. Consequently, the COVID-19 pandemic that ravaged the world's economies has led to the disruption of construction activities and millions of lives lost.

In its 2021 sectorial brief on the impact of COVID-19 on construction, the ILO (2021) posits that the pandemic and its disruption impacted negatively on the construction sector, particularly on the HSW of site workers. Recent studies conducted in Nigeria and Malaysia (Alozie et al., 2020; Zakaria and Singh, 2021) on the effects of COVID-19 on the construction industry indicated that pandemic resulted in projects experiencing suspensions, delays, time and cost overruns. At the same time, the ILO (2021) suggests that the industry has been impacted by shortages of construction materials and other inputs due to disruption of the global supply chain, as well as loss of revenue to contractors and subcontractors. Undoubtedly, the devastating effects of COVID-19 have had severe consequences on human health and the global economy (WHO, 2020a; ILO, 2021).

DOI: 10.1201/9781003278368-6

The case of construction site workers' health, safety and well-being (HSW) in Nigeria worsened during the COVID-19 pandemic. According to Okorie and Musonda (2020), the construction industry in developing countries is typically underdeveloped and dysfunctional. In addition, several of the developing countries, especially those in Sub-Saharan Africa, do not have the capabilities and technologies to cope with such global threatening diseases as COVID-19 (WHO, 2020a; ILO, 2020). Thus, construction site workers' HSW in developing countries like Nigeria did not receive the desired attention, particularly the small and medium construction enterprises when compared with what obtained in developed countries like the United Kingdom (UK), United States of America (US), Germany, Russia etc., during the peak of COVID-19 (ILO, 2021).

Globally, construction enterprises consist of different classes, sizes and types (Hinze, 2006). Thus, larger contractors may have different perspectives than SMEs when it comes to the handling of COVID-19 cases, as different mechanisms are put in place to overcome the problems (WHO, 2020b). Alara (2021) argues that a large construction enterprise is better equipped to combat the spread of COVID-19 infections. However, in handling a pandemic like COVID-19, its spread must be contained to reduce the impact on the economy, society and human health. This called for in-depth research on the adaptability, effects and prospects, consequences, potential risks, control measures and impacts of COVID-19 on the construction industry. This study is conducted to investigate the various measures taken to reduce the spread of COVID-19 among small, medium and large construction enterprises in the South-South geo-political zone of Nigeria, and how the transmission and infection affects construction site workers' performance.

## Theoretical perspectives and background

### *COVID-19 measures by the Nigerian government*

The WHO (2020b) initiated the Public Health and Social Measures (PHSMs) embedded in specific protocols, rules or guidelines as necessary steps and undertakings by countries, territories and areas in order to limit the spread of COVID-19. The PHSMs includes rules and guidelines such as facial mask-wearing; limits and restrictions on public and private gathering, domestic movement and transport; stay-at-home orders; closure of schools and businesses; and international travel restrictions including entry restrictions, quarantining and testing (WHO, 2020b). As with the rest of the world, the Federal Government of Nigeria imposed guidelines on activities of all economic sectors, and signed the COVID-19 Disease Health Protection (DHP) into law (Federal Republic of Nigeria (FRN, 2021). Regardless of these rules, regulations and imposed Movement Control Order (MCO) in line with PHSM guidelines, the health impacts of COVID-19 among the construction workers in the study area were on the increase in terms of number of deaths and spread of the virus.

However, the strictness of MCO is dependent on the severity of the public health crisis of each country. Nonetheless, in some countries, construction activities were deemed essential. For instance, the timely construction of emergency facilities and hospitals was given priority in some countries (ILO, 2020). For example, in China and Italy, the construction sector was exempted from lockdown to meet up with the timing and construction of emergency facilities and hospitals (ILO, 2020). Following the imposition of MCO in Nigeria, there was a serious economic downturn in investment, loss of revenue and reduced income in all aspects of human enterprises, including the construction industry.

In fact, the negative impact of the COVID-19 pandemic on global economies and the loss of human lives is unquantifiable. In Nigeria, the case of construction site workers' HSW became worse. In addition, construction projects encountered delays in the completion period, and suspension, loss in revenue to clients and contractors, cases of disruption in material supply chains and shortages in the workforce are the corresponding negative impacts of the COVID-19 pandemic in Nigeria's construction industry. The COVID-19 impact varies from one sector to another but has been significant in the construction industry due to its peculiar nature (Alozie et al., 2020). The truth of the matter is that construction activities in developing countries like Nigeria are less mechanized and labour-intensive, while most of their operations are carried out in enclosed environments. The ILO (2021) states that the industry is known for employing a large number of people with a diverse range of skills to achieve the aim of the projects. Consequently, the people in construction (PiC), materials suppliers' merchants and society at large were negatively impacted by the COVID-19 pandemic. The ILO (2020) and WHO (2020a) noted that the COVID-19 outbreak exacerbated the poor health and safety (H&S) that the construction industry is known for.

### Impact of COVID-19 measures on construction enterprises

The impact of the COVID-19 pandemic on construction enterprises has been significant, with many facing liquidity problems (ILO, 2021). There is a drastic reduction in spending and consumption capacity among enterprises and other stakeholders due to restrictions on the movement of goods and services for fear of infection. The International Monetary Fund (IMF, 2021) reports on Policy Responses to COVID-19 state that liquidity shortages threaten the sustainability of small and medium enterprises (SMEs), especially in developing countries like Nigeria. The ILO (2021) identifies SMEs' bankruptcy as one of the growing negative impacts of COVID-19 on the global economy if the pandemic continues.

In Nigeria, SMEs and large construction enterprises were impacted seriously because of the MCO. While in some Nigerian states the control measures involved total or partial lockdowns of construction sites, contractors were restricted from travelling to cities where their projects were located. Construction projects encountered delays, suspensions and loss of revenue to project developers. According to the ILO (2021), many contractors around the world have had to activate specific contractual provisions giving entitlements to additional time and financial resources. Therefore, construction enterprises had to pay higher prices on wages and salaries due to COVID-19, in addition to facing other issues such as high rates of mortality and morbidity among workers (Alara, 2021; ILO, 2021).

Enterprises of all sizes are looking at ways to manage the impacts on their projects, businesses and employees. The ILO (2021) identifies measures such as general contractual provisions and legal principles that excuse liability for non-performance (force majeure), as well as specific contractual provisions that allow adjustments in time and financial resources, particularly for SMEs in developing countries. The ILO further adds that some financial institutions could support construction enterprises in managing COVID-19-related risks, such as repayment delays, which are particularly relevant for SMEs' survival. In the absence of relief packages for SME construction enterprises, the effects may have a long-term impact, as it will take time for construction activities to return to pre-COVID-19 levels, particularly in developing countries.

### *Resultant effects of COVID-19 restrictive measures on the construction materials supply chain*

Construction activities are severely impacted by the COVID-19 pandemic and the disruption of global supply chains, with shortages of building raw materials and other inputs (ILO, 2021; WHO, 2021). Some building material supply chains have suspended production and distribution (Alara, 2021). According to Kukoyi et al. (2021), managing the risks and challenges occasioned by COVID-19 among SMEs and large construction enterprises in Nigeria includes delays and increasing costs of imported raw materials and off-site construction components, as many factories have been closed down. In addition, bans on the transportation of goods and persons across the 36 states of the Nigerian Federation slowed down the project delivery period, equipment manufacturers and equipment rental services (Alara, 2021; Kukoyi et al., 2021).

It was noted by Kukoyi et al. (2021) that in many cases, there were shortages of plants, equipment and construction materials due to changes and delays in importation orders and the global supply chain. The global lockdowns occasioned by COVID-19 undoubtedly triggered shortages of construction materials supplies, particularly in developing countries (ILO, 2021).

### *Disruptive outcomes emanated from COVID-19 measures among construction professionals/consultants*

Globally, the PiC and Builders render both tangible and intangible services to clients and contractors for efficient and timely delivery of construction projects. According to the ILO (2021), disruption of construction activities occasioned by the global COVID-19 pandemic has severely impacted the ongoing projects in different countries, which led to cancelling or suspension of the project during the MCO period. In Nigeria, approximately 12,786 different consultants were contacted for work; regrettably only 2,120 submitted quotations within the period (Alara, 2021).

Luo et al. (2020) identified challenges facing the design and construction of the Leishenshan hospital building in Malaysia during the COVID-19 pandemic as project delay, and design optimization and communication of project information among project stakeholders. Sharing crucial project information among professionals was hampered by the limitation on the movement of people, products and services brought on by the pandemic. Similarly, due to the MCO order enforced by the Nigerian government, consultants hired by the clients for efficient site supervision may not be on the project's site. Projects will be put on hold, there will be time and cost overruns, the client or property developer will lose money and suppliers and contractors will also be negatively impacted.

### Measures to control the spread of COVID-19 disease among the construction site workforce and its impact

Rural migrant workers have always been a source of regular and cheap labour for the construction industry in urban cities (Okorie and Smallwood, 2011). The use of unskilled rural migrant workers for construction work in urban cities is a global phenomenon. These groups of rural migrants migrate to urban areas in pursuit of better opportunities. Consequently, COVID-19 changed the narrative, as the HSW of construction site workers was seriously impacted.

Following this, the Nigerian government saw the urgent need to protect the HSW of the PiC in the face of a widespread and increasing number of deaths caused by COVID-19 in the country. Subsequently, the government signed the COVID-19 Disease Health Protection Regulations into law. The regulations require the use of face masks in the workplace, restrictions on gatherings, require a physical distance of at least 2 metres between workers, restrictions on more than 50 people to work in an enclosed work environment and permit access to only critical personnel on-site, and prohibit entry to a construction site by a worker with a body temperature above 38 degrees Celsius, while such a worker may be advised to seek medical attention at the time. Construction sites' peculiarities, which cluster employees together and put them in danger of exposure to and infection with COVID-19, are found all over the world. SMEs must closely follow COVID-19 H&S procedures in order to prevent the COVID-19 virus from spreading to construction site personnel.

Therefore, in line with the WHO (2020a) and ILO (2020), the COVID-19 global response strategies for workplaces and the Federal Government of Nigeria COVID-19 regulations, the basic requirements for COVID-19 H&S procedures should be strictly observed by both the SMEs and large construction enterprises in Nigeria. Thus, some of the basic measures and regulations in accordance with the PHSM guidelines are discussed here.

#### Temperature testing and health screening of workers

The WHO (2020a) and ILO (2020) in response to the COVID-19 global pandemic came up with health policies to contain the transmission and infection of COVID-19. In response to the devastating effects of COVID-19 in Nigeria, the federal government signed the COVID-19 Disease Health Protection Regulations into law. One of the policies is testing the temperature and health screening of workers as pre-conditions for entry into the work sites, business premises, restaurants, offices, schools, etc. Thus, this code of practice becomes the norm that a person can only be admitted into any work environment with a temperature of 38 degrees Celsius. In addition, it is compulsory for rural migrant workers to undergo temperature screening to ensure they are free from COVID-19 infection. Consequently, the resultant effect will be an increase in workforce shortages on site.

According to the ILO (2020), construction site operations by their very nature are labour-intensive; therefore, workforce shortages translate to a high cost of labour, delay in project completion time and loss of revenue to property developers.

### *Wearing of a nose mask as an element of PHSM guidelines*

Nose mask-wearing has become the new norm on construction sites, in addition to other personal protective equipment (PPE). In order to reduce the spread of COVID-19 in work environments, employers must provide and educate workers on the need to put on their nose masks as the requirement of the hygienic standard and H&S work practices. The construction site is notorious for its poor H&S practices; the use of nose masks on-site could improve workers' H&S performance. Thus, the face or nose mask measure is in line with the PHSM guidelines as prescribed by the WHO (2020b).

### *Social distance as a necessary restrictive measure to control the spread of COVID-19*

Social distancing in work environments came as a result of the COVID-19 pandemic outbreak. This deadly disease devastated world economies and caused untimely deaths to millions of people globally. Thus, COVID-19 has significantly impacted the way humans interact and socialize in their daily activities and in the workplace environment (Onubi et al., 2021). The quick spread of COVID-19 spirals out of control, causing complete lockdowns of all human activities as well as disruptions to the country's SMEs and major construction firms. The infected counties developed a variety of preventative and containment measures against the development of COVID-19 in order to slow the rapid spread of this deadly disease. As a result, SMEs and large construction companies must deal with new legal and nonpharmaceutical interventions, including social distancing.

By their very nature, construction site operations require a huge workforce to complete assigned duties in a timely manner. The WHO (2020a), ILO (2020) and FRN (2021) mandate that workers should maintain social distancing. Reducing the workforce on construction sites to comply with social distancing requirements, according to Zakaria and Singh (2021), will undoubtedly have a negative effect on the time it takes to complete projects. Additionally, there might be delays brought on by cutting back on staff members owing to social distance, which would result in cost and time overruns.

However, the government's judgements on matters involving personal protective equipment (PPE), such as social distancing, face masks, gloves and hand sanitizers, must consider people's attitudes (Esmaeilzadeh, 2022). Therefore, rules that encourage the use of small work teams to reduce interpersonal contact, restrict the use of changing rooms on construction sites to ensure workers' safety, designate a single entry/exit point to ensure safe interpersonal space, limit movements to and from the construction site and make sure that site meetings are conducted in a private setting are all examples of effective social distancing as a protective and preventive measure on construction sites (Onubi et al., 2021).

### An illustrated impact of COVID-19 restrictive measures on Nigerian construction sites

The outbreak of COVID-19 brought untold hardship to the world economy and human health. According to the WHO (2020c), people died in millions daily, particularly the elderly, and the world's economy was brought to a standstill. Consequently, there is a drastic reduction in consumption of goods and services, a hike in business operating costs, disruption of the labour supply chain and poor health and safety of people. The devastating effects of COVID-19 have negative impacts on construction enterprises, the building materials supply chain and the HSW of construction site workers (ILO, 2020). Alara (2021) and Kukoyi et al. (2021) observed that COVID-19 caused the closure of workplaces, poor economic prospects, travel restrictions of persons, goods and services, low productivity, hardship to families, rise in H&S management budget to governments at all levels and high cost of operations.

   In the face of these global calamities, the WHO (2020c) and ILO (2020) came up with policy guidelines on H&S measures to adequately contain the COVID-19 pandemic globally. In a similar line, COVID-19 Regulations of Disease Health Protection were released by the FRN (2021). However, the nature of construction site operations and the setting that brings workers together could put them at high risk of exposure to COVID-19. Consequently, small, medium and large construction enterprises in Nigeria are impacted negatively as a result of COVID-19. Government restrictive measures are illustrated in Figure 5.1.

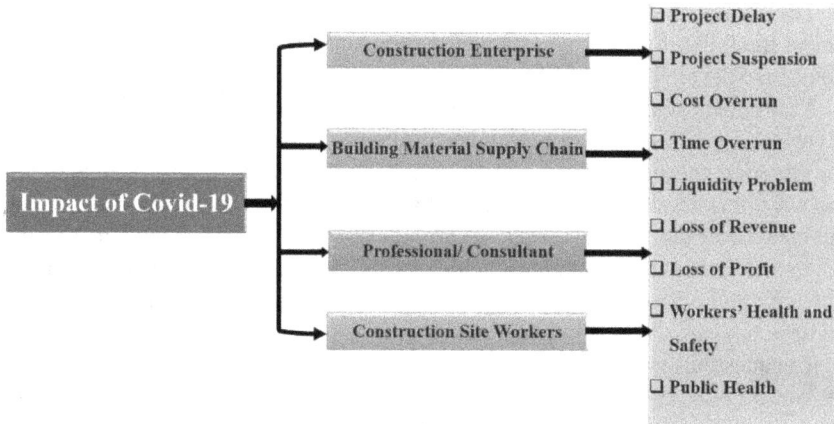

*Figure 5.1* An illustration of the impact of COVID-19 disease in Nigeria.

## Methodology

The sample for the interviews was purposively selected among 24 SMEs from PiC to facilitate an in-depth discussion of the subject matter under investigation. The sample selection criteria include interviewees' involvement and participation in their construction fields, i.e., actively/currently working at a construction site in the study area: the South-South geo-political zone of Nigeria. The South-South political zone of Nigeria is made up of 6 States: Akwa Ibom, Bayelsa, Cross River, Delta, Edo and Rivers. The 6 States are imbued with oil and gas minerals; thus, exploration of these natural minerals attracts infrastructure developments to the area. In addition, major urban cities like Port Harcourt, Warri, Asaba, Calabar, Benin City and Uyo always have ongoing renovation and construction projects. Therefore, the sample criteria were in line with the research topic, which seeks to investigate the various measures taken to reduce the spread of COVID-19 among SMEs and large construction enterprises in the South-South geo-political zone of Nigeria and how the transmission and infection affect workers' performance. The purposive sampling technique was used to draw participants from SMEs and large construction enterprises within the study area. It is notable that participants who worked for large firms were managers saddled with contract administration responsibilities that include workers' HSW, whereas participants from the SMEs were owners and site supervisors whose responsibilities included staffs' HSW. Although 24 construction enterprises (small, medium and large) were contacted at the beginning of the fieldwork, only 12 firms agreed to take part in the study. The decision to proceed with the 12 participants was made based on the fact that the study at this stage is exploratory, and that a phenomenology-based study can be conducted with 12 participants (Flick, 2014). The details of the 12 participants are provided in Table 5.1. In addition, the limitation on social gathering as a result of the COVID-19 protocol and the peculiar nature of construction projects' operations result in adopting an interview protocol for the study (Okorie et al., 2014). Thus, the interviews and discussions were conducted with due regard to ethical considerations governing this type of study.

The choice of the unstructured interview was employed because it offers sufficient flexibility to approach different respondents. Unstructured interview questions were developed from relevant literature to guide the questions.

The primary sources of the interview questions included an exhaustive literature review on COVID-19 restrictive and control measures and their compliance within the Nigerian construction industry (Alara, 2021; Kukoyi et al., 2021). In addition, the questions allowed participating contractors, managers and supervisors to discuss the use of the thermal reader, the attitude of construction site workers towards the use of face masks on-site, social distancing, the impact of COVID-19 on productivity and obstacles in reducing COVID-19 transmission and infection among construction site workers in Nigeria.

The questions were structured to elicit responses from the PiC on ways COVID-19 can be effectively managed by SMEs in the Nigerian construction industry. Interviewees were informed of the voluntary nature of their participation, and they

*Table 5.1* Interviewees' profile outlook (small, medium and large construction enterprises in the South-South geo-political zone of Nigeria).

| S/n | Name of city | Category of business entity | | | |
|---|---|---|---|---|---|
| | | Large (8 firms) | Medium (8 firms) | Small (8 firms) | Total |
| 1 | Port Harcourt | L1 & L2 | M1 | S1 | 2 |
| 2 | Warri | L3 | M2 & M3 | S2 | 2 |
| 3 | Asaba | L4 | M4 & M5 | S3 | 2 |
| 4 | Calabar | L5 | M6 | S4 & S5 | 2 |
| 5 | Benin City | L6 & L7 | M7 | S6 | 2 |
| 6 | Uyo | L8 | M8 | S7 & S8 | 2 |
| | **Total** | **4** | **4** | **4** | **12** |

*Note:* L= Large firms, M= Medium firms, S= Small firms respectively

were assured of the confidentiality of their comments. The discussions with each interviewee, as well as their opinions and suggestions, were recorded on iPhone with the permission of the interviewee before transcription.

The researchers then captured the data on the computer after each interview. The principal investigator listened several times to the recorded opinions and suggestions and personally transcribed them. To enhance the validity of the findings, the transcribed versions were sent to the participants/interviewees who agreed that accurate versions of discussions were obtained. After the transcription of the data, the analysis thereof brought about the identification of major themes in the form of:

- Lack of thermometer temperature reading equipment;
- The poor attitude of construction site workers towards the use of nose masks;
- Social distancing and construction site workers' productivity, and
- Obstacles in reducing COVID-19 transmission and infection among construction site workers.

## Results and discussion

The findings presented in this section are based on the perceptions of contractors and the PiC on the impacts of COVID-19 in the Nigerian construction industry.

### Lack of thermometer temperature testing equipment
### among construction enterprises

The use of thermal readers has become a norm for entry into general workplaces and construction sites. When asked whether their companies employed experienced medical personnel for thermal reading, one of the managers from the large company answered in the affirmative:

My company has thermometer temperature testing equipment used by our medical trained personnel on-site.

- L3

In contrast to this answer, a supervisor from one of the small construction enterprises said the opposite. S2 reported that: "Our company does not have thermometer temperature testing equipment for screening of workers before entry site for work". Another supervisor from one of the medium enterprises, M2, corroborated this and went further to say that: "My company does not have thermometer testing equipment and trained medical team for COVID-19 disease surveillance".

The International Monetary Fund (IMF, 2021) reports on Policy Responses to COVID-19 state that SMEs, especially in developing countries, lack the capacity and technology to contain the COVID-19 pandemic. The WHO (2020a) describes the COVID-19 pandemic as a desert to the global economy and a threat to human existence.

### *The poor attitude of construction site workers towards the use of face masks*

The need for a drastic attitude and behavioural change among people to prevent and minimize the wide spread of COVID-19 was a necessity, especially with the mandatory wearing of face masks in public spaces.

A question was posed to the interviewees: Does your company fully comply with the Nigeria Federal Government regulation for compulsory face mask-wearing in public spaces? One of the site managers from large firms responded and stated: "Yes, we are compliant with the government rules on wearing face masks"- L2. "Our company is very strict in ensuring that everybody on site is wearing their face mask, because it is helping us to reduce the spread of COVID-19 among our site workers"- L2. "In addition, I am personally aware of a person who has died of COVID-19 disease, so it is not a joke or conspiracy theory"- L2. L1 explained that, "If I found anybody on-site without a face mask, I will order the person to leave our site immediately and report the matter to management".

Statements of construction site workers from SMEs were different. S4 reported that:

> For me, I am just wearing the face mask because my supervisor made it compulsory for site workers. Wearing a face mask is not because of the Nigerian government rules on COVID-19 disease. M1 stated that: I don't care about COVID-19; I am only interested [in] work[ing] and earn[ing] money.
> In addition, a site supervisor from one of the small firms responded with these statements. S8 reported that:

> COVID-19 disease is a rich men's disease and it has nothing to do with us because we are poor. COVID-19 kills only rich men in Nigeria. Let me tell you something: once I leave this construction site, I don't wear any face masks because it is difficult for me to breathe properly, and I don't believe even that COVID-19 exists.

COVID-19 has posed a serious threat to people's health and countries' healthcare systems.

Despite several academic studies substantiating that wearing a face mask can effectively reduce infection and mortality rates resulting from COVID-19, some individuals still believe that COVID-19 is a White man's trick to drastically reduce the African population (Esmaeilzadeh, 2022).

### *Social distancing and construction site workers' productivity*

Government compulsory regulation on social distancing in places of gathering and workplaces was adopted as one of the proactive measures towards minimizing the rate of COVID-19 transmission and infection. The question was posed: How does your company enforce social distancing among construction site workers and its impact on productivity? L8, a project manager from one of the large firms made the following statements:

 In our company, we strive earnestly to maintain a reasonable social-physical distancing in accordance with the government regulations, but occasionally it was very difficult to maintain social distancing on-site due to the nature of our work. Let me tell you, site productivity and project delivery timeline has been affected greatly because we only employed a few site workers in order to keep with the social distance rules.

Two site supervisors from SMEs expressed their views this way:

M3 reported that: "The issues of social distancing within construction sites have made it very difficult to effectively control site workers to optimal productivity and to keep projects on track since the COVID-19 saga".

M2, one of the supervisors went on to state that:

 Our site operations have been negatively impacted since the outbreak of COVID-19. There are great loss[es:] huge hours of the workforce, low productivity, and challenging financial sustainability as a result of maintaining social distancing regulations on our project activities.

The construction industry depends on the high productivity of site workers to remain financially sustainable. Undoubtedly, COVID-19 has significantly disrupted how construction projects and the workforce are organized and managed. Onubi et al. (2021) posit that the construction industry globally witnessed low worker productivity as a result of adhering to mandatory preventive measures such as social distancing, which resulted in delays in project completion time and cost overruns.

### *Obstacles in reducing COVID-19 transmission and*
### *infection among construction site workers*

The peculiarity of construction site operations posed serious challenges to effective control and management of COVID-19 transmission and infection, as its spread invokes direct human contact with infected persons and through airborne transmission when talking, coughing or sneezing. A question was then asked: What are some of the key barriers and obstacles towards effective control of COVID-19 transmission and infection in your construction site? A site manager from one of the large construction firms made the following statements:

> Enforcing face mask-wearing on-site sometimes makes it difficult for workers to effectively communicate orally and occasionally some workers would consciously or unconsciously remove their face masks, therefore endangering and posing a health risk to themselves and other workers.
>
> - L4

> For me, I don't believe in this COVID-19 stuff and forcing workers to wear face masks doesn't make sense because there is no COVID-19 in Nigeria. All these measures in place are tools state governments are using to get money from the Federal Government.
>
> - L5

A site supervisor from one of the SMEs made the following statements:

> In my company, we do not have trained medical surveillance team, and thermal testing equipment are inadequate for testing everybody entering the site"- S5. S5 further stated that: "Also, occasionally we may be in shortage of face masks and hand sanitisers". Thus, M6- project manager from a medium firm reported that: "We understand that these lapses are potential ways COVID-19 infection can spread among us, but there is nothing we can do because management and clients want us to deliver their projects".

The prior statements made by interviewees validate ILO's (2020) sectorial brief on the impact of COVID on the construction sector. Some notable critical barriers while implementing COVID-19 preventive measures included poor safety culture, absence of medical personnel, particularly among the SMEs, and inadequate resources like thermal testing equipment. Esmaeilzadeh (2022), noted that many people in the Sub-Saharan African countries did believe that coronavirus is not a serious threat to their life as a result of various propaganda and perceptions due to misinformation and disinformation usually spread by social media about the transmission and infection of COVID-19 disease.

## Implications

It is an imperative measure for all construction industry stakeholders and role players, especially among small, medium, and large construction enterprises in Nigeria, to undertake a holistic approach towards resolving issues with the poor site workers' health, safety, and well-being (HSW). Thus, effective management of construction site workers' health, safety, and well-being would significantly enhance the Nigerian construction industry's performance and competitiveness outlook. Therefore, the experience and lessons learned during the COVID-19 pandemic with regard to the management of construction workers' health, safety, and well-being protocol should be internalized and integrated as a good or best practice among small, medium, and large construction enterprises in Nigeria.

## Conclusions

There were concerns about the extent and nature of compliance of COVID-19 preventive and protective measures among SMEs and large construction enterprises in the South-South geo-political zone of Nigeria. There is evidence from the study findings that SME construction firms and their workers lack adequate resources and critical knowledge to effectively manage and control the spread of COVID-19 in comparison with large firms that are moderately resourceful and knowledgeable regarding effective measures to reduce the spread of COVID-19 in line with PHSM guidelines (WHO, 2020b).

The study findings revealed that there are general inadequate safety measures as a result of culture, and poor attitudinal and behaviour changes among SME construction firms and their site workers towards adjusting to the COVID-19 protocol and preventive measure in terms of wearing face masks. Many complain of the discomfort of face masks and their conviction that COVID-19 is a conspiracy, whilst the large firms are seen mostly as strict in undertaking preventive measures such as enforcing wearing face masks among their workers. Thus, the study has alluded to those challenges faced by SMEs for not adhering to wearing face masks, which may be linked to a lack of business structure and chain of command among them. However, the study advocates that SMEs especially should be encouraged to leverage on experiences gained from COVID-19 challenges to ensure that site workers' HSW are adequately protected.

The issue that social distancing as a preventive measure against the spread of COVID-19 has negatively impacted construction productivity was generally acknowledged by both SMEs and large construction firms in the South-South geo-political zone, as it was difficult to effectively control project activities. The idea to drastically minimize the spread of COVID-19 transmission and infection among PiC in Nigeria through the adoption of COVID-19 protective and preventive measures proved challenging, as its implementation met barriers such as lack of adequate resources, poor safety culture, lack of trust in public/government regulations, misinterpretation and misinformation of the seriousness of the threat of COVID-19 and its devastating impacts on human HSW.

## Acknowledgement

In reflection of this research study, we immensely recognize and acknowledge all the construction firms and their employees that granted and assisted with their time and inputs during the interview sessions within the South-South political zone of Nigeria.

## References

Alara, S.A. (2021). Organisational characteristics and COVID-19 safety practices among small and medium construction enterprises in Nigeria. *Frontiers in Engineering and Built Environment*, 1(1), 4154.

Alozie, C.E., Ideh, A.O., & Ifelunini, I. (2020, September 21). Coronavirus COVID-19 pandemic economic consequences and strategies for ameliorating macroeconomic shocks in Nigeria. *Economy*.

Esmaeilzadeh, P. (2022). Public concerns and burdens associated with face mask-wearing: Lessons learned from the COVID-19 pandemic. *Progress in Disaster Science*, 13, 100215, 1–11.

Federal Republic of Nigeria. (2021). Coronavirus disease (COVID-19) health protection regulations 2021. *Nigeria Centre for Disease Control, Federal Republic of Nigeria*. Available at https//covid19.ncdc.gov.ng/media/files/Coronavirus_Disease_COVID19_Health_ProtectionRegulations_2021.pdf (Accessed 21 April 2022).

Flick, U. (2014). *An introduction to qualitative research* (5th ed.). London: Sage.

Hinze, J.W. (2006). *Construction safety*. Hoboken: Prentice-Hall Inc.

International Labour Organisation. (2020). *Monitor COVID-19 and world of work*. Geneva: ILO.

International Labour Organisation. (2021). *Impact of COVID-19 on construction sector: ILO Sectorial Brief*. Geneva: ILO.

International Monetary Fund. (2021). Policy responses to COVID-19 pandemic (Accessed 12 April 2922).

Kukoyi, P.O., Simpeh, F., Adebowale, O.J., & Agumba, J.N. (2021). Managing the risk and challenges of COVID-19 on construction sites in Lagos, Nigeria. *Journal of Engineering Design and Technology*, 20 (1), 99–144.

Luo, H., Liu, J., Li, C., Chen, K., & Zhang, M. (2020). Ultra-rapid delivery of specialty field hospitals to combat COVID-19: Lessons learned from the Leishenshan Hospital project in Wuhan. *Automation in Construction* (Elsevier Ltd), 119(103345), 1–10.

Okorie, V.N., Emuze, F.A., Smallwood, J.J., & van Wyk, J.J. (2014). A qualitative view of the health and safety: Leadership roles of managers in South African construction firms. *Journal of Construction Project Management and Innovation*, 4(2), 950–965.

Okorie, V.N., & Musonda, I. (2020). An investigation on supervisor's ability and competency to conduct construction site health and safety induction training in Nigeria. *International Journal of Construction Management*. doi: 10.1080/15623599.2018.1531808.

Okorie, V.N., & Smallwood, J.J. (2011). Impact of rural migrant workers on construction health and safety. In *Proceedings of ASOCSA 6th built environment conference* (pp. 128–140). Johannesburg: Association of Schools of Construction of Southern Africa.

Onubi, H.O., Yusof, N., Hassan, A.S., & Bahdad, A.A.S. (2021). Forecasting the schedule performance resulting from the adoption of social distancing in construction projects. *Engineering, Construction and Architectural Management*. doi: 10.1108/ECAM-07-2021-0632.

World Health Organization (WHO). (2020a). *Coronavirus disease COVID-19 health and safety in workplace*. Available at www.who.int/newsroom/q-a-detail/coronavirus-diseas-covid19health-safety-in the workplace (Accessed April 2022).

World Health Organization. (2020b). *WHO COVID-19 dashboard*. Geneva: World Health Organization. Available at https://covid19.who.int/ (Accessed April 2022).

WHO Health Organization (WHO). (2020c). *Coronavirus disease COVID-19 dashboard, world health organization.* Available at www.who.int.newsroom/q-a-detail/coronavirus. disease-covid19health (Accessed April 2022).

Zakaria, S.A., & Singh, A.M. (2021). Impact of COVID-19 outbreak on civil engineering activities in the Malaysia construction industry: A review. *Journal of Social Sciences and Humanities Open Access*, (1), 1000074.

# 6 COVID-19 pandemic

## Challenges in practising new norms for construction workers

*Mohd Amizan Mohamed @ Arifin, Raja Muhamad Amir Hamzah Raja Mohd Azlan, Syahirah Intan Mohd Sheffie and Nazirah Mohd Apandi*

### Introduction

This virus has already expanded globally, with China being the first infected. The World Health Organization declared COVID-19 a pandemic on March 11, 2020. A pandemic is a disease that has swept over multiple countries, regions, or perhaps the entire globe (Sharma, 2020). On March 18, 2020, the Malaysian authorities announced a first movement control order (MCO), which was extended until mid-April. These rules were placed for a specific reason (Abdullah et al., 2020). Aside from the inherent dangers of the job, construction workers and specialists face a significant risk of exposure (Zhang et al., 2020). The Occupational Safety and Health Administration published COVID-19 Guidance for the Construction Workforce (OSHA). To avoid the spread of COVID-19, it is critical to develop rules for construction workers on the job site. Companies need to consider any COVID-19 safety standards imposed by the state or municipality where the project is being built on behalf of construction employees. On the building site, all workers must adhere to the SOP. Some worker safety precautions may be beneficial to prevent COVID-19 and similar crises.

Even though the construction industry is widely recognised as one that poses significant risks to workers' health and safety, the beginning of COVID-19 presents an additional risk that has the potential to have a significant and negative impact on the health and safety of workers in the construction industry. Because this is a once-in-a-century occurrence, several unheard-of precautions have been made to prevent COVID-19 from spreading throughout the business and to lessen the impact it will have on the overall progression of the company and its workers. Therefore, construction sites must protect their workers during the COVID-19 pandemic by taking actions to decrease the risk of infection and dissemination. Cleaning, disinfection, and other care and security services provided by building service workers are critical to protecting public health by reducing COVID-19 infections. In response to the Malaysian government's official statement of the National Recovery Plan, which is the country's exit strategy regarding the COVID-19 pandemic, the Construction Industry Development Board of

DOI: 10.1201/9781003278368-7

Malaysia (CIDB) has published the standard operating procedure (SOP) for the construction industry.

Evaluating the perceptions of fieldworkers regarding COVID-19-related strategies that the construction industry has implemented is essential. This is because the COVID-19 pandemic is a dynamic event, and there is a need to support the effective implementation of strategies both during and after the pandemic. This evaluation needs to consider the possible variations across the various demographic aspects of the critical organisation. However, there is a lack of information regarding the viewpoints of fieldworkers regarding safety and health interventions implemented in response to a pandemic such as COVID-19. This void in both theory and practice is what the current investigation aims to address, and it will do so in the following ways:

a) To determine new standards and practices for construction workers that are applicable in light of the COVID-19 pandemic.
b) To explore construction employees' difficulties while attempting to implement new standards during the COVID-19 pandemic.
c) To determine the most effective methods for normalising the new standards of practice for construction workers affected by the COVID-19 pandemic.

The research was conducted in the Klang Valley state. The Klang Valley is a Malaysian urban conglomeration centred in Kuala Lumpur and comprising Selangor's adjacent cities and villages. The scope of this study will be limited to construction employees on-site during the COVID-19 pandemic. The data were gathered via a survey using Google Forms given to construction employees to gather reliable information about their issues and experiences with the new norms in the workplace during the COVID-19 pandemic.

**Perspectives and concepts**

On January 25, 2020, Malaysia's first three cases of COVID-19 were verified to be imported cases. Following notification from the Singapore Ministry of Health that eight close contacts of a confirmed case of Chinese nationality in Singapore had travelled into Johor, Malaysia, the three cases were discovered through tracing and screening. The number of cases in Malaysia had risen to 22, including 12 people under investigation (PUI), eight close contacts of confirmed cases, and two Malaysian evacuees from a humanitarian relief mission in Wuhan, China, as of February 15 (Hashim, 2021).

Many nations, including Malaysia, ordered lockdowns just three months after the first confirmed case to curb this pandemic. The Malaysian government issued an initial movement control order (MCO) on March 18, 2020, extending it until mid-April. These regulations were put in place for a purpose. MCO enforcement became increasingly strict, with roadblocks around the nation and armed units recruited to increase MCO enforcement (Abdullah et al., 2020).

The Food and Drug Administration (FDA) has authorised various medications to treat severe COVID-19, yet no particular and effective therapy is available. As a result, all nations strive to stem the spread of the disease by instituting lockdowns and quarantines, community-wide usage of face masks, social distancing measures, and travel restrictions. Unfortunately, these attempts have resulted in significant bodily and psychological harm to individuals and a global economic downturn. As a result, developing and deploying a COVID-19 vaccine is one of the most cost-efficient and effective ways to combat the pandemic. Several vaccines have been approved for use in Malaysia, such as AstraZeneca, Pfizer, Sinovac, Johnson & Johnson, Moderna, and CanSino (Marzo, 2021).

After that, Malaysia will open additional industries to fully vaccinated persons to reconstruct portions of the economy that have been closed due to the COVID-19 pandemic. Manufacturing sector restrictions have also been loosened, with no limit on the operational capacity for enterprises with a staff between 80% and 100% vaccinated. Companies with an immunisation rate between 60% and 79% will be subject to an 80% workforce limit (Hermesaouto, 2021).

Practising new norms during COVID-19, such as following the SOPs for construction workers, are the ways to prevent the risk of COVID-19 spread. Employers should use a mix of engineering and administrative controls, safe work practices, and personal protective equipment (PPE) to prevent worker exposures based on a complete workplace hazard assessment.

According to Dato' Sri Haji Fadillah, Senior Ministry of Works, the CIDB recently took a survey to determine why these firms have failed to operate. According to the surveys, they confronted five key challenges, including existing industry conditions and the expense of COVID-19 screening. Hence, extensive steps to minimise COVID-19 transmission from person to person is essential to managing the present outbreak. Several efficient ways prevented the construction workers from getting COVID-19 spread. For example, employers should provide free COVID-19 swab tests for their construction workers. Other than that, workers should be trained in appropriate hand-washing techniques and other preventive measures. Employers should supply workers with soap, clean running water, and equipment for drying their hands. Also, employers must provide their workers with information on COVID-19, how it spreads, and the risk of exposure (in a language they understand). Based on a summary provided by Assaad and El-adaway (2021), the short-term and long-term impacts that the COVID-19 virus will have on the construction industry include the following: (1) workforce-related issues, such as worker shortages because of infections and preventive quarantines and worker layoffs caused by project cancellations and delays; (2) project and workplace considerations, such as implementing new workplace practises and policies; (3) procurement and supply chain implications, such as the restriction of movement of materials, and to successfully navigate these obstacles, the construction sector must devise and put into action efficient techniques. Researchers have repeatedly emphasised the importance of prioritising worker safety, health, and well-being at this challenging time to mitigate the anticipated workforce problem in the construction sector (Ogunnusi et al., 2020; Alsharef et al., 2021; Assaad and El-adaway, 2021).

This study evaluates the health and safety precautions the construction industry took during the COVID-19 outbreak and the perceived challenges and effectiveness of the COVID-19 countermeasures that have been applied in practice on construction job sites. To be more specific, this study responds to the following research questions from the point of view of construction field workers:

a) In the context of the COVID-19 pandemic, what are the most up-to-date standards and best practices for those who work in the construction industry?
b) What difficulties may arise when implementing new standards among construction workers during the COVID-19 pandemic?
c) What are the most effective methods for standardising the new rules and practises for construction workers in the wake of the COVID-19 pandemic?

Finally, this research can provide a positive outcome for construction employees by allowing them to normalise new practices during the COVID-19 pandemic. They will comprehend the significance of the MOH (Ministry of Health) Malaysia's SOP (Standard Operating Procedure) at construction sites. So, to evaluate the impact on project performance and supplier chains, existing research has depended chiefly on surveys and interviews with construction companies. However, no research on construction workers has yet been conducted. This study fills the gap by quantitatively analysing OSHA's COVID-19 complaints data collected from construction sites. The study's findings provide insight into current construction site safety and health trends, lay the framework for future academic and practitioner work to address construction workers' concerns, and serve as lessons learned for the industry in the event of a future pandemic.

## Methodology

This research used quantitative techniques to analyse the data. The first strategy at this step was choosing a research area at Klang Valley. Next is finding the problem statement. The problems can be formulated after reviewing the construction workers' situation during the COVID-19 pandemic. The research questions will guide the data collection towards the study's aims. After determining the problem statement, the next step would be to settle on the research objective. A lack of grasp of the research objective will influence the written substance of the paperwork, hindering the objective from being fulfilled. Because of this, it was essential to have a solid understanding of the goals of the research. This is because having clearly stated goals assists in the identification and prioritising of the study, in addition to ensuring that the findings are pertinent.

After that, conduct a literature review and decide on data collection methods. The study approach begins with background reading about the COVID-19 pandemic. It has been done to see if there is a need for the research. To choose a topic, it must go through this process. After the chosen topic, the literature review for this research begins. The researcher will gather data using the redesigned questionnaire. The sample size was crucial in determining the total number of respondents in the research area. The respondents in this study were among the construction workers who worked on COVID-19 construction projects. CIDB provided the information for the reported construction project. Based on the research scope, the research area is focused on Klang Valley (Selangor and Kuala Lumpur). The total number of local construction workers in was 8,677, while for foreigners it was 32,973. In Kuala Lumpur, the total number of local construction workers was 8,184, while for foreigners it was 36,018. So, the total number of local and foreign workers in Klang Valley was 85,852. Then, the researcher will get the sample size from the sample population using the Krejcie and Morgan Table. To overcome the discrepancy, a table for determining the sample size for a particular population was created as a simple reference. The Krejcie and Morgan Table assists the researcher in determining sample size. As for this research, the population size is 85,852; then, by referring to the Krejcie and Morgan Table, the sample size for actual data is 382.87 or 383 after interpolating the data by using a calculator. The responder will receive the questionnaire based on a sample size of 383. The targeted respondents are construction workers who work during the COVID-19 pandemic.

The questionnaire was given to the construction workers. The Statistical Package for Social Sciences (SPSS) and Microsoft Excel were used to evaluate the data collected from the questionnaire. The software generated results for every question in the survey, which must be analysed to receive accurate findings. As a result, it is crucial to estimate the fundamental research to determine whether it would be accepted. The objectives of this research will be achieved after performing the data analysis. After deciding on a data collection approach, which will be quantitative, the final phase will be spent collecting primary data. The researcher will create a questionnaire based on the study's objective. The question will be in four sections: Section A for demographic information, Section B for new norms practices, Section C for challenges, and Section D for efficient ways of normalising the new norms. Then, there will be a pilot study that needs to distribute the questionnaire to the targeted respondents, which are construction workers. After that, the reliability test is to know the level of acceptance for any errors and the results from reliability that refer to the Cronbach Alpha. Lastly, the questionnaire must be rechecked so that the collected actual data will ease smoothly.

Lastly, the data gathered from the questionnaire were analysed. Section A has three questions about demographic information gained from the personal information from the respondents. Then, Section B analyses the first objective, which is to investigate the construction workers' new COVID-19 norms and practices. Section C identifies the challenges construction workers face in practising new norms during the COVID-19 pandemic. Lastly, Section D is to identify the efficient ways that will help the construction workers normalise the new norms in the COVID-19 pandemic.

**Results and discussion**

Table 6.1 illustrates the reliability test result on the new norms and practices for construction workers during the COVID-19 pandemic. By referring to the rule of reliability, the value of 0.946 with 11 no. of items lies in the excellent range with a > 0.9. Thus, the questionnaire that has been distributed has high validity and consistency for actual data collection. The reliability test result on the challenges of practising new norms among construction workers in COVID-19 is shown in Table 6.1. By referring to the rule of reliability, the value of 0.961 with 9 no. of items lies in the excellent range with a > 0.9. The questionnaires were reliable because the coefficient was larger than 0.9, and Cronbach's Alpha table confirmed it as a rule of thumb. As a result, the reliability and correlation of this part are appropriate for use in actual data collecting. Table 6.1 shows the reliability test result on the effective ways of normalising the new norms and practices for construction workers during the COVID-19 pandemic. By referring to the rule of reliability, the value of 0.965 with 10 no. of items lies in the excellent range with a > 0.9. This value is based on the responses of respondents who have been constant throughout time. Therefore, because the findings demonstrate validity and consistency, actual data gathering in this study will be successful.

The first objective focuses on the new norms that construction workers followed during the COVID-19 pandemic. For example, all construction workers will need to do a COVID-19 swab test every two weeks, sanitise everything they have used, and maintain social distance among themselves. With a mean value of 4.83, most construction workers agreed with the statement that if they followed the COVID-19 SOPs, they would have the least likelihood of becoming infected with the COVID-19 virus. According to OSHA, implementing new COVID-19 regulations, such as following SOPs for construction workers, is one approach to reducing the risk of COVID-19 spreading to them. The construction employees are then informed that, with a mean value of 4.73, they must perform a COVID-19 swab test once a week to begin their work. According to Dayak Daily, all construction employees, whether local or international, must take a COVID-19 swab test every two weeks by 2021. Construction workers ranked third, with a mean value of 4.58, and agreed to maintain hygiene by regularly cleaning and disinfecting places they have touched. Besides that, the construction workers' use of a face mask ranks third lowest, with a mean value of 4.39. Social distancing must always be used at work, during breaks, and travelling. Finally, with a mean value of 4.32, employers should use a mix of engineering and administrative controls, safe work practices, and personal protective equipment (PPE) to prevent worker exposure, as shown in Table 6.2.

During the COVID-19 pandemic, construction employees will have obstacles to practising new norms, which will be the focus of Objective 2. According to the survey's findings, CIDB faces five significant problems, including the existing state of the sector and the cost of COVID-19 screening. Other issues include SOP compliance, worker difficulty, and SOP complexity. After analysing the data with

*Table 6.1* Reliability test result for Sections B, C, and D

| Section | Cronbach's Alpha | Cronbach's Alpha based on standardized items | N of items |
|---------|-----------------|---------------------------------------------|------------|
| B | 0.946 | 0.934 | 11 |
| C | 0.961 | 0.959 | 9 |
| D | 0.965 | 0.965 | 8 |

*Table 6.2* Questionnaire, mean and rank for Objective 1.

| Question | Mean | Rank |
| --- | --- | --- |
| Practising new rules for COVID-19, such as following SOPs for construction workers, are approaches to reduce the chance of COVID-19 spreading to them. | 4.83 | 1 |
| Before being permitted to work on construction projects, all local and foreign workers must do COVID-19 swab tests every two weeks. | 4.73 | 2 |
| Clean and disinfect frequently touched surfaces throughout and at the start and end of each shift. | 4.58 | 3 |
| For example, closer contact between personnel or indoor work may require a more protective mask than outside activity. | 4.57 | 4 |
| A 1.5 m or 2 m physical distance between construction workers should be implemented to decrease in-person contact. | 4.55 | 5 |
| Improve cleaning procedures for shared equipment and common areas, particularly surface sanitation. | 4.52 | 6 |
| Use an alcohol-based hand sanitiser with at least 60% alcohol, or wash your hands for at least 20 seconds with soap and water. | 4.48 | 7 |
| Regularly touched items such as handrails, ladders, doorknobs, and portable toilets should all be cleaned and disinfected. | 4.47 | 8 |
| For construction workers, face masks should be part of their first line of defence. | 4.39 | 9 |
| Physical distancing should always be practised at work, during breaks, and in automobiles. | 4.37 | 10 |
| Employers should utilise engineering and administrative controls, safe work practices, and personal protective equipment (PPE) to avoid worker exposure. | 4.32 | 11 |

SPSS, it was shown that construction employees, who ranked first with a mean value of 4.82, find it challenging to follow all the Ministry of Health's SOPs. This is because they felt out of the ordinary while on the job. Following that, workers in the second rank, with a mean value of 4.64, found it difficult to maintain social distance while carrying an enormous burden together. Then, because they remained in congested settings such as labour camps, some immigrants were more easily exposed to COVID-19, with a mean value of 4.61. Apart from that, the difficulty in convincing construction employees, mainly immigrant labourers, to follow the newly formed SOPs ranks second-worst with a mean score of 4.37, as shown in Table 6.3. Finally, social distancing is one of the SOPs guidelines that construction employees may find challenging.

During the COVID-19 pandemic, Objective 3 identifies the most effective approaches to assist construction workers in establishing new norms, as shown in Table 6.4. Significant steps must be taken to prevent COVID-19 from spreading from person to person to contain the current outbreak. Employers must provide free COVID-19 swab tests for their workers, according to the SPSS result, which ranks best with a mean value of 4.84. This will help construction workers with their financial problems. Employers should provide construction workers with extra time to thoroughly wash their hands regularly, according to the second rank, which has a mean value of 4.73. Following that, the construction workers believed that

*Table 6.3* Questionnaire, mean, and rank for Objective 2.

| Question | Mean | Rank |
| --- | --- | --- |
| Construction workers found it difficult to comply with COVID-19 SOPs. | 4.82 | 1 |
| When workers are required to handle bigger items than they should be managing alone, it is difficult to adapt to the two-meter distance rule. | 4.64 | 2 |
| Some immigrant construction workers are exposed to COVID-19 as they stay in crowded labour camps. | 4.61 | 3 |
| Immigrant workers sometimes had to live in filthy conditions. | 4.57 | 4 |
| Different rules and regulations create a great deal of confusion among industry players who must follow the rules. | 4.52 | 5 |
| Even within the same state, individual local councils and agencies may have their own rules and laws. | 4.47 | 6 |
| Immigrant workers sometimes had to live in filthy conditions. | 4.45 | 7 |
| It wasn't easy to persuade foreign staff to adopt the new SOPs that had been established. | 4.37 | 8 |
| Social distancing among workers is one of the SOP compliances that might be challenging for construction workers. | 4.35 | 9 |

*Table 6.4* Questionnaire, mean, and rank for Objective 3.

| Question | Mean | Rank |
| --- | --- | --- |
| Employers should supply their construction workers with a free COVID-19 swab test. | 4.84 | 1 |
| Employers could also change performance objectives to pay their workers more time to wash their hands properly and regularly. | 4.73 | 2 |
| Hand-washing stations or hand sanitisers should be placed in various locations, including in or near portable bathrooms. | 4.65 | 3 |
| Deliver basic information to your workers, explain the preventative processes in place regarding the new COVID-19 SOPs, and perform toolbox briefings at all job sites. | 4.61 | 4 |
| Determine that there is an adequate quantity of gloves and that they are readily available. | 4.60 | 5 |
| Post posters at the entrance to the workplace and other areas where they're likely to be seen advising workers to stay home whenever they're sick, cough and sneeze etiquette, COVID-19 signs and symptoms, and proper hand hygiene procedures. | 4.54 | 6 |
| Employers must advise their employees about COVID-19, how it spreads, and the danger of infection (in a language they understand). | 4.45 | 7 |
| If workers do not have access to hand-washing or hand sanitiser, use disposable gloves as the last option to reduce hand contact with highly infected surfaces. | 4.44 | 8 |
| Employers should install soaps, clean running water, and tools for drying workers' hands or provide alcohol-based hand sanitisers with around 60% alcohol at workstations throughout the facility for workers and clients. | 4.35 | 9 |
| Hand-washing routines and other preventive measures should be taught to construction workers. | 4.29 | 10 |

proper hand-washing units and hand sanitisers should be placed in various areas so that they could conveniently utilise them, with a mean value of 4.65. Other than that, with a mean value of 4.35, employers should place soaps, clean water, and tools for drying workers' hands at workspaces throughout the facility for workers and clients to use. Employers should also provide alcohol-based hand sanitisers, including around 60% alcohol at workstations across the facility for workers and clients. Finally, with a mean score of 4.29, construction workers must be taught proper hand-washing techniques and other preventative measures.

**Implications for practice or research**

This chapter presents various recommendations to enhance and persuade construction companies and the government to reduce COVID-19 disease among construction workers. Several parties, including the government, construction firms, and future researchers, have received advice from the researchers. During the COVID-19 outbreak, construction workers in the Klang Valley had difficulty implementing the new standards. As a result, future academics should investigate how the government and other agencies dealt with the issues in the past so that future research can see if the construction industry is functioning normally. Aside from that, because this study was conducted during the COVID-19 pandemic, future researchers should conduct biological research and analyse construction workers during the COVID-19 endemic. As a result, they can compare the outcomes and discussions of the COVID-19 pandemic and endemic eras.

**Conclusions**

The main objective of this study was to look into how construction workers implemented new norms during the COVID-19 outbreak. The Klang Valley was chosen as the research location. For the record, the widespread nature of COVID-19 posed many issues for the building sector, particularly for construction workers, as the project progressed. To reduce their chances of contracting the disease, they must follow all the new SOPs issued by the government and OSHA. For example, every two weeks, all local and foreign workers must take the COVID-19 swab test. They must also clean and disinfect all items they utilise before and after their shift. The research's next goal was to explore the problems of implementing new norms among construction workers during the COVID-19 pandemic. When the COVID-19 epidemic hit, construction workers encountered many obstacles as they started their projects. As they became used to their jobs, COVID-19 cases spread, making it increasingly difficult for them to follow the new SOPs. In addition, several of them will have been sued for not implementing the SOPs throughout their job. The problem stemmed from the workers' lack of enthusiasm for the new COVID-19 criteria.

Finally, this study aims to determine the most effective methods for normalising the new normative practices for construction workers affected by the COVID-19 pandemic. The government, ministry of health, CIDB, and other agencies have devised several effective methods for construction workers to avoid becoming infected with COVID-19, allowing them to continue working as usual. Employers can help their employees by providing a free COVID-19 swab test to alleviate stress. The cleaning and disinfection products should then be upgraded or increased at the site or workplace. In addition, construction workers can be taught how to disinfect and clean the items that have been utilised. If all workplaces were green, it would be valuable and practical. It is expected that the findings of this investigation will provide much-needed information to professionals involved in incorporating adequate COVID-19 safety and health measures into their regular health and safety management plan and will also assist professionals in adopting measures that field-workers recognise to be effective.

Adopting health and safety measures that are regarded to be effective by employees minimises employee opposition to implementing such measures and encourages employees to take part in and adhere to the safety plan. Contractors could use the findings of this study to improve the effectiveness of their safety programmes and prevent the spread of infectious diseases like COVID-19 on their projects by integrating multiple practices and technologies into their existing safety programmes. These practices and technologies could be integrated using the findings of this study. Construction companies should develop a comprehensive safety and health plan that includes a training programme on infectious diseases, a policy for collecting and communicating knowledge, and training to encourage adopting and implementing safety and health management technology. In conclusion, it is essential to remember that general contractors often determine the safety culture and the criteria and that subcontractors are frequently obliged to carry out particular safety programmes.

In this study, subcontractors were not questioned regarding whether the methods employed on their respective projects were mandated by the general contractor or their direct line employer (sub/specialty contractor). Knowing whether specific methods were implemented by the general contractor (or their direct employer) could provide additional insights into how they feel about these strategies if they were implemented. In the end, the current research defined "small organisations" as establishments with fewer than 100 staff members. Further research might investigate the attitudes of workers employed by micro-organizations (those with fewer than 10 staff members) concerning COVID-19 safety and health measures. It is workable that various micro-organizations could have varied perceptions of the practical actions that can be taken to prevent the spread of COVID-19.

## References

Abdullah, J.M., Wan Ismail, W.F.N., Mohamad, I., Ab Razak, A., Harun, A., Musa, K.I., Lee, Y., & Sharma, Y. (2020). A critical appraisal of COVID-19 in Malaysia and beyond. *The Malaysian Journal of Medical Sciences*, 27(2), 1–9.

Alsharef, A., Banerjee, S., Uddin, S.J., Albert, A., & Jaselskis, E. (2021). Early impacts of the COVID-19 pandemic on the United States construction industry. *International Journal of Environmental Research and Public Health*, 18(4), 1559.

Assaad, R., & El-adaway, I.H. (2021). Guidelines for responding to COVID-19 pandemic: Best practices, impacts, and future research directions. *Journal of Management in Engineering*, 37(3), 06021001.

Hashim, J.H., Adman, M.A., Hashim, Z., Mohd Radi, M.F., & Kwan, S.C. (2021, May 7). COVID-19 epidemic in Malaysia: Epidemic progression, challenges, and response. *Frontiers in Public Health*. Frontiers Media S.A. https://doi.org/10.3389/fpubh.2021.560592.

Hermesauto. (2021, August 15). Malaysia relaxes COVID-19 curbs further for fully vaccinated individuals. *The Straits Times*. Available at www.straitstimes.com/asia/se-asia/malaysia-relaxes-COVID-19-curbs-further-for-fully-vaccinated-individuals (Accessed 28 October 2021).

Marzo, R.R., Ahmad, A., Abid, K., Khatiwada, A.P., Ahmed, A., Kyaw, T.M., . . . Shrestha, S. (2021). Factors influencing the acceptability of COVID-19 vaccination: A cross-sectional study from Malaysia. *Vacunas*. https://doi.org/10.1016/j.vacun.2021.07.007.

Ogunnusi, M., Hamma-Adama, M., Salman, H., & Kouider, T. (2020). COVID-19 pandemic: The effects and prospects in the construction industry. *International Journal of Real Estate Studies*, 14(Special Issue 2).

Sharma, A.K. (2020). Novel coronavirus disease (COVID-19). *Resonance*, 25(5), 647–668. https://doi.org/10.1007/s12045-020-0981-3.

Zhang, J., Xiang, P., Zhang, R., Chen, D., & Ren, Y. (2020). Mediating effect of risk propensity between personality traits and unsafe behavioral intention of construction workers. *Journal of Construction Engineering and Management*, 146(4), 04020023.

# 7 Health and safety in the construction industry during the Covid-19 pandemic
## Case study of Vietnam

*Hai Chien Pham, Nghia Hoai Nguyen and Thi-Thanh-Mai Pham*

## 1. Introduction

The construction industry has been considered dangerous due to the high number of occupational accidents (Huynh et al., 2021; Bao et al., 2022; Pedro et al., 2020). Worldwide statistics show construction accidents constitute the highest rate compared to other industries (Hussain et al., 2018; Pham et al., 2015). Many studies have demonstrated that health, safety, and environment (HSE) practices are important in reducing fatal accidents and severe injuries on construction sites (Pedro et al., 2018; Pham et al., 2021; Hussain et al., 2017). Moreover, accidents have caused project delay and cost overrun, negatively impacting construction performance (Pham et al., 2018; Le et al., 2016; Pham et al., 2019).

The Covid-19 pandemic has spread worldwide and caused negative impacts to people's health and safety since the end of 2019 until now. Many countries must lock down to minimize the Covid-19 spread (Ezeokoli et al., 2020; Dennerlein et al., 2020; Simpeh et al., 2021). Therefore, many construction projects must be cancelled or delayed (Gashahun, 2020; Kabiru et al., 2020). For crucial construction projects that need to deploy during the pandemic, such as new hospitals, roads, and infrastructure, the construction stakeholders must comply with strict Covid-19 prevention regulations approved by government authorities (Hollingsworth et al., 2020; Choudhari et al., 2020). For instance, Ebekozien et al. (2021) identified the eight Covid-19 safety rules adopted on construction sites: stay at home if one is sick; use of face mask; place wash stations or hand sanitizers in multiple locations at sites; provision of personal protective equipment (PPE) for workers; practise social distancing; post in areas visible to all workers the required hygienic practices; clean and disinfect frequently touched places; designate site-based Covid-19 supervisors. Similarly, Assaad and El-adaway (2021) recommend HSE practices based on key aspects, including personal responsibilities; social distancing; jobsite/office practices; management of sick employees; engineering controls; administrative controls; safe work practices; and PPE.

Similar to other countries, the Vietnam government has quickly issued regulations (e.g., the directive No.15/CT-TTg and the directive No.16/CT-TTg) to curb the spread of Covid-19. Directive No.16/CT-TTg requires strict social

DOI: 10.1201/9781003278368-8

distancing and isolation, including critical points: (1) limit only two people at the same place, (2) keep the 2-metre minimum safe distance among people when the direct conversation, (3) suspend all business and construction; and (4) immediately isolate those who are infected with Covid-19. Otherwise, Directive No.15/CT-TTg reduces strict regulations compared to Directive No.16/CT-TTg. For instance, it limits ten people at the same place, and allows businesses or construction to continue operating if their HSE plans are approved by government inspectors (Le et al., 2021). This flexible approach supports construction stakeholders to decide whether projects should continue and what Directive should be applied.

Based on government policies, construction owners and contractors must issue new strict regulations on construction sites, and then submit them to government authorities for approval before implementation. For example, these regulations require stakeholders always to wear face masks, disinfect, measure body temperature, and conduct Covid-19 tests with negative results before entering construction sites, limit the number of workers, and ensure a minimum distance of two metres among workers, etc. Thanks to these regulations, Vietnam achieved the lowest rate of infections and zero deaths in the world in 2020 (Van Nguyen et al., 2021), even though Vietnam is geographically close to China, where Covid-19 emerged. Despite good preliminary achievements, new pandemic outbreaks in 2021 led to new strict policy changes (La et al., 2020). Thus, the implementation of HSE practices on construction sites always faces challenges.

Therefore, this chapter studies the compliance and effectiveness levels of measures to prevent and control Covid-19 spread on construction sites and evaluates the influence level of the directives on HSE practices. The study surveyed two stages: 1) a pilot study with construction experts to ensure the clarity of the questionnaire, and 2) an industry-wide survey of key stakeholders who have much experience in carrying out construction projects to collect their opinions about implementing Covid-19 prevention regulations, and their recommendations for best HSE practices. The research results showed that construction projects have strictly complied with the government's regulations, and they confirmed that the government's policies support curbing the spread of Covid-19 on construction sites. Finally, a thorough discussion provides lessons learned to help the Vietnam construction industry recover quickly after the Covid-19 pandemic.

## 2. Methodology

The research methodology is illustrated in Figure 7.1. First, this study investigates measures to prevent Covid-19 infection during the pandemic. Based on the literature and Vietnam policy review, a list of measures to prevent Covid-19 infection is proposed to design the questionnaire for a survey. After that, to minimize bias during data collection, a pilot study is carried out to ensure the clarity of the questionnaire so that respondents can answer all questions. The pilot study is conducted with five experts (two directors, a project manager, a head of the department, and one senior university lecturer actively involved in industry practice) who have over 20 years of experience in construction practice. The experts are invited to give their comments focusing on the clarity and adequacy of the list of measures. The experts suggest one measure, "eliminate the night shifts," to the proposed question-naire. They state that owners usually require night shifts to complete projects as scheduled due to government regulations reducing the number of workers. After correcting the questionnaire, including 12 measures to prevent Covid-19 infection, an industry-wide survey is carried out to collect data.

The questionnaire consists of three parts. The first part aims to collect general information about respondents. According to the five-point Likert scale, the sec-ond part requests the respondents to assess their perceptions on the compliance level of measures (i.e., from 1 – not compliance to 5 – strong compliance); and the effectiveness levels of measures (i.e., from 1 – not effectiveness to 5 – strong effectiveness) to prevent Covid-19 infection at jobsites. Moreover, participants are also asked to evaluate how government policies (e.g., the directive No.15/CT-TTg, and directive No.16/CT-TTg) influence the HSE practices on construction sites by using five-point Likert scales (i.e., from 1 – not influence to 5 – strong influence). In the final part, respondents are required to provide their suggestions to effectively cooperate with the measures to prevent Covid-19 infection and HSE practices.

The collected data is then tested to confirm the normality variables using the skewness and kurtosis values. Standardized scores (z-score) tests are also used to detect outliers. Levene's and Welch's tests evaluate the equality of variances before analysis of variance (ANOVA) to assess the difference in mean between groups for population categories (Aczel and Sounderpandian, 2008).

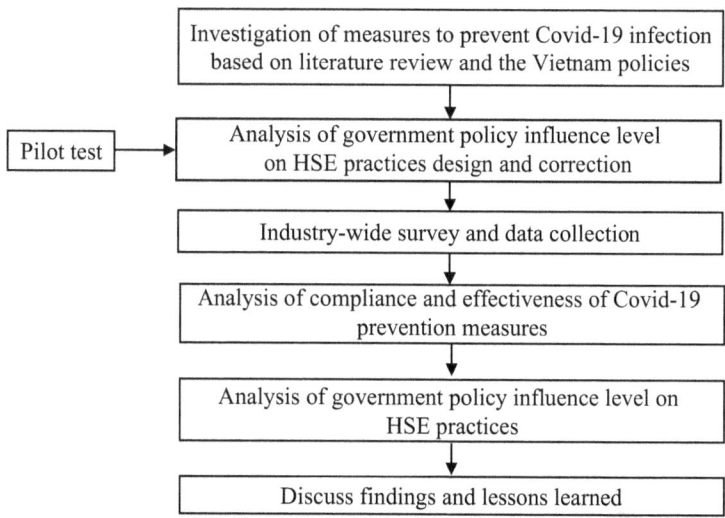

*Figure 7.1* Research methodology.

### 3.   Data collection and analysis

This study collects data by using the convenient sampling method. Through Google Forms, the questionnaires are delivered directly to the owners, consultants, contractors, and government inspectors, who are the principal stakeholders in construction projects. A total of 56 feedbacks are received. The sample size (56 respondents) is a bit less than the statistical requirement that should be at least five times the number of variables (12 items) analysed (Zhang et al., 2015). However, it is adequate to conduct the statistical analysis in this research because many studies (Reinaldo et al., 2021; Wu et al., 2018; Zhang et al., 2015) have accepted these similar small sample sizes to analyse data. Out of 56 responses, 10 respondents (17.9%) are owners, 15 respondents (26.8%) are consultants, 25 respondents (44.6%) are contractors, and six respondents (10.7%) are government inspectors. In terms of experience, 12 respondents (21.4%) are less than five years, 12 are between 5 and 10 years (21.4%), and 32 are over 10 years (57.2%). All respondents are working on high-rise building projects. The results show that all data follow a normal distribution, with all the skewness and kurtosis values in acceptable ranges of $\leq \pm 2$ and $\leq \pm 7$, respectively. The z-score values of the data set are also confirmed with all values $\leq \pm 3.29$ that are acceptable range (Nguyen and Chinda, 2018).

Levene's test at the significance level of 0.05 is employed to assess the equality of variances for the compliance and effectiveness levels of measures to prevent Covid-19 infection on construction sites based on stakeholders and working positions. For the items with the sig. of Levene's test $\leq 0.05$, the Welch test is then conducted to assess the equality of variances.

After conducting the Levene and Welch tests, the ANOVA is performed to examine the differences in the mean between groups. A probability value (significance level) of the ANOVA test below 0.05 suggests a high degree of difference of opinions between groups on the items. The Levene test results of consistency for the compliance and effectiveness levels of 12 measures to prevent Covid-19 infection on construction sites based on stakeholders confirmed that there were some measures with the sig. values were smaller than 0.05. The Welch test was then conducted with these four measures in compliance levels (measure the body temperature periodically, always wear the face mask, must make the Covid-19 declaration before entering construction sites, and clean hands by using sanitizers) and four measures in the effectiveness levels (measure the body temperature periodically, clean hands by using sanitizers, eliminate to work in the night shifts, and reduce the number of workers at the same place). The Welch test result of these measures was used for the ANOVA.

Similarly, the Levene test results confirmed that further test (the Welch test) should be conducted with one measure in compliance levels (provide adequate medical materials and equipment) and two measures in the effectiveness levels (eliminate to work in the night shifts and comply strictly with the lane specialized for movement of workers) as evaluating the compliance and effectiveness levels of measures to prevent Covid-19 infection based on positions.

To prevent the spread of the Covid-19 pandemic, the Vietnamese government has issued Directive No.15/CT-TTg, and Directive 16/CT-TTg. Based on these directives, all construction stakeholders (e.g., owners, contractors, consultants) must issue the revised HSE plans, including new special regulations for Covid-19 prevention, and then submit them to government authorities for approval before construction. The influences of government Directives on HSE practices are also examined in the stakeholders' perspectives based on the ANOVA analysis. The Levene test results of consistency for the effect of Directives confirmed all the sig. values were higher than 0.05. Therefore, the ANOVA was able to analyze based on these test results.

## 4. Results

The analysis results (Table 7.1) show that the compliance levels of measures to prevent Covid-19 infection on construction sites has no statistically significant difference in terms of stakeholders (i.e., owners, consultants, contractors, and government inspectors). Most of the respondents agree that the five measures which have the highest compliance at sites include: (1) measure the body temperature periodically; (2) always wear the face mask; (3) must make the Covid-19 declaration before entering construction sites; (4) clean hands by using sanitizers; and (5) establish new strict hygiene protocols to prevent Covid-19 infection. Ranking results based on stakeholders (Table 7.1) are similar to those based on positions (Table 7.2).

As described in Table 7.1, the contractors comply the most strictly with the approved HSE regulations compared to owners and consultants because they suffer a lot of damages due to significant increases in direct costs (e.g. materials, labour, and machines), which are caused by severe supply chain disruption during the Covid-19 pandemic. Moreover, as illustrated in Table 7.2, workers at construction sites strictly comply with the HSE regulations because the possibility of Covid-19 infection in this group is very high due to the group working closely.

Similar to the compliance levels of measures, the analysis results of the effectiveness levels confirm that there are no statistically significant differences in the mean between groups except for the effectiveness levels of the measure "must make the Covid-19 declaration before entering construction sites." (Tables 7.3 and Table 7.4). The five most crucial measures affecting the HSE practices are confirmed by the stakeholders, including: (1) reduce the number of workers at the same place; (2) comply social distancing among workers on site; (3) eliminate to work in the night shifts; (4) must make the Covid-19 declaration before entering construction sites; and (5) always wear the face mask.

Moreover, all stakeholders agreed that Directive No.16/CT-TTg has a more substantial influence on the HSE practices than the No.15/CT-TTg due to its strict requirements (Table 7.5). The result also confirmed the same perspective of all positions (Table 7.6). This finding determined the compliance of all stakeholders with the Government regulations on Covid-19 spreading prevention. This firm compliance led to the quick recovery of Vietnam's construction industry.

*Table 7.1* The compliance levels of measures to prevent Covid-19 infection based on stakeholders.

| ID | Measures | Mean | | | | | ANOVA | |
|----|----------|------|--|--|--|--|-------|--|
| | | Overall | Contractor | Consultant | Owner | Government inspector | F statistics | Significant |
| 1 | Measure the body temperature periodically | 4.36 | 4.68 | 4.27 | 3.80 | 4.17 | 1.986* W = 0.196 | 0.127 |
| 2 | Always wear the face mask | 4.34 | 4.68 | 4.27 | 3.80 | 4.00 | 2.195* W = 0.192 | 0.100 |
| 3 | Must make the Covid-19 declaration before entering construction sites | 4.23 | 4.44 | 4.13 | 3.80 | 4.33 | 0.844* W = 0.635 | 0.476 |
| 4 | Clean hands by using sanitizers | 4.09 | 4.48 | 3.87 | 3.40 | 4.17 | 3.045* W = 0.113 | 0.037 |
| 5 | Establish new strict hygiene protocols to prevent Covid-19 infection | 3.89 | 4.16 | 3.80 | 3.80 | 3.17 | 1.394 | 0.255 |
| 6 | Reduce the number of workers during safety training | 3.77 | 4.00 | 3.67 | 3.50 | 3.50 | 0.703 | 0.555 |
| 7 | Provide adequate medical materials and equipment | 3.59 | 3.60 | 3.67 | 3.30 | 3.83 | 0.232 | 0.874 |
| 8 | Eliminate to work in the night shifts | 3.45 | 3.72 | 3.13 | 3.00 | 3.83 | 1.179 | 0.327 |
| 9 | Reduce the number of workers at the same place | 3.43 | 3.68 | 3.27 | 2.90 | 3.67 | 1.219 | 0.312 |
| 10 | Comply strictly with the lane specialized for movement of workers | 3.38 | 3.56 | 3.13 | 3.50 | 3.00 | 0.561 | 0.643 |
| 11 | Comply social distancing among workers on site | 3.29 | 3.60 | 3.13 | 2.90 | 3.00 | 0.878 | 0.458 |
| 12 | Disinfect tools, equipment, and construction workplace | 2.91 | 3.16 | 2.73 | 2.40 | 3.17 | 0.858 | 0.469 |

*Note:* the sig. of Welch $\geq 0.05$ means there is no statistically significant differences in mean between groups.

Table 7.2 The compliance levels of measures to prevent Covid-19 infection based on positions.

| ID | Measures | Mean | | | | | ANOVA | |
|---|---|---|---|---|---|---|---|---|
| | | Overall | Staff | Head of department | Project manager | General manager | F statistics | Significant |
| 1 | Measure the body temperature periodically | 4.36 | 4.65 | 4.27 | 4.22 | 4.13 | 0.872 | 0.462 |
| 2 | Always wear the face mask | 4.34 | 4.70 | 4.18 | 4.22 | 4.06 | 1.348 | 0.269 |
| 3 | Must make the Covid-19 declaration before entering construction sites | 4.23 | 4.40 | 4.18 | 4.22 | 4.06 | 0.273 | 0.845 |
| 4 | Clean hands by using sanitizers | 4.09 | 4.25 | 3.91 | 3.89 | 4.13 | 0.355 | 0.786 |
| 5 | Establish new strict hygiene protocols to prevent Covid-19 infection | 3.89 | 4.05 | 3.45 | 3.67 | 4.13 | 1.041 | 0.382 |
| 6 | Reduce the number of workers during safety training | 3.77 | 4.05 | 3.18 | 4.00 | 3.69 | 1.665 | 0.186 |
| 7 | Provide adequate medical materials and equipment | 3.59 | 3.75 | 3.18 | 4.00 | 3.44 | 0.786* $W=0.621$ | 0.507 |
| 8 | Eliminate to work in the night shifts | 3.45 | 3.65 | 2.55 | 3.78 | 3.63 | 2.253 | 0.093 |
| 9 | Reduce the number of workers at the same place | 3.43 | 3.70 | 2.64 | 3.56 | 3.43 | 2.216 | 0.097 |
| 10 | Comply strictly with the lane specialized for movement of workers | 3.38 | 3.75 | 2.55 | 3.44 | 3.44 | 2.372 | 0.081 |
| 11 | Comply social distancing among workers on site | 3.29 | 3.40 | 2.55 | 3.44 | 3.56 | 1.464 | 0.235 |
| 12 | Disinfect tools, equipment, and construction workplace | 2.91 | 3.45 | 2.09 | 3.00 | 2.75 | 2.556 | 0.065 |

*Note*: the sig. of Welch $\geq 0.05$ means there is no statistically significant differences in mean between groups.

*Table 7.3* The effectiveness levels of measures to prevent Covid-19 infection on HSE practices based on stakeholders.

| ID | Measures | Mean | | | | | ANOVA | |
|---|---|---|---|---|---|---|---|---|
| | | Overall | Contractor | Consultant | Owner | Government inspector | F statistics | Significant |
| 1 | Reduce the number of workers at the same place | 3.61 | 3.76 | 3.33 | 3.90 | 3.17 | 0.985* W = 0.297 | 0.407 |
| 2 | Comply social distancing among workers on site | 3.57 | 3.96 | 3.13 | 3.70 | 2.83 | 2.441 | 0.075 |
| 3 | Eliminate to work in the night shifts | 3.46 | 3.84 | 2.73 | 3.70 | 3.33 | 2.721* W = 0.115 | 0.054 |
| 4 | Must make the Covid-19 declaration before entering construction sites | 3.36 | 3.48 | 2.47 | 4.10 | 3.83 | 3.397 | 0.024 |
| 5 | Always wear the face mask | 3.27 | 3.48 | 2.67 | 3.30 | 3.83 | 1.092 | 0.361 |
| 6 | Provide adequate medical materials and equipment | 3.11 | 3.44 | 2.40 | 3.10 | 3.50 | 2.934 | 0.042 |
| 7 | Measure the body temperature periodically | 3.07 | 3.28 | 2.27 | 3.50 | 3.07 | 1.921* W = 0.067 | 0.138 |
| 8 | Comply strictly with the lane specialized for movement of workers | 3.05 | 3.40 | 2.07 | 3.80 | 2.83 | 8.242 | 0.000 |
| 9 | Clean hands by using sanitizer | 3.02 | 3.32 | 2.27 | 3.20 | 3.33 | 1.590* W = 0.123 | 0.203 |
| 10 | Reduce the number of workers during safety training | 3.00 | 3.28 | 2.00 | 3.70 | 3.17 | 6.586 | 0.001 |
| 11 | Disinfect tools, equipment, and construction workplace | 2.93 | 3.16 | 2.53 | 2.90 | 3.00 | 0.849 | 0.474 |
| 12 | Establish new strict hygiene protocols to prevent Covid-19 infection | 2.84 | 3.08 | 2.07 | 3.40 | 2.83 | 2.935 | 0.042 |

*Note*: the sig. of Welch $\geq 0.05$ means there is no statistically significant differences in mean between groups.

*Table 7.4* The effectiveness levels of measures to prevent Covid-19 infection on HSE practices based on positions.

| ID | Measures | Mean | | | | | ANOVA | |
|---|---|---|---|---|---|---|---|---|
| | | Total | Staff | Head of department | Project manager | General manager | F statistics | Significant |
| 1 | Reduce the number of workers at the same place | 3.61 | 3.55 | 3.64 | 4.11 | 3.38 | 0.845 | 0.476 |
| 2 | Comply social distancing among workers on site | 3.57 | 3.55 | 3.55 | 4.00 | 3.38 | 0.499 | 0.685 |
| 3 | Eliminate to work in the night shifts | 3.46 | 3.50 | 3.45 | 4.00 | 3.13 | 0.903* W = 0.346 | 0.446 |
| 4 | Must make the Covid-19 declaration before entering construction sites | 3.36 | 3.10 | 3.64 | 4.44 | 2.88 | 2.858 | 0.046 |
| 5 | Always wear the face mask | 3.27 | 3.00 | 3.09 | 4.44 | 3.06 | 2.018 | 0.123 |
| 6 | Provide adequate medical materials and equipment | 3.11 | 2.80 | 3.45 | 3.67 | 2.94 | 1.588 | 0.203 |
| 7 | Measure the body temperature periodically | 3.07 | 2.70 | 3.09 | 4.00 | 3.00 | 1.446 | 0.240 |
| 8 | Comply strictly with the lane specialized for movement of workers | 3.05 | 3.00 | 3.09 | 3.67 | 2.75 | 1.258* W = 0.430 | 0.298 |
| 9 | Clean hands by using sanitizers | 3.02 | 2.85 | 2.64 | 3.89 | 3.00 | 1.200 | 0.319 |
| 10 | Reduce the number of workers during safety training | 3.00 | 2.80 | 3.27 | 3.78 | 2.63 | 2.284 | 0.090 |
| 11 | Disinfect tools, equipment, and construction workplace | 2.93 | 2.85 | 2.91 | 3.44 | 2.75 | 0.686 | 0.565 |
| 12 | Establish new strict hygiene protocols to prevent Covid-19 infection | 2.84 | 2.70 | 3.09 | 3.56 | 2.44 | 1.684 | 0.182 |

*Note*: the sig. of Welch $\geq$ 0.05 means there is no statistically significant differences in mean between groups.

*Table 7.5* The influence levels of the Directives on HSE practices based on stakeholders.

| Directive | Mean | | | | | ANOVA | |
|---|---|---|---|---|---|---|---|
| | Total | Contractor | Consultant | Owner | Government inspector | F statistics | Significant |
| Directive No.15/ CT-TTg | 3.70 | 3.88 | 3.07 | 4.10 | 3.83 | 2.265 | 0.092 |
| Directive No.16/ CT-TTg | 4.13 | 4.40 | 3.47 | 4.40 | 4.17 | 2.370 | 0.081 |

*Table 7.6* The influence levels of the Directives on HSE practices based on positions.

| Directive | Mean | | | | | ANOVA | |
|---|---|---|---|---|---|---|---|
| | Total | Staff | Head of department | Project manager | General manager | F statistics | Significant |
| Directive No.15/ CT-TTg | 3.70 | 3.80 | 3.55 | 4.11 | 3.44 | 0.756 | 0.524 |
| Directive No.16/ CT-TTg | 4.13 | 4.20 | 4.28 | 4.56 | 3.75 | 0.978 | 0.410 |

## 5.  Discussion

### Strict compliance with government policies

Vietnam has a high risk of the Covid-19 pandemic due to a lack of vaccines and its geographical proximity to China, where Covid-19 has emerged (Van Nguyen et al., 2021). However, Vietnam has been acknowledged as one of the few countries to effectively prevent the spread of the Covid-19 pandemic (La et al., 2020). This success can be explained by strict compliance with government policies, including public support for Covid-19 prevention measures, financial relief, economic stimulus, and sufficient vaccines for all citizens (Vu, 2021). At the early stage of the Covid-19 outbreak, when the Vietnamese are not vaccinated enough, they must comply with very strict social distancing and isolation for Covid-confirmed cases to stop the spread of coronavirus. Therefore, most construction sites must be closed to comply with Directive No.16/CT-TTg, which is acknowledged as the strictest policy. In Vietnam, many projects, after being approved by the government authorities to continue construction, have outbreaks from construction workers; as a result, these projects have been forced to suspend, disinfect, and isolate all infections. The high compliance levels in this study confirm that Vietnam construction sites strictly comply with all government policies in reality.

*Strict but flexible policies*

Vietnam applies flexible prevention policies by classifying three areas, which include the red area (Covid-19 infected cases), the orange area (suspected cases of Covid-19), and the green area (no confirmed cases). All construction sites must close in the red areas, while all projects in the green areas can continue construction as planned. For the orange areas, only a few important construction projects (e.g., new hospitals, national roads, etc.), in which stakeholders are fully vaccinated, continue construction based on the approved HSE plans, including measures and guidelines to prevent Covid-19 infection similar to previous studies (Gan and Koh, 2021; Ding et al., 2020; Stiles et al., 2021). Depending on the dangerous level of Covid-19 spread in a specific province, the provincial government must decide what directive would be applied (Pham et al., 2022). For example, construction projects in the orange areas must comply the Directive No.16/CT-TTg, while construction sites in the green regions usually apply Directive No.15/CT-TTg. The flexible approach of Vietnam would minimize the number of projects that must be closed. In other words, the effectiveness levels of measures to prevent Covid-19 would be increased.

*Strong commitments of project stakeholders*

Strong commitments of project stakeholders are important for HSE practices (Fruhen et al., 2019; Pedro et al., 2022; Pham and Pham-Hang, 2020). In Vietnam, if a construction project violates its commitments, the approval of the HSE plan would be withdrawn, and the construction works would be forced to close immediately. In fact, the owners have the highest responsibility to the local government for Covid-19 prevention, while the contractors must pay all costs incurred if a Covid-19 outbreak occurs at the jobsite during construction (Pham et al., 2022). Therefore, owners and contractors strongly commit to the effectiveness of the 12 measures for Covid-19 infection prevention compared with the consultant group (Table 7.3). Regarding the job position (Table 7.4), project managers highly commit to the effectiveness levels of measures because they are the highest responsibility for the project's success and the approved HSE compliance.

## 6. Conclusion

The Covid-19 pandemic has seriously impacted HSE practices on construction sites. However, Vietnam has been acknowledged as one of the few countries to prevent the Covid-19 pandemic successfully. Therefore, this research investigates practical measures of Covid-19 infection prevention at the jobsites in Vietnam by surveying 56 construction experts and professionals working for owners, consultants, contractors, and government authorities. The research findings revealed 12 critical solutions implemented in construction projects during the pandemic. In addition, the study evaluates the compliance and effectiveness levels of measures contributing to the successful implementation of HSE practices on construction sites. This Vietnam case study provides practical lessons (e.g., strict compliance with government policies, the need for a flexible approach in policy implementation, and strong commitments of project stakeholders) for developing countries to cope with the Covid-19 pandemic. Due to the government's strict regulation during the Covid-19 pandemic, the research limitation is small samples focusing on high-rise building projects. Therefore, future work would survey different construction projects, such as bridges, roads, tunnels, etc., to comprehensively evaluate the effectiveness of government regulations in preventing Covid-19 transmission in construction projects. Through this, experts' recommendations would support governments to establish comprehensive and effective policies to overcome this dangerous pandemic and recover the construction industry.

### Acknowledgement

The authors would like to thank all interviewees and experts for their useful information and recommendations of HSE practices on construction sites.

### References

Aczel, A., & Sounderpandian, J. (2008). *Complete business statistics* (7th ed.). Irvine: McGraw-Hill.

Assaad, R., & El-adaway, I.H. (2021). Guidelines for responding to COVID-19 pandemic: Best practices, impacts, and future research directions. *Journal of Management in Engineering*, 37(3), 06021001.

Bao, L., Tran, S.V.T., Nguyen, T.L., Pham, H.C., Lee, D., & Park, C. (2022). Cross-platform virtual reality for real-time construction safety training using immersive web and industry foundation classes. *Automation in Construction*, 143, 104565.

Choudhari, R. (2020). COVID 19 pandemic: Mental health challenges of internal migrant workers of India. *Asian Journal of Psychiatry*, 54, 102254.

Dennerlein, J.T., Burke, L., Sabbath, E.L., Williams, J.A., Peters, S.E., Wallace, L., . . . Sorensen, G. (2020). An integrative total worker health framework for keeping workers safe and healthy during the COVID-19 pandemic. *Human Factors*, 62(5), 689–696.

Ding, Z., Xie, L., Guan, A., Huang, D., Mao, Z., & Liang, X. (2020). Global COVID-19: Warnings and suggestions based on experience of China. *Journal of Global Health*, 10(1).

Ebekozien, A., Aigbavboa, C., & Aigbedion, M. (2021). Construction industry post-COVID-19 recovery: Stakeholders perspective on achieving sustainable development goals. *International Journal of Construction Management*, 1–11.

Ezeokoli, F.O., Okongwu, M.I., & Fadumo, D.O. (2020). Adaptability of COVID-19 safety guidelines in building construction sites in Anambra state, Nigeria. *Archives of Current Research International*, 69–77.

Fruhen, L.S., Griffin, M.A., & Andrei, D.M. (2019). What does safety commitment mean to leaders? A multi-method investigation. *Journal of Safety Research*, 68, 203–214.

Gan, W.H., & Koh, D. (2021). COVID-19 and return-to-work for the construction sector: Lessons from Singapore. *Safety and Health at Work*, 12(2), 277–281.

Gashahun, A.D. (2020). Assessmenton impact of Covid-19 on Ethiopian construction industry. *International Journal of Engineering Science and Computing*, 10(7), 26891–26894.

Hollingsworth, J. (2020). Construction safety practices for covid-19. *Professional Safety*, 65(6), 32–34.

Hussain, R., Lee, D.Y., Pham, H.C., & Park, C.S. (2017). Safety regulation classification system to support BIM based safety management: In ISARC. Proceedings of the International Symposium on Automation and Robotics in Construction (Vol. 34). IAARC Publications.

Hussain, R., Pedro, A., Lee, D.Y., Pham, H.C., & Park, C.S. (2018). Impact of safety training and interventions on training-transfer: Targeting migrant construction workers. *International Journal of Occupational Safety and Ergonomics*, 26(2), 272–284.

Huynh, V.H., Nguyen, T.H., Pham, H.C., Huynh, T.M.D., Nguyen, T.C., & Tran, D.H. (2021). Multiple objective social group optimization for time-cost-quality-carbon dioxide in generalized construction projects. *International Journal of Civil Engineering*, 19(7), 805–822.

Kabiru, J.M., & Yahaya, B.H. (2020). Can Covid-19 considered as force majeure event in the Nigeria construction industry. *International Journal of Scientific Engineering and Science*, 4(6), 34–39.

La, V.P., Pham, T.H., Ho, M.T., Nguyen, M.H.P., Nguyen, K.L., Vuong, T.T., . . . Vuong, Q.H. (2020). Policy response, social media and science journalism for the sustainability of the public health system amid the COVID-19 outbreak: The Vietnam lessons. *Sustainability*, 12(7), 2931.

Le, Q.T., Pedro, A., Pham, H.C., & Park, C.S. (2016). A virtual world based construction defect game for interactive and experiential learning. *International Journal of Engineering Educcation*, 32, 457–467.

Le, T.A.T., Vodden, K., Wu, J., & Atiwesh, G. (2021). Policy responses to the COVID-19 pandemic in Vietnam. *International Journal of Environmental Research and Public Health*, 18(2), 559.

Nguyen, N.H., & Chinda, T. (2018). Interrelationship among key profit factors of Vietnamese residential projects using structural equation modeling. *Sonklanakarin Journal of Science and Technology*, 40(2), 467–474.

Pedro, A., Chien, P.H., & Park, C.S. (2018, April). Towards a competency-based vision for construction safety education. IOP Conference Series: Earth and Environmental Science (Vol. 143, No. 1, p. 012051). IOP Publishing.

Pedro, A., Hussain, R., Pham-Hang, A.T., & Pham, H.C. (2022). Visualization technologies in construction education: A comprehensive review of recent advances. *Engineering Education for Sustainability*, 67–101.

Pedro, A., Pham, H.C., Kim, J.U., & Park, C. (2020). Development and evaluation of context-based assessment system for visualization-enhanced construction safety education. *International Journal of Occupational Safety and Ergonomics*, 26(4), 811–823.

Pham, H.C., Dao, N.N., Kim, J.U., Cho, S., & Park, C.S. (2018). Energy-efficient learning system using web-based panoramic virtual photoreality for interactive construction safety education. *Sustainability*, 10(7), 2262.

Pham, H.C., Le, Q.T., Pedro, A., & Park, C.S. (2015, October). Visualization based building anatomy model for construction safety education. Proceedings of the 6th International Conference on Construction Engineering and Project Management (ICCEPM), Busan, Korea (pp. 11–14).

Pham, H.C., Pedro, A., Le, Q.T., Lee, D.Y., & Park, C.S. (2019). Interactive safety education using building anatomy modelling. *Universal Access in the Information Society*, 18(2), 269–285.

Pham, H.C., & Pham-Hang, A.T. (2020). Virtual photoreality for safety education. In *New perspectives on virtual and augmented reality* (pp. 211–223). Abingdon, UK: Routledge.

Pham, Q.D., Dao, N.N., Nguyen-Thanh, T., Cho, S., & Pham, H.C. (2021). Detachable web-based learning framework to overcome immature ICT infrastructure toward smart education. *IEEE Access*, 9, 34951–34961.

Pham, Q.V., Pham-Hang, A.T., & Pham, H.C. (2022). A legal framework and compliance with construction safety laws and regulations in Vietnam. In *Engineering education for sustainability* (pp. 103–140). New York: River Publishers.

Reinaldo, L.D.S.P., Neto, J.V., Caiado, R.G.G., & Quelhas, O.L.G. (2021). Critical factors for total quality management implementation in the Brazilian construction industry. *The TQM Journal*, 33(5), 1001–1019. https://doi.org/10.1108/TQM-05-2020-0108.

Simpeh, F., & Amoah, C. (2021). Assessment of measures instituted to curb the spread of COVID-19 on construction site. *International Journal of Construction Management*, 1–19.

Stiles, S., Golightly, D., & Ryan, B. (2021). Impact of COVID-19 on health and safety in the construction sector. Human Factors and Ergonomics in Manufacturing & Service Industries.

Van Nguyen, Q., Cao, D.A., & Nghiem, S.H. (2021). Spread of COVID-19 and policy responses in Vietnam: An overview. *International Journal of Infectious Diseases*, 103, 157–161.

Vu, V.T. (2021). Public trust in government and compliance with policy during COVID-19 pandemic: Empirical evidence from Vietnam. *Public Organization Review*, 21(4), 779–796.

Wu, P., Zhao, X., Baller, J.H., & Wang, X. (2018). Developing a conceptual framework to improve the implementation of 3D printing technology in the construction industry. *Architectural Science Review*, 61(3), 133–142.

Zhang, R.P., Lingard, H., & Nevin, S. (2015). Development and validation of a multilevel safety climate measurement tool in the construction industry. *Construction Management and Economics*, 33(10), 818–883.

# 8 Construction safety culture management during the COVID-19 pandemic

*Thanwadee Chinda*

## Introduction

Construction safety culture (CSC) represents the product of individual and group behaviours, attitudes, norms and values, perceptions, and thoughts that determine the commitment to, and style and proficiency of, a company's system and how its personnel act and react in terms of the company's ongoing safety performance in construction site environments (Choudhry et al., 2007; Kim et al., 2021). It guides the safety practices for all levels in the company.

Construction sites involve various parties, such as management, supervisors, workers, and contractors who perform interdependent and interrelated activities that involve frequent changes. Strong coordination among the parties is therefore required to achieve high levels of CSC in this dynamic environment. All stakeholders should take part in the process of aligning the company's safety culture to achieve long-term sustainability. This should be applied to all construction projects, regardless of location or project size, because it focuses on the actions of the stakeholders, not the project characteristics (Abosede et al., 2019).

Chinda and Mohamed (2008) identified five key enablers necessary for successful CSC implementation in Thailand, namely Leadership, Policy and Strategy, People, Resources, and Processes. Leadership is the main driver of effective safety culture, and the strong commitment of leaders is crucial in promoting safety culture (Chinda and Mohamed, 2008). Leaders should be a role model in promoting healthy and safe work behaviour, ensure that workers accept their safety responsibilities, and set a realistic safety policy and communicate this policy throughout companies. People enabling plays a key role in successful safety culture implementation in construction companies. Thai construction managers believe that human resources and teamwork are more crucial to successful safety implementation than the provision of safety resources (Aksorn and Hadikusumo, 2007). Excellent safety outcomes, i.e., reduced number and cost of accidents, higher work morale, and enhanced industry image, can be achieved through the rigorous implementation of safety-related policies and processes, which are directed by the efficient CSC management of Leadership and People enablers.

The COVID-19 pandemic affects the work practices of all industries, including the construction industry. Various research studies have been conducted to examine

DOI: 10.1201/9781003278368-9

the effects of the pandemic on work practices. Hansen and Kolokotronis (2020), for example, investigated how safety communication can affect safety in the building industry during the COVID-19 pandemic and concluded that the use of digitalization and digital tools for communication within construction sites are necessary during the pandemic to support social distancing at the workplace and survive in the market. Stiles et al. (2020) presented a commentary on safe construction in the UK during and beyond COVID-19, covering the human factor challenges and practicality of implementing COVID-19 measures. The study results emphasize the role of safety leadership to ensure safe application of COVID-19 working practices.

CSC during the COVID-19 pandemic has also been mentioned in various construction literature. Celoch and Smolag (2021), for example, conducted the questionnaire survey on construction companies in Poland to determine whether the pandemic influenced the work safety culture in the construction industry during the COVID-19 pandemic. The results confirm the positive effects of the pandemic on work safety culture in the physical environment, employee behaviour, and internal characteristics of employees. It is commented that the provision of personal and collective protective equipment, implementation of new employee protective measures, provision of knowledge regarding occupational health and safety (OHS), and employee involvement in OHS issues should be encouraged within the companies to maintain safety standards on construction sites during the pandemic. Hansen and Kolokotronis (2020) stated that safety communication among staff is a crucial tool to achieve positive safety culture in the building industry, especially during the COVID-19 pandemic. Various communication tools may be used to raise safety concerns, such as the use of safety training, safety weeks, safety posters, newsletters, email, intranet, boards, and safety campaigns. Tei Expert (2021) mentioned that safety culture is crucial during the COVID-19 pandemic and suggested that the companies review current safety policies with employees and update additional protocols that have arisen due to the pandemic. Leaders should engage with safety practices, demonstrate safe behaviours, encourage and acknowledge employees' feedback, and enhance communication in the companies during the pandemic. Dakota Software (2020) stated that COVID-19 presents the greatest health and safety challenge in the construction industry, and that construction organizations must maintain their healthy safety cultures during the pandemic. Leaders must demonstrate safe behaviours, support two-way communication, clearly set safety procedures and expectations during the pandemic, and educate employees on how to keep themselves and co-workers safe.

In Thailand, various literature mentions the management of the COVID-19 pandemic in the construction industry. SCG (2020), for example, implemented strict preventive measures in compliance with the government's COVID-19 control measures in offices, manufacturing facilities, stores, and at construction sites to ensure maximum safety of employees, trading partners, and customers during the COVID-19 outbreak. Extra hygiene precautions were also taken in providing customer services, along with sharing knowledge and precautions against COVID-19 to partners in the construction industry including developers, contractors, builders, and dealers. Chaisaard et al. (2020) proposed guidelines for the management of construction projects in the pre-construction, construction, and post-construction phases during the COVID-19 outbreak in Thailand.

The management of CSC during the COVID-19 pandemic is crucial to ensure health and safety of workers of all parties on construction sites. In this chapter, in-depth interviews are conducted to gather perceptions and practices of CSC management of small-, medium-, and large-sized construction companies during the COVID-19 pandemic utilizing five key CSC enablers proposed by Chinda and Mohamed (2008). It is expected that the study results suggest practical guidelines for construction companies to manage their safety and health practices during and after the pandemic.

In summary, this chapter sets the research question, "How do construction companies cope with CSC on sites during the COVID-19 pandemic?" Research objectives, including examination of CSC practices on sites during the COVID-19 pandemic and suggestion of safety guidelines to be used during and after the pandemic are also set to answer the research question. Research flow is shown in Figure 8.1.

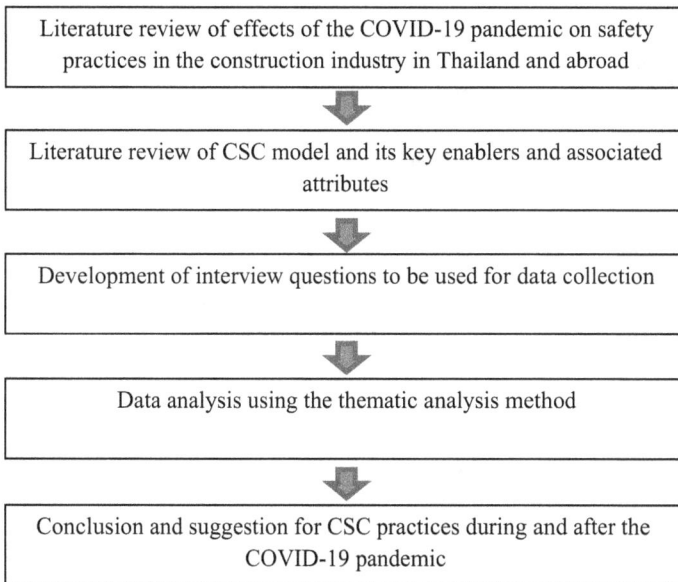

| Literature review of effects of the COVID-19 pandemic on safety practices in the construction industry in Thailand and abroad |
| Literature review of CSC model and its key enablers and associated attributes |
| Development of interview questions to be used for data collection |
| Data analysis using the thematic analysis method |
| Conclusion and suggestion for CSC practices during and after the COVID-19 pandemic |

*Figure 8.1* Research flow of this study.

## CSC enablers

Five key CSC enablers are as shown in Figure 8.2 (Chinda and Mohamed, 2008). They are associated with 20 attributes (see Table 8.1). Leadership enabler consists of five attributes. Lingard and Blismas (2006) stated that companies whose top management gave high levels of safety support and commitment had better safety performance. Teo and Fang (2006) found that to enhance safety culture performance and progress through to higher safety culture maturity levels, companies need more face-to-face communications, both formal and informal, between management and frontline staff. Policy and Strategy enabling consists of four attributes. Othman et al. (2020) stated that safety policy and regulations are the foundation of safety management. Safety rules and regulations as defined in international safety standards should be adopted to improve safety culture in the companies. Vongvitayapirom et al. (2013) commented that to improve safety in construction companies, various campaigns should be initiated by utilizing incident statistics, increasing employee awareness, and creating a common safety culture understanding.

Three attributes are associated with People enabling. Cooperation about safety and joint responsibility between managers and workers is one of the cornerstones of health and safety work (Grytnes et al., 2020). Al-Bayati (2021) mentioned that safety behaviour will not be achieved without cooperation from workers. Resources enabling consists of four associated attributes. Sufficient safety resources should be allocated to carry out day-to-day activities to accomplish short- and long-term safety goals (Aksorn and Hadikusumo, 2007). Vitharana and Chinda (2017) stated that a training program is a low-cost feasible first step towards the reduction of site accidents that should be encouraged through policy and regulations. Four attributes are associated with Processes enabling. Tam et al. (2004) revealed that the safety score in a company where feedback is given is higher than that in companies where no feedback is given. Vongvitayapirom et al. (2013) stated that to comply with the safety management system, implementing safety documentation e.g., standards, procedures, and guidelines must cover all operations for employees to understand the nature and cautions required for each work task beforehand, and then appropriately follow the given instruction.

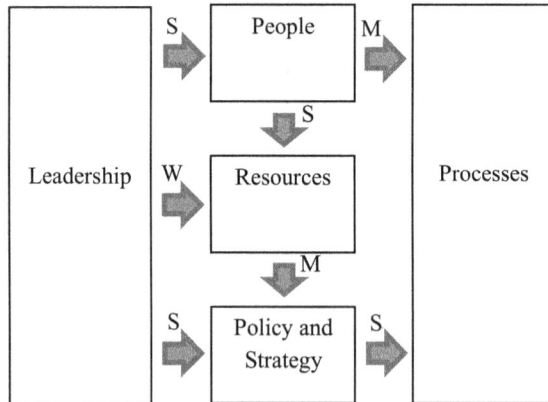

**Note:** W = weak relationship, M = medium relationship, S = strong relationship

*Figure 8.2* CSC enablers.

*Source:* (Adapted from Chinda and Mohamed, 2008)

*Table 8.1* CSC enablers and their associated attributes (Chinda and Mohamed, 2008).

| CSC enabler | Associated attribute |
| --- | --- |
| Leadership | • Top management commitment<br>• Effective two-way communication<br>• Management accountability<br>• Management leading by example<br>• Alignment of productivity and safety targets |
| People | • Safety empowerment and responsibilities<br>• Project participants and stakeholders' cooperation<br>• Human resources management |
| Resources | • Adequacy of financial resources dedicated to safety<br>• Availability of necessary safety-related resources<br>• Worker involvement<br>• Safety training |
| Policy and strategy | • Safety awareness and promotion<br>• Safety standards, laws, regulations<br>• Safety initiatives to improve safety standards<br>• Relationships among workers |
| Processes | • Feedback on safety implementation<br>• Site safety documentations<br>• Having an effective benchmarking system,<br>• Safety as an integral part of business goal settings |

The five CSC enablers relate to each other with strong, medium, and weak relationships. Chinda (2020) mentioned that strong, medium, and weak relationships show path coefficients of more than 0.5, 0.3–0.5, and less than 0.3, respectively. Chinda and Mohamed (2008) concluded that Leadership enablers strongly influences People and Policy and Strategy enablers (see Figure 8.2). Leaders should therefore be a role model in promoting healthy and safe work behaviour, ensure that workers accept their safety responsibilities, and set a realistic safety policy and communicate this policy throughout their companies. It is clear that Leadership is the main driver to effective safety culture, and the strong commitment of leaders is crucial in promoting safety culture. Leadership enablers also have an indirect effect to Resources enablers through People enablers. This indirect effect corroborates well with the overall perception of Thai construction managers, where human resources and teamwork are believed to be more crucial to successful safety implementation than the provision of safety resources (Aksorn and Hadikusumo, 2007). Safety policy and strategy should reflect the need of safety resources requested by the workers; this is reflected by direct and indirect relationships between Resources and Policy and Strategy enablers, and between People and Policy and Strategy enablers, respectively. People and Policy and Strategy enablers play a key role in successful safety implementation, as verified by the strong links from these two enablers to Processes enabler.

## Research method

The in-depth interviews are conducted to gather primary data and safety culture practices of construction companies during the COVID-19 pandemic using the five key CSC enablers and their associated attributes. Personal interview, or face-to-face interview, has a major advantage in that it allows the researcher to record not only verbal responses, but also any facial or bodily expressions (Jackson, 2003). These nonverbal responses may give the researcher greater insight into the respondents' true opinions and beliefs. The other advantages include: 1) the respondents can ask for the questions to be clarified, 2) the researchers can ask follow-up questions, if they think they will provide more reliable data, 3) supplementary material, such as audio/video materials, can be used to increase the respondents understanding of the questions, and 4) the response rates are generally high (Jackson, 2003).

Six interviewees from six construction companies located in Bangkok, Thailand participate in the interviews. They are from small-, medium-, and large-sized construction companies (Bank of Thailand, 2022). Details of the interviewees are summarized in Table 8.2.

Each interviewee is asked to provide CSC practices on construction sites during the COVID-19 pandemic using the open-ended questions. The questions are based on the associated attributes of the five key CSC enablers. Examples of questions are:

- Do your leaders assign additional safety accountability to employees to ensure safety and health practices on construction sites during the COVID-19 pandemic, and if yes, how?
- Does your company have a new safety and health regulation to be used during the COVID-19 pandemic? If yes, what are the main differences compared with the previous one?
- Does your company adjust the number of employees on construction sites to suit the pandemic situation and ensure safety and health of employees? If yes, what is the adjustment (e.g., hiring more employees to substitute with the high-risk employees)?
- Does your company provide extra safety and health budget to deal with the COVID-19 pandemic? If yes, how is this extra budget utilized (e.g., for mask and alcohol gel purchasing, separate zone installation for high-risk employees etc.)?
- Does your company utilize the feedback system on how to work safely during the COVID-19 pandemic to improve the work practices on construction sites? If yes, please give some examples of the improvement activities.

The interviewees can ask for clarifications during the interviews if needed and can also provide comments and suggestions on how to further improve safety standards during the pandemic and achieve sustainable CSC in the long term.

The interview data are analysed using the thematic analysis method. It is a qualitative research analysis method used to identify, analyse, organize, describe, and report themes found within a data set (Novell et al., 2017). It is a useful method for examining the perspectives of different research participants, highlighting similarities and differences, and generating unanticipated insights.

Table 8.2 Details of the interviewees.

| No. | Position | Size of company | Experience in the construction industry (years) | Experience in the current company (years) | Safety policy in the company | Safety involvement |
|---|---|---|---|---|---|---|
| 1 | Manager | Large | 17 | 20 | Yes | • Safety audit |
| 2 | Chief commander | Large | 20 | 10 | Yes | • Revise safety policy and safety implementation plan<br>• Assign safety responsibilities to the staff |
| 3 | Senior manager | Medium | 14 | 11 | Yes | • Supervise and monitor safety activities on sites |
| 4 | Sales manager | Small | 20 | 5 | Yes | — |
| 5 | Manager | Small | 15 | 11 | Yes | • Revise safety policy and safety implementation plan |
| 6 | Engineering director | Small | 18 | 6 | Yes | • Revise safety policy and safety implementation plan<br>• Assign safety responsibilities to the staff |

## Interview results

The interviewees provided valuable information of safety and health implementation during the COVID-19 outbreak. Details of safety practices in each CSC enabler are provided.

## Leadership enabler

The interview results show that leaders take safety and health actions seriously during the pandemic. Safety policy is adjusted, and safety accountabilities are assigned to all employees.

### Top management commitment

The interview results reveal that top management, regardless of company sizes, commit to maintain and enhance CSC standard during the pandemic. Rigorous CSC policy is set to ensure the health and safety of employees. Interviewee #1 and interviewee #5 suggest the use of work-from-home (WFH) strategy, if possible. Only small groups of workers are allowed to work together, and social distancing must be strictly conformed. All interviewees mention that their employees must be tested with the antigen test kids (ATKs) weekly before entering the construction sites.

### Alignment of productivity and safety targets

All the interviewees mention that during the COVID-19 outbreak, a large portion of employees work from home, and that only small groups of employees are assigned to work on sites. This is to reduce the risks and ensure employees' safety and health, though it may lower productivity and may delay the work schedule.

### Effective two-way communication

Interviewee #1, interviewee #2, and interviewee #3 from large- and medium-sized companies state that the work plan during the pandemic is adjusted based on the suggestions from both management and operational levels. Online meetings are set to solve onsite problems. Interviewee #2 comments that suggestions from onsite employees and stakeholders, such as the provision of alcohol gel, the bring-your-own lunch and water bottle strategy, and the onsite toilet renovation are implemented to reduce the chance of the virus spreading.

### Management accountability

All interviewees mention that supervisors and/or safety staff are empowered to, for example, make decisions to stop the work, separate the affected workers, and allow high-risk workers to self-quarantine to ensure safety and health of employees during the pandemic. Interviewee #2 also states that the assigned supervisor must report the spreading of COVID-19 on sites in terms of number of new cases, number of high-risk workers, as well as their symptoms on a regular basis.

### Management leading by example

All interviewees mentioned that all levels in the company, from management to operational levels, must strictly follow the safety and health rules and implementation plans during the COVID-19 pandemic.

## Policy and Strategy enabler

The interview results show that safety-related policies are adjusted to support safe work practices during the pandemic and maintain CSC standards.

### Safety standards, laws, regulations

Safety regulations during the pandemic are officially announced and implemented on sites. All the interviewees state that additional safe work practices, such as the use of face masks, the ATK test before entering the sites, the social distancing concept, and the separation of contaminated wastes are used on sites. All employees are also encouraged to receive the COVID-19 vaccination. Interviewee #2 suggests the use of a so-called "bubble and seal strategy" to minimize the risks by not allowing workers on sites to go outside of the construction sites, and people from outside to enter the construction sites. While doing this, the company provides food and a temporary dormitory for the employees.

### Safety initiatives to improve safety standards

According to interviewee #1, interviewee #2 and interviewee #6, safety meetings are organized on a regular basis to monitor safety practices and adjust safety plans to suit with the situations and severities of the COVID-19 pandemic.

### Safety awareness and promotion

All interviewees mentioned that safety plan during the pandemic is announced to all employees and stakeholders through various channels, such as email, line chat, safety meeting, and in person.

### Workers' relationship strategy

Surprisingly, almost all the interviewees mention that employees are not encouraged to give advice on how to work safely during the pandemic. This may be because of the social distancing concept that does not allow employees to have close contact with others. However, interviewee #6 from a small-sized company states that during the pandemic, his company separates the employees into small teams of five to 10 persons, and that team members help each other to minimize risks and ensure safety implementation on sites.

## People enabler

The interview results reveal that employees cooperate and follow safety rules and regulations during the COVID-19 outbreak.

### *Safety empowerment and responsibilities*

Employees are empowered to make safety-related decisions based on their roles and responsibilities. Operation workers may decide to stop working if they show COVID-19 symptoms or are in high-risk groups. Interviewee #1 from a large-sized company states that the project manager is responsible to develop the tier 1 (affected employees), tier 2 (high-risk employees), and tier 3 (low-risk employees) lists and decide on work schedule adjustment to suit with the employees.

### *Project participants and stakeholders' cooperation*

All stakeholders cooperate and follow safety rules and regulations to ensure safety on sites. All of them must be tested with ATKs before entering the sites. Moreover, interviewee #1 from a large-sized company adds that subcontractors must also show the proof of COVID-19 vaccination (called the COVID-19 passport) to enter the construction sites.

### *Adequacy of workers*

Half of the interviewees (interviewee #1, interviewee #2, and interviewee #4) state that their companies have adequate employees to work during the pandemic. By using the bubble and seal strategy and the proactive plan, work schedules are adjusted to match with on-site and WFH employees. Half of the interviewees (interviewee #3, interviewee #5, and interviewee #6), however, agree that the COVID-19 outbreak forces the construction sites to reduce the number of employees to follow the social distancing concept. Moreover, several employees are COVID-19 patients, bringing a high number of high-risk employees who have to be quarantined for a period of time.

## Resources enabler

Financial and safety-related resources are provided to support the safety practices during the COVID-19 pandemic.

### *Adequacy of financial resources dedicated to safety*

All interviewees state that additional budgeting is provided to purchase safety-related equipment. Interviewee #6 from a small-sized company mentions that his company provided budget for employees to purchase laptops and printers, if necessary, for effective WFH implementation. Additional health insurance is also provided for onsite employees.

### *Availability of necessary safety-related resources*

All interviewees state that their companies provide adequate safety-related equipment, such as ATKs, alcohol gel, face masks, thermometers, and oximeters to support safe work during the COVID-19 pandemic.

### *Human resource management*

Two interviewees from large-sized companies (interviewee #1 and interviewee #2) and an interviewee from a small-sized company (interviewee #6) mentions that their companies provide their employees the guidelines for safe work during the pandemic.

### *Provision of safe work training*

The majority of the interviewees state that their companies do not provide special safe work training during the COVID-19 outbreak. However, safety officers in some companies are assigned to provide safe work practices during the pandemic to their employees through online and onsite channels. Interviewee #6 from a small-sized company mentions that the safety training for safe work during the pandemic is sometimes provided by the main contractor.

## Processes enabler

The interview results show that leaders, regardless of company size, take safety and health actions seriously during the pandemic.

### *Feedback on safety implementation*

Feedback on safety implementation is used to improve and adjust safety practices on sites during the pandemic. Two interviewees from large-sized companies (interviewee #1 and interviewee #2) mention that safety feedback is crucial during the pandemic as the COVID-19 virus often mutates from alpha to delta and omicron variants. Therefore, safe work practices must be adjusted to suit the outbreak situations.

### *Site safety documentation*

Interviewees from large- and medium-sized companies (interviewee #1, interviewee #2, and interviewee #3) state that reports of COVID-19 patients on sites, including timelines and treatment histories, are kept and used for future references.

Two interviewees from small-sized companies (interviewee #4 and interviewee #5), however, mention no reporting and safety documentation system on sites.

### Effective benchmarking system

Interviewees from large- and medium-sized companies (interviewee #1, interviewee #2, and interviewee #3) mention the benchmarking system among the partner companies to improve CSC standard during the pandemic. Small-sized companies, however, have no benchmarking system in use.

### Safety as an integral part of business goal settings

Interviewees from large- and medium-sized companies (interviewee #1, interviewee #2, and interviewee #3) agree that employees' safety is a part of business goals, especially in the outbreak of COVID-19.

## Implications for the construction industry

Based on the in-depth interview results, strategies for CSC management during and after the COVID-19 pandemic can be established as follows.

## Leadership enabler

Safety commitment from leaders is crucial to continue safe work on sites during the COVID-19 outbreak. As the Leadership enabler influences the Policy and Strategy, Resources, and People enablers, leaders must take safety actions seriously and be a role model on how to work safely during the COVID-19 outbreak. Various online communication channels, such as email, line chat, and online meeting platforms should be encouraged to avoid or reduce the in-person contacts. Online meetings could also be continued after the pandemic, if possible, to reduce the travel time and cost. Safety accountability should be clearly set to employees at all levels to reduce possible risks and enhance their own and others' safety on sites during and after the pandemic.

## Policy and Strategy enabler

CSC rules and regulations must be established, promoted, and enforced in all construction companies, regardless of company sizes, to ensure the health and safety of the employees. As the Policy and Strategy enabler strongly influences the Processes enabler, these CSC rules and regulations must be practical and effectively implemented in real practices. Simple safety rules and regulations, such as wearing face masks, receiving the vaccination, and disposing of contaminated wastes must be announced and followed by all employees. CSC rules and regulations should also be consistently updated to effectively tackle COVID-19 and other diseases. Opinions and suggestions from the employees, especially those who were directly affected by the COVID-19, are vital and should be carefully considered when adjusting the CSC rules and regulations.

### People enabler

Cooperation of employees is crucial in successful CSC implementation during the COVID-19 outbreak as the People enabler influences the Resources and Processes enablers. Employees at all levels must be responsible for their own and others' safety. They should be empowered to make safety-related decisions based on their roles and responsibilities to reduce risks. Appropriate CSC resources should be provided upon request. A mixture of WFH and on-site-work strategy or flexible work scheduling (e.g., fewer workdays with longer work hours) may be allowed for employees after the pandemic, if possible, to provide work flexibility, reduce the employees' expenses, enhance family time (i.e., less time in traffic), and reduce chances of spreading the diseases; all of these may lead to higher work productivity. The bubble and seal concept may be applied for high-risk or contaminated work to reduce risks and ensure employees' safety.

### Resources enabler

All construction companies should continue to provide basic safety equipment and materials, such as alcohol gel, face masks, first aid kits, and personal protective equipment to ensure employees' safety during and after the pandemic. Provision of safety-related training should be regularly scheduled to enhance safety knowledge and update with the spreading of the diseases. Small-sized companies with possibly less safety budgeting may, instead of organizing the safety training, cooperate with their stakeholders through, for example, online channels to share tips on how to work safely during and after the pandemic to improve CSC standard in the long term.

### Processes enabler

Feedback on safety implementation is crucial to enhance CSC standards in the long term. Records on site accidents and illnesses must be kept and examined to avoid recurrences. Management of contagious patients and high-risk employees should strictly follow the Ministry's health and safety guidelines to ensure safety on sites. The safety action plans should be monitored and benchmarked, internally, nationally, and internationally, on a regular basis to update with the new diseases and proactive plans to maintain and improve the companies' CSC standards.

### Conclusion

CSC received more attention in construction companies, regardless of company sizes, during the COVID-19 outbreak as it highly affects employees' health and safety and may reduce the company's productivity and performance. To ensure CSC performance during and after the COVID-19 pandemic, it is important that construction companies focus on five key CSC enablers, including Leadership, Policy and Strategy, People, Resources, and Processes enablers. Leaders should be role models and lead safety implementation by, for example, wearing masks on sites, following social distancing rules, and monitoring and updating the COVID-19 situations. Leaders must also ensure that safety policies and strategies are up to date to deal with current situations of the COVID-19 pandemic. These policies and strategies need to be practical and cover suggestions from government authorities, partners, and companies' employees, especially those who are directly affected by the COVID-19 disease. Disease protection should be integrated into safety and health policy even after the COVID-19 pandemic to ensure safety and health of employees. Some strategies, such as WFH and bubble and seal strategies may be continued after the pandemic with some adjustments. The WFH strategy, for example, may be applied when working on paperwork and does not require being present on sites. Bubble and seal strategies, together with specific safety equipment and materials, may be applied when having contagious diseases to ensure safety and health of workers both on and off sites.

Employees are crucial in safety implementation, and great employees' cooperation in safety responsibilities and empowerment are needed to maintain CSC standards in the companies. Leaders must ensure that safety responsibilities and empowerment related to the COVID-19 pandemic are properly assigned and monitored to all working levels. Financial and safety resources must be adequately provided to support safe work during and after the pandemic. Face masks, alcohol gel, and other hygiene supplies should continue to be provided even after the pandemic to ensure CSC standards on sites. Apart from the regular safety training, employees should be educated and trained in how to protect themselves from contagious diseases.

The COVID-19 pandemic raises concerns about safety and health in the construction industry. Safety must be integrated into working culture to ensure health and safety of workers, both physically and mentally, reduce chances of workforce shortage, and maintain overall company's performance. Good safety practices must be sustained, embedded into rules and regulation, and enforced to be used even after a pandemic.

This research study has a limitation. The number of interviewees from different sizes and types of companies may be increased to achieve more reliable results. Further research of CSC practice after the pandemic may be conducted and compared with previous implementation to highlight positive and negative issues for long-term improvement.

### Acknowledgement

The author would like to thank all interviewees for useful information about safety and health practices on construction sites.

# References

Abosede, A.O., Opawole, A., Olubola, B., Ojo, G.K., & Kajimo-Shakantu, K. (2019). Performance analysis of small and medium-sized construction firms in Oyo State, Nigeria. *Acta Structilia*, 26(1), 66–96.

Aksorn, T., & Hadikusumo, B.H.W. (2007). Critical success factors influencing safety program performance in Thai construction projects. *Safety Science*, 46(4), 709–727.

Al-Bayati, S.J. (2021). Impact of construction safety culture and construction safety climate on safety behaviour and safety motivation. *Safety*, 7(41), 1–13.

Bank of Thailand. (2022). *Criteria for company sizes from ministry of industrial, Thailand* [in Thai]. Available at www.bot.or.th/Thai/ConsumerInfo/List_InfoImage/SMEs.jpg.

Celoch, A., & Smolag, K. (2021). The impact of the COVID-19 pandemic on managing the work safety culture in the construction industry companies in Poland. *Quality Production Improvement*, 3, 105–119.

Chaisaard, N., Ngowtanasuwan, G., & Doungpan, S. (2020, August 28). A review of construction project management guidelines under the impact of COVID-19 epidemic dispersal: A case study of Thai construction projects. SUT International Virtual Conference on Science and Technology, Nakorn-Ratchasima, Thailand, IVCST-2020-0073.

Chinda, T. (2020). Factors affecting cost in pre-construction and construction phases: Structural equation modelling. *International Journal of Construction Supply Chain Management*, 10(3), 21, 115–140.

Chinda, T., & Mohamed, S. (2008). Structural equation model of construction safety culture. *Engineering, Construction and Architectural Management*, 15(2), 114–131.

Choudhry, R.M., Fang, D., & Mohamed, S. (2007). Developing a model of construction safety culture. *Journal of Management in Engineering*, 23(4), 207–212.

Dakota Software. (2020). *Keeping your safety culture healthy during COVID-19*. Available at https://ehsdailyadvisor.blr.com/2020/08/keeping-your-safety-culture-healthy-during-covid-19/.

Grytnes, R., Tutt, D.E., & Anderson, L.P.S. (2020). Developing safety cooperation in construction: Between facilitating independence and tightening the grip. *Construction Management and Economics*, 38(11), 977–992.

Hansen, A.C.S., & Kolokotronis, I. (2020). Managing health and safety on the building site: A study on communication issues between the involved actors. Student Report. Denmark: Aalborg University.

Jackson, S.L. (2003). *Research methods and statistics: A critical thinking approach*. Boston: Thomson Wadsworth.

Kim, S., Lee, H., Hwang, S., Yi, J.S., & Son, J.W. (2021). Construction workers' awareness of safety information depending on physical and mental load. *Journal of Asian Architecture and Building Engineering*, 21(3), 1067–1077.

Lingard, H., & Blismas, N. (2006). Building a safety culture: The importance of shared mental models in the Australian construction industry. In D. Fang, R.M. Choudhry, & J.W. Hinze (eds.), *Proceedings of the CIB W99 2006 international conference on global unity for safety and health in construction, 28–30 June 2006, Beijing, China* (pp. 201–208). Beijing: Tsinghua University Press.

Novell, L.S., Norris, J.M., White, D.E., & Moules, N.J. (2017). Thematic analysis: Striving to meet the trustworthiness criteria. *International Journal of Qualitative Methods*, 16(1), 1–13.

Othman, I., Kamil, M., Sunindijo, R.Y., Alnsour, M., & Kineber, A.F. (2020). Critical success factors influencing construction safety program implementation in developing countries. *Journal of Physics: Conference Series*, 1529(042079), 1–8.

SCG. (2020). Building resilience for sustainability leadership. Sustainability Report 2020. The Siam Cement Public Company Limited, Bangkok, Thailand. https://www.scg.com/pdf/en/SD2020.pdf.

Stiles, S., Golightly, D., & Ryan, B. (2020). Impact of COVID-19 in health and safety in the construction sector. *Human Factor Management*, 1–13. doi: 10.1002/hfm.20882.

Tam, C.M., Zeng, S.X., & Deng, Z.M. (2004). Identifying elements of poor construction safety management in China. *Safety Science*, 42(7), 569–586.

Tei Expert. (2021). *Why building safety culture during the coronavirus pandemic is more important than ever?* Available at www.triumvirate.com/blog/why-building-safety-culture-during-the-coronavirus-pandemic-is-more-important-than-ever.

Teo, A.L., & Fang, D. (2006). Measurement of safety climate in construction industry: Studies in Singapore and Hong Kong. In D. Fang, R.M. Choudhry, & J.W. Hinze (eds.), *Proceedings of the CIB W99 2006 international conference on global unity for safety and health in construction, 28–30 June 2006, Beijing, China* (pp. 157–164). Beijing: Tsinghua University Press.

Vitharana, V.H.P., & Chinda, T. (2017). Policy analysis of the budget used in training program for reducing lower back pain among heavy equipment operators in the construction industry: System dynamics approach. *IOP Conference Series: Earth and Environmental Science*, 140(012114), 1–9.

Vongvitayapirom, B., Sachakamol, P., Kropsu-Vehkapera, H., & Kess, P. (2013). Lessons learned from applying safety culture maturity model in Thailand. *International Journal of Synergy and Research*, 2(1), 5–21.

# 9 Policy assessment framework to measure the efficacy of mask-wearing arrangements during the COVID-19 outbreak

## Case studies from Jakarta, Indonesia

*Seng Hansen, Ferdinand Fassa and Marcelino Danu Egardy*

### Introduction

Starting in late 2019, the COVID-19 outbreak has spread around the world, including Indonesia. This is actually not the first outbreak with unprecedented impact on peoples' lives. Other outbreaks by airborne viruses have also occurred in various parts of the world, such as severe acute respiratory syndrome (SARS) in 2002 and H1N1 swine flu in 2009. Various steps have been taken by the governments to prevent the spread of COVID-19, such as lockdowns, social and physical distancing, isolation centres, case tracing, and testing facilities (Hansen, 2020a; Irfan et al., 2021). These efforts not only have an impact on socio-economic activities but also on the sustainability of construction projects (Fauziyah et al., 2022).

One of the efforts promoted by the governments to prevent the spread of COVID-19 is the use of masks. Experts believe that mask-wearing is an effective intervention in controlling the spread of airborne viruses like COVID-19 (Irfan et al., 2021; Lima et al., 2020; O'Kelly et al., 2021). In Indonesia, the mandatory use of masks outside the home has been enforced since April 9, 2020 through the issuance of the Ministry of Health Circular Letter No. HK.02.02/I/385/2020 concerning the Use of Masks and the Provision of Handwashing Facilities with Soap to Prevent Transmission of Corona Virus Disease 2019. It was strengthened by the issuance of the Decree of the Ministry of Health of the Republic of Indonesia No. HK.01.07/MENKES/328/2020 concerning Guidelines for the Prevention and Control of Corona Virus Disease 2019 on May 20, 2020.

The mask-wearing obligation also applies to construction projects. In the Ministry of Public Works and Housing Instruction No. 02/In/M/2020 concerning the Protocol for Preventing the Spread of COVID-19 in the Execution of Construction Services, one of the instructions confirms that contractors are obliged to provide masks for all workers and guests on construction projects. In response to these regulations, Indonesian contractors have been trying to create and implement mask-wearing policies in their projects. However, there has been no research that

DOI: 10.1201/9781003278368-10

examines the effectiveness of mask-wearing policy on construction projects, espe-cially in Indonesia. The successful implementation of this policy is very important to study to control and prevent the risk of COVID-19 in the construction environ-ment. This study answers this challenge by developing a framework to assess the mask-wearing policy based on the four policy dimensions.

## Mask-wearing policy in construction projects

Masks are respiratory protection used as a method to protect individuals from inhaling hazardous substances or contaminants in the air. Masks are not intended to replace the preferred method that can eliminate disease, but are used to adequately protect the wearers (Cohen and Birkner, 2012). In the context of the COVID-19 pandemic, mask-wearing aims to protect a healthy person when in contact with an infected person or to control the source by preventing further transmission (Kris-mantoro and Susilo, 2021).

The use of masks is not new in construction projects. Masks are one of the per-sonal protective equipment items that provide respiratory protection for construc-tion workers against dust or hazardous substances in the air (Egardy, 2022). The use and types of masks in construction projects generally depend on the type of activity and the characteristics of the pollutant. For example, the use of N95 masks by masons to prevent Portland cement dust is recommended by Pranata (2019), while specific welding respiratory masks are recommended to control the impact of welding activities such as UV rays (Purnomo et al., 2016) and fumes (AWS, 2021). Cohen and Birkner (2012) distinguish masks into three types, namely quar-ter mask, half mask, and full-face mask.

On the other hand, O'Kelly et al. (2021) highlighted the importance of wear-ing masks that fit the wearer's face. Although N95 masks offer higher levels of protection than surgical masks and cloth masks, most N95 masks fail to fit the wearer adequately. Meanwhile, research on the effectiveness of cloth masks shows moderate efficacy in preventing the spread of respiratory infections. However, this effectiveness also depends on the type of cloth used, the number of layers, and the frequency of washing cloth masks (Lima et al., 2020). Therefore, double masking is recommended to improve the fit of the mask (Sickbert-Bennett et al., 2021). The types of masks that can be used are three-layer surgical masks and cloth masks. The use of these two types effectively limits the possibility of the COVID-19 transmis-sion (Cheng et al., 2021; Chua et al., 2020; Lima et al., 2020; O'Kelly et al., 2021).

## Indonesian construction industry during the COVID-19 pandemic

The COVID-19 pandemic has been declared a national disaster by the Indonesian government through Presidential Decree No. 12/2020. This pandemic has weak-ened various sectors in Indonesia including the construction sector, which has been a priority sector for development. The Indonesian Contractors Association revealed that the Indonesian construction sector has experienced a slowdown dur-ing the pandemic, which requires a fast response (Fitriani, 2020). The impact on the construction industry is not only related to the health aspects of construction workers but also the economy, including reduced profits, labour and material shortages, and reallocation of government budgets, resulting in the suspension and/or termination of construction project tenders (Suraji, 2021).

On the other hand, the Ministry of Public Works and Housing is committed to continuing infrastructure development in order to maintain economic sustainability in the midst of a pandemic by issuing regulations and guidelines related to preventing the spread of COVID-19 in the construction project environment. This is reinforced by the inclusion of the construction sector as one of the 11 essential sectors that are allowed to remain operational during the pandemic. Various strategies have been carried out in an attempt to maintain the productivity of the construction industry (Suraji, 2021).

In an effort to control and prevent the transmission of COVID-19 in construction projects, contractors are required to comply with government regulations and recommendations regarding the use of masks (Egardy, 2022), especially considering that construction projects are labour-intensive (Farihin et al., 2021) and many construction activities must be carried out in groups so that the implementation of physical distancing becomes difficult. Previous studies have indicated cases of COVID-19 among Indonesian construction workers, as happened in Surakarta (Susila and Arbianto, 2021) and Semarang (Siswanto et al., 2022). Thus, the enforcement of mask-wearing policy among construction workers is a must.

## Methodology

This study adopts a qualitative approach to observe and evaluate the implementation of mask-wearing policy at two different construction projects in Jakarta, Indonesia. The selection of these case studies is based on consideration of the diversity of project types. Project A is a high-rise building project located in Menteng district, Jakarta. It consists of three towers and has a contract value of more than IDR 900 billion, with a total number of 1200 workers. Meanwhile, Project B is an elite housing project located in Pasar Minggu district, Jakarta. This project has a contract value of IDR 10 billion, and a total number of 100 workers.

Data collection techniques were carried out by observations and interviews. A field observation is a direct examination related to the research phenomenon at the project sites. The data was recorded in the form of on-site photographs. Meanwhile, semi-structured interviews were conducted face-to-face with each respondent and recorded. According to Hansen (2020b), respondent diversity is important to determine. Respondents in this study are heterogeneous, consisting of construction workers and HSE (health, safety and environment) officers from two different projects. The criteria for respondents are a minimum of three years of working experience for construction workers and a minimum of five years of experience for HSE officers.

Two pilot interviews were conducted on March 8 and 14, 2022 to validate the designed interview questions with two HSE experts. Meanwhile, actual observations and interviews were conducted on April 12 and 14, 2022. A total of 21 respondents were successfully interviewed. Project A respondents consisted of three HSE officers and seven workers while Project B respondents consisted of one HSE officer and 10 workers. The interview data was analysed using content analysis to draw conclusions from the respondents' answers. Thus, this study fulfils four criteria for the credibility of qualitative research, namely truth value, consistency, applicability, and neutrality.

**Development of policy assessment framework**

This study modifies Pradhan et al.'s framework (2017) to analyse the effectiveness of mask-wearing policy implementation at construction projects. As illustrated in Figure 9.1, the policy assessment framework consists of four dimensions: policy issue, policy creation, policy implementation, and policy evaluation. The issue is a crucial topic faced by policy makers to overcome a phenomenon. It must be identified and served as a purpose to be achieved in the implementation of a policy. Policy creation emphasises the formulation of policy content by identifying assessment indicators, developing the required procedures, and finalisation by policy makers. The policy that has been approved is then implemented on project sites. Policy implementation describes the practices that occur when the policy is implemented. Meanwhile, policy evaluation is a systematic analysis to evaluate the

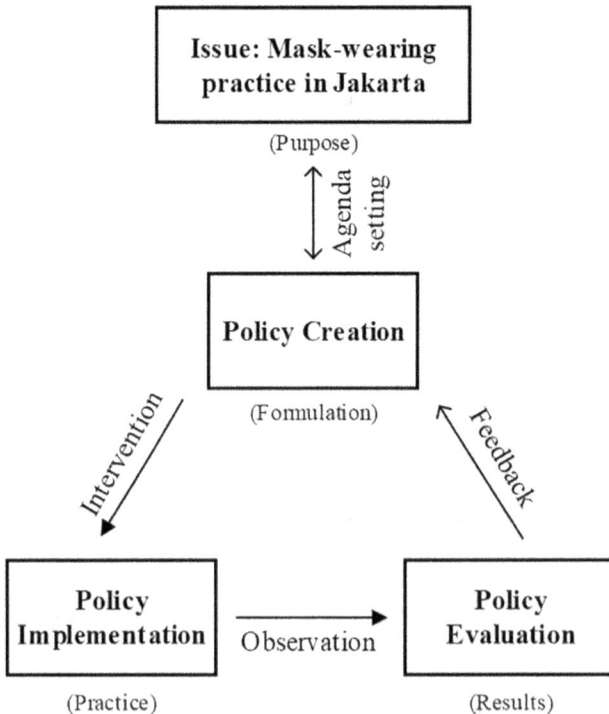

*Figure 9.1* Policy assessment framework.

success and results of implementing the policy. The feedback generated is useful as input for policy improvements until the policy objectives are achieved. This framework utilises feedback loops between policy creation, implementation, and evaluation to provide inputs to policy makers for planning and implementing the policy.

To validate this framework, three validation criteria were applied: real case study implementation, an uncontrolled environment, and expert practitioner involvement. Two project case studies in Jakarta were considered. In the context of this research, the identified issue focuses on mask-wearing practices in order to control the spread of COVID-19 outbreak in construction projects. The policies that have been made by contractors are observed for their implementation and evaluated qualitatively, which includes the four dimensions of this framework. Several interview questions were determined to collect qualitative data from the expert respondents. The collected data was processed and interpreted to provide feedback for policy improvements in these two case studies.

**Results and discussion**

The results of observations and interviews of the two case studies are presented in Table 9.1 and Figure 9.2. The following subsections provide detailed discussions for each dimension.

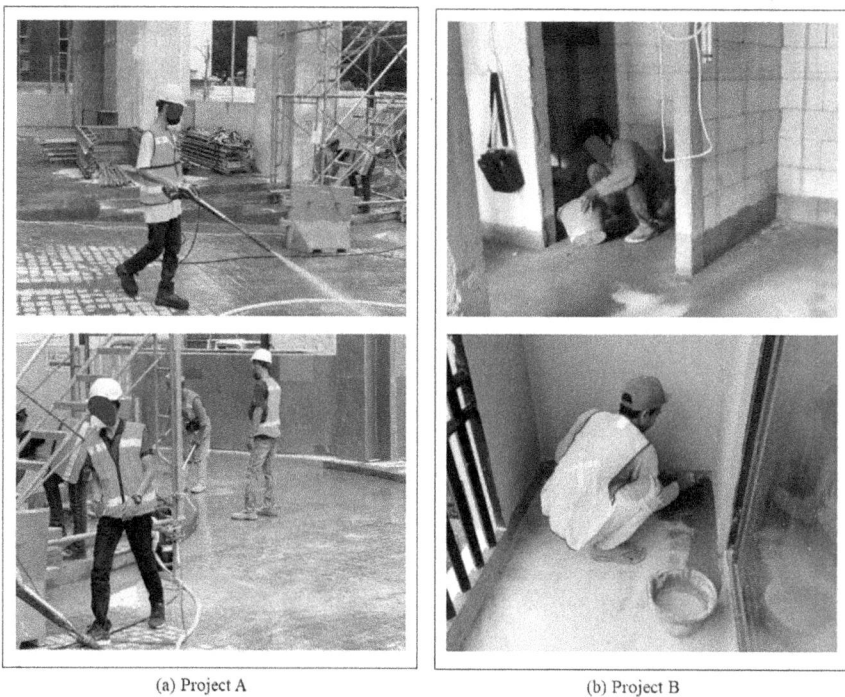

(a) Project A          (b) Project B

*Figure 9.2* Field observations.

Table 9.1 Observation and interview findings.

| No | Indicators | Response option | Case study Project A | Project B |
|---|---|---|---|---|
| *Observation findings* | | | | |
| 1 | Is there a mask-wearing policy in the project? | Yes/No | Yes, as part of the COVID-19 Health protocol regulations in the project | Yes, as part of the COVID-19 Health protocol regulations in the project |
| 2 | Are masks provided? | Yes/No | Yes, masks are provided by subcontractors | No |
| 3 | Do workers wear masks? | Yes/No | Yes, workers are seen wearing surgical masks and some are wearing double masks | No, workers are reluctant to follow the policy |
| *Interview findings from HSE officers* | | | | |
| 4 | Does the contractor provide masks for workers on site? | Yes/No | Yes, but this only happens at the beginning of the pandemic. Currently, several subcontractors on the project still provide masks for their workers | Yes, but this only happens at the beginning of the pandemic |
| 5 | What types of masks do they wear? | Text | 3-ply surgical mask (provided by the subcontractors) and cloth mask (by the workers) | 3-ply surgical mask (only when provided) |
| 6 | How many times does the contractor instruct workers to change/wash the masks regularly? | Text | Replace it at least once a day | Replace it at least once a day |
| 7 | Does the use of masks affect the productivity of workers on site? | Yes/No | Yes, but only affected at the beginning due to adjustment | Yes, but only affected at the beginning due to adjustment |
| 8 | Are there sanctions for workers who violate the mask-wearing policy? | Yes/No | No, only verbal reprimand when found violations during patrol. Besides that, those who don't wear masks are not allowed to enter the project site | No, only verbal reprimand |

| | | | | |
|---|---|---|---|---|
| 9 | Has there ever been a positive case of COVID-19 in this project? | Yes/No | Yes, when the cases of delta variant are <10% and the omicron variant are <2% | No (perhaps due to lack of data) |
| 10 | How do contractor ensure workers to wear masks? | Text | Implement screening when entering the project site by security (only those who wear masks are allowed to enter) and patrol the project regularly | Occupational Health and Safety (OHS) briefing in the morning |
| 11 | Is this mask-wearing policy also a stipulation in the labour or main contract? | Yes/No | No | No |

*Interview findings from the workers*

| | | | | |
|---|---|---|---|---|
| 12 | How often do workers wear masks? | Text | Always wear masks every day | Workers rarely wear masks |
| 13 | Do workers regularly change masks? | Yes/No | Yes, replaced every day | No |
| 14 | Do workers regularly clean their cloth masks? | Yes/No | Yes, the cloth masks are washed every day | Not wearing a cloth mask |
| 15 | Do workers feel comfortable wearing masks while working? | Text | Depending on the type of activity being carried out, sometimes it is hard to breathe | Depending on the type of activity being carried out, sometimes it is hard to breathe |
| 16 | Are workers having trouble wearing a mask? | Yes/No | No | No |
| 17 | How important is wearing a mask for workers? | Scale 1 to 5 | From a scale of 1 to 5, all builders chose a scale of 5 (very important) | From a scale of 1 to 5, most workers chose a scale of 3 |

**Policy creation**

The issue of health and safety in Indonesian construction projects has long been a major challenge. This is exacerbated by the COVID-19 pandemic, which is very easy to transmit between workers. For example, Project A has experienced difficulties due to the outbreak of positive cases of COVID-19. Therefore, a policy is needed that regulates efforts to prevent COVID-19 outbreak in construction projects. In this context, a policy is defined as the ability to control the COVID-19 pandemic through mask-wearing by construction workers. Experts argue that the use of masks should be mandatory to prevent the spread of COVID-19 in construction projects (Kim et al., 2021; Oerther and Shattell, 2020; Waluyo, 2020).

The policy planning process could be top-down or bottom-up (Pradhan et al., 2017). Based on the analysis, the mask-wearing policy planning process in the two observed projects was carried out through a top-down approach. According to HSE officers in both projects, these policies refer to the holding company policies derived from the government regulations. In an effort to overcome the spread of the COVID-19 outbreak, which is a force majeure event and a disruptor to construction activity (Hansen, 2020a), this approach is considered more appropriate because it can be implemented immediately. In addition to regulating the mandatory use of masks by construction workers, this policy should provide technical instructions such as the recommended types of masks and procedures for replacing and washing cloth masks.

**Policy implementation**

The mask-wearing policy is the right effort because it is inexpensive and easy to implement (Koebele et al., 2021). To be effective, it requires an enabling policy environment (Pradhan et al., 2017). Based on the analysis, there are significant differences in the implementation of the mask-wearing policy between the two projects observed. In Project A, this policy can be implemented comprehensively and consistently. This can also be seen from the results of observations, where workers wear masks according to instructions. However, in Project B, the situation looks different because many workers are not wearing masks. Likewise, the instructions for changing surgical masks and washing cloth masks are routinely carried out by Project A workers but not Project B workers.

Regarding the effect of wearing masks on workers' performance, workers in both projects agreed that the use of masks had an effect during the adjustment period. However, in general there are no obstacles to wearing masks. While it has become a habit in Project A, many workers in Project B do not wear masks due to a lack of understanding and enforcement. In Project A, the main contractor applies screening and regular patrols to ensure every worker wears a mask. This is not implemented in Project B.

**Policy evaluation**

From various indicators, it can be evaluated whether the objectives of implementing the mask-wearing policy are achieved. The results of this evaluation are useful for policy makers to analyse workers' perceptions of policy implementation which will provide feedback for policy improvement (Chen et al., 2014; Pradhan et al., 2017). Based on the analysis, it can be seen that the awareness of Project B workers about the importance of wearing masks is still low. This is in line with the findings of Pattisinai et al. (2020), which also highlighted the low understanding of workers regarding health and safety aspects and the use of masks in construction projects in Indonesia. This is indicated by the perception of Project B workers, who mostly chose a scale of 3 out of 5 regarding the importance of wearing masks. Even though the availability of masks is one of the identified risks as explained in the research of Fauziyah et al. (2022), this study found that the main contractors no longer provide free masks in order to reduce cost overruns. This has an impact on the enforcement of mask-wearing policy as well. Therefore, the control of the contractor management plays an important role in enforcing this policy (Wati et al., 2021).

As observed in Project A, there was a spike in positive cases of COVID-19 before the mask-wearing policy was implemented. However, along with the implementation of the mask-wearing policy, there have not been any cases of COVID-19. Meanwhile, Project B respondents stated that there had never been a case of COVID-19. This can be due to the absence of testing facilities so that there is no data on positive COVID cases in Project B. Furthermore, the evaluation also found that workers sometimes feel short of breath while wearing a mask when doing their activities. Therefore, it is also necessary to consider the types of activities and workers who should and should not wear masks as a policy improvement in the future. If the type of construction activity is heavy and requires a lot of oxygen intake and the use of masks is not recommended, then other strategies such as physical distancing can be considered when carrying out the work. The same applies to workers who have respiratory-related diseases.

Policy enforcement also relies heavily on sanctions for policy violators. Unfortunately, from the two case studies, no strict sanctions were applied to workers who did not wear masks. For this reason, it is recommended that the policy improvement includes strict sanctions for violations of the mask-wearing policy. In addition, it is also recommended to consider mask-wearing as one of the points in the employment contract and in the main contract.

**Overall effectiveness**

The overall effectiveness is determined by understanding the framework elements. Based on these findings, Table 9.2 is a policy assessment typology which presents a summary of the efficacy of mask-wearing policy implementation as observed in the two case studies. It can be concluded that the implementation of mask-wearing policies may differ between projects and depends on the policy enforcement strategy undertaken by the contractors. This study found that the implementation of mask-wearing policy in Project A is better than Project B. The mask-wearing policy needs to be enforced in an effort to create the mask-wearing behaviour of construction workers (Wati et al., 2021). However, this is a major challenge, especially considering that changing behaviour requires a long period of policy intervention (Pradhan et al., 2017). A prior study by Susila and Arbianto (2021) found that only 60% of construction projects in the city of Surakarta have a COVID-19 task force to enforce the implementation of this policy. In addition, it is important to socialise existing policies to create safe and healthy work places (Kim et al., 2021; Sari, 2021). Although it is not always easy, socialisation of this policy must continue to be conveyed periodically in an effort to raise worker awareness. Finally, this study looks at the easing of the mask-wearing policy implementation (especially in Project B), even though the policy is still in effect. Thus, it is necessary to make improvements to the policy and its implementation strategy to ensure that the policy objectives are achieved.

*Table 9.2* Policy assessment typology.

| *Issue: Mask-wearing practice* | | *Case study* | |
|---|---|---|---|
| *Framework elements** | *Points of discussion** | *Project A* | *Project B* |
| Purpose | What are the priority issues? | To control and prevent the COVID-19 transmission on project site through mask-wearing behaviour | To control and prevent the COVID-19 transmission on project site through mask-wearing policy implementation |
| Policy | What are the measures taken? | Focus on creating a mask-wearing behaviour | Focus on creating mask-wearing policy |
| Planning | What is the policy-making process? | Top-down approach based on government regulations | Top-down approach based on government regulations |
| Practice | What happened? | Contractor is responsible for creating a mask-wearing behaviour | Contractor is responsible for the implementation of mask-wearing policy |
| Implementation | How do workers adapt to the policy? | Although initially forced by regulations, workers became aware of the importance of wearing masks and voluntarily wear them | Workers have not realised the importance of wearing masks and often do not wear them |
| Performance | What were the results? | There is a continuous enforcement of mask-wearing policy so that workers' awareness to continue wearing masks occurs | There is support from the contractor to enforce the mask-wearing policy; however, long-term adaptation was not their priority |
| Evaluation/ feedback | What are the recommend-dations? | The policy may be updated. The use of masks can become an HSE culture in the project environment | The policy should be updated. The contractor must establish a mask-wearing behaviour by raising the workers' awareness |

*adopted from Pradhan et al. (2017)

**Implications for practice**

Construction health and safety is essential, especially responding to the COVID-19 pandemic when contractors are responsible for creating a safe workplace (Fauziyah et al., 2022). The COVID-19 pandemic is caused by a mutation in the SARS-CoV virus which is very easily transmitted. The use of masks is highly recommended to control the spread of the virus. In the context of construction projects, the mask-wearing policy becomes important considering that construction activities are generally carried out in groups (Egardy, 2022). In addition, mask-wearing is one of the best solutions because it is economical, easy to apply, and effective in suppressing the spread of COVID-19 (Farihin et al., 2021; Kim et al., 2021; Koebele et al., 2021).

This study was successful in evaluating the effectiveness of mask-wearing policy implementation in two construction projects. The results of this study imply that the enforcement of mask-wearing policy is very dependent on the contractor's ability and strategy to regulate the attitude of his workers. Even if a policy is in effect, its implementation can be varied. As proper policy planning leads to good practices and results in better performance (Pradhan et al., 2017), this study suggests policy improvements based on these findings. In addition, this study also highlights the importance of socialising the mask-wearing policy to foster self-awareness of workers in wearing masks. Although it requires a variety of programs and long interventions, this can become a health culture in construction projects.

In general, this study contributes by providing a policy assessment framework. Policy makers can adopt the framework to assess their mask-wearing policy effectiveness. This framework is flexible and can be modified for other contexts as well. For instance, it can be used to assess the effectiveness of other project policies. In addition, the findings of this study can be considered in the future management of HSE in construction projects. For example, it is necessary to have mask-wearing as one of the points of consideration in employment contracts. Since this study is qualitative in nature, it is also recommended that further studies focus on an experimental approach to see how effective the use of masks in preventing COVID-19 is in construction projects quantitatively, or how much effect wearing a mask has on workers' productivity.

**Conclusions**

This chapter observes the mask-wearing policy and behaviour as practiced by construction workers during the COVID-19 pandemic. To assess the effectiveness of this policy, a policy assessment framework is developed by incorporating four dimensions of policy issue, creation, implementation, and evaluation. This framework was validated by two case studies to comprehensively analyse all indicators influencing policy implementation. The results indicate that there are differences in policy implementation between the two observed case studies. The two case studies provide empirical evidence that workers' perception of the effectiveness of mask-wearing policy implementation is guided by enforcement control and strategies (such as awareness-raising socialisation, incentives, etc.) by contractors. The findings also reveal the need to update the mask-wearing policy in both projects for future improvements. Finally, policy makers can take advantage of this policy assessment framework directly or with necessary adjustments. They should pay close attention to the four assessment dimensions and their indicators to successfully evaluate and improve the mask-wearing policy.

**References**

Australian Welding Supplies (AWS). (2021). *A practical guide to welding fume control.* Artarmon, NSW: Australian Welding Supplies Pty Ltd.

Chen, H., Wang, J., & Huang, J. (2014). Policy support, social capital, and farmers' adaptation to drought in China. *Global Environmental Change*, 24, 193–202.

Cheng, Y., Ma, N., Witt, C., Rapp, S., Wild, P.S., Andreae, M.O., Poschl, U., & Su, H. (2021). Face masks effectively limit the probability of SARS-CoV-2 transmission. *Science*, 372(6549), 1439–1443.

Chua, M.H., Cheng, W., Goh, S.S., Kong, J., Li, B., Lim, J.Y.C., Mao, L., Wang, S., Xue, K., Yang, L., Ye, E., Zhang, K., Cheong, W.C.D., Tan, B.H., Li, Z., Tan, B.H., & Loh, X.J. (2020). Face masks in the new COVID-19 normal: Materials, testing, and perspectives. *Research*, 2020(6), 1–40.

Cohen, H.J., & Birkner, J.S. (2012). Respiratory protection. *Clinics in Chest Medicine*, 33(4), 783–793.

Decree of the Minister of Health of the Republic of Indonesia No. HK.01.07/MEN-KES/328/2020 concerning Guidelines for the Prevention and Control of Corona Virus Disease 2019 on 20 May 2020.

Egardy, M.D. (2022). *Identifikasi Masker sebagai Alat Pelindung Diri (APD) dan Alat Pencegah Virus COVID-19 pada Proyek Konstruksi di Jakarta.* Bachelor Thesis, Construction Engineering & Management Program, Universitas Agung Podomoro, Jakarta.

Farihin, W.A., Alamsyah, D.F., & Pudjihardjo, H.S. (2021). *Analisis Resiko Pelaksanaan Pembangunan Proyek Konstruksi Bangunan Gedung IGD RSUD Ajibarang pada Saat Pandemi COVID-19.* Bachelor Thesis, Civil Engineering Program, Universitas Semarang, Semarang.

Fauziyah, S., Susanti, R., & Lukman. (2022). The mitigation of Covid-19 in the perspective of contractor for sustainable construction in Indonesia. *IOP Conference Series: Earth and Environmental Science*, 969, 012071.

Fitriani, R. (2020). Mengintip Panduan Pengendalian COVID-19 Sektor Konstruksi oleh OSHA. *Buletin Konstruksi*, 4, 4–6.

Hansen, S. (2020a). Does the COVID-19 outbreak constitute a force majeure event? A pandemic impact on construction contracts. *Journal of the Civil Engineering Forum*, 6(2), 201–214.

Hansen, S. (2020b). Investigasi Teknik Wawancara dalam Penelitian Kualitatif Manajemen Konstruksi. *Jurnal Teknik Sipil*, 27(3), 283–294.

Irfan, M., Akhtar, N., Ahmad, M., Shahzad, F., Elavarasan, R.M., Wu, H., & Yang, C. (2021). Assessing public willingness to wear face masks during the COVID-19 pandemic: Fresh insights from the theory of planned behavior. *International Journal of Environmental Research and Public Health*, 18(9), 4577, 1–22.

Kim, Y.J., Choi, S., & Nam, B.H. (2021). Developing advanced data-driven models to understand the complex patterns of mask wearing amid the COVID-19 pandemic: Efforts to accelerate collective cognition of shared risk. *Natural Hazards Review*, 22(2), 02521001.

Koebele, E.A., Albright, E.A., Dickinson, K.L., Blanch-Hartigan, D., Neuberger, L., DeLeo, R.A., Shanahan, E.A., & Roberts, J.D. (2021). Perceptions of efficacy are key determinants of mask-wearing behavior during the COVID-19 pandemic. *Natural Hazards Review*, 22(3), 06021002.

Krismantoro, & Susilo, W.H. (2021). Study of customer demand for cloth masks during the COVID-19 pandemic and an affecting the performance: Insight the industrial organization theory in management research. *International Journal of Research in Commerce and Management Studies*, 3(5), 1–12.

Lima, M.M.Ds., Cavalcante, F.M.L., Macedo, T.S., Galindo-Neto, N.M., Caetano, J.A., & Barros, L.M. (2020). Cloth face masks to prevent Covid-19 and other respiratory infections. *Revista Latino-Americana de Enfermagen*, 28, 1–8.

Ministry of Health Circular Letter No. HK.02.02/I/385/2020 concerning the Use of Masks and the Provision of Handwashing Facilities with Soap to Prevent Transmission of Corona Virus Disease 2019.

Ministry of Public Works and Housing Instruction No. 02/In/M/2020 concerning the Protocol for Preventing the Spread of COVID-19 in the Execution of Construction Services.

Oerther, D.B., & Shattell, M. (2020). Environmental hygiene for COVID-19: It's all about the mask. *Journal of Environmental Engineering*, 146(12), 01820004.

O'Kelly, E., Arora, A., Pirog, S., Ward, J., & Clarkson, P.J. (2021). Comparing the fit of N95, KN95, surgical, and cloth masks and assessing the accuracy of fit checking. *PLoS One*, 16(1), e0245688.

Pattisinai, A.R., Widayanti, F.R., Nusantara, D.A.D., & Nadiar, F. (2020). The importance of occupational safety and health in the construction project site in the era pandemic COVID-19. *PROTEKSI*, 2(2), 84–89.

Pradhan, N.S., Su, Y., Fu, Y., Zhang, L., & Yang, Y. (2017). Analyzing the effectiveness of policy implementation at the local level: A case study of management of the 2009–2010 drought in Yunnan Province, China. *International Journal of Disaster Risk Science*, 8, 64–77.

Pranata, Y.H. (2019). *Kajian terhadap Semen Portland sebagai Material Berbahaya bagi Pekerja Proyek Konstruksi*. Bachelor Thesis, Construction Engineering & Management Program, Universitas Agung Podomoro, Jakarta.

Presidential Decree No. 12 of 2020 concerning the Determination of Non-Natural Disasters for the Spread of COVID-19 as a National Disaster.

Purnomo, M.R.A., Shinta, R.C., Ramadhani, R., Yassaruddin, A.R., & Sabit, M.I. (2016). Automatic polarizing filter system for welding mask. Proceeding of 9th International Seminar on Industrial Engineering and Management, September 20–22, Padang, West Sumatera, Indonesia, pp. 1–7.

Sari, H.M. (2021). Penerapan Protokol Pencegahan Penyebaran Corona Virus Disease 2019 (COVID-19) Pada Penyelenggaraan Proyek Konstruksi. *Mecha Jurnal Teknik Mesin*, 3(2), 16–22.

Sickbert-Bennett, E.E., Samet, J.M., Prince, S.E., Chen, H., Zeman, K.L., Tong, H., & Bennett, W.D. (2021). Fitted filtration efficiency of double masking during the COVID-19 pandemic. *JAMA Internal Medicine*, 181(8), 1126–1128.

Siswanto, A.B., Salim, M.A., & Ramawati, D. (2022). Analisis Penerapan K3 Masa Pandemi COVID-19 pada Proyek Dermaga Samudera Semarang. *Teras Jurnal: Jurnal Teknik Sipil*, 12(1), 229–244.

Suraji, A. (2021). Dampak, Adaptasi dan Mitigasi Pandemi COVID-19 di Sektor Konstruksi Indonesia. In *Buku 3 Konstruksi Indonesia 2021* (pp. 574–592). Jakarta: Kementerian Pekerjaan Umum dan Perumahan Rakyat.

Susila, H., & Arbianto, R. (2021). Penerapan Protokol Pencegahan COVID-19 dalam Pelaksanaan Proyek Konstruksi. *Jurnal Teknik Sipil dan Arsitektur*, 26(2), 10–17.

Waluyo, P. (2020). Penerapan Pekerjaan Proyek Konstruksi pada Masa Pandemi COVID-19 Menggunakan Pendekatan OHSAS 18001. *Jurnal Konstruksia*, 12(1), 69–80.

Wati, E.T., Muda, C.A.K., Rusdy, M.D.R., & Handayani, P. (2021). Factors related to the behaviour of the use of mask in workers in the era of covid-19 pandemic in project. *Majalah Ilmu Keperawatan dan Kesehatan Indonesia*, 10(2), 185–195.

# 10 Construction sector in Indonesia

## Occupational health and safety during the outbreak of COVID-19

*Harijanto Setiawan, Agustina Kiky Anggraini and Gumbert Maylda Pratama*

### Introduction

The Covid-19 pandemic has had a profoundly significant impact on various aspects of human life in all countries of the world. Many countries around the globe have experienced economic downturns and recessions. Business activities in all fields have been severely restricted or locked down. In this situation, the working from home (WFH) concept has been introduced in dealing with businesses locked down in various fields (Gamil and Alhagar, 2020). However, not all business activities can be run remotely. Many activities require the interaction of the people carrying out the activities.

The construction industry is different compared to other sectors. The business in this industry is based on labor-intensive projects requiring the involvement of all project members on-site. Therefore, construction projects include activities that cannot be executed remotely. In addition, activities on construction projects are activities that contain a substantial risk of accidents. According to Badan Penyelenggara Jaminan Sosial (BPJS), or the Social Insurance Administration Organization in Indonesia, occupational accidents are increasing yearly. In 2017, the number of accidents reported was 123,041 cases, and in 2020 it reached 177,000 cases. Among all industrial sectors, the construction sector is the most significant contributor to the number of occupational accidents. The contribution from year to year is around 30% of the total number of occupational accidents. This risk increased during the Covid-19 pandemic because coronavirus is extremely easy and fast to spread, primarily through human interaction. Moreover, the coronavirus has a hazardous impact and even can lead to death. From January to September 2021, the number of occupational illnesses reported was 179 cases, and coronaviruses was identified as causing 65% of them.

Working safely and healthily in construction projects is particularly important in this situation. However, it is hard to implement for several reasons, such as working conditions and worker awareness. Most construction project activities are outdoor activities and are strongly influenced by the weather. Meanwhile, as a tropical country, Indonesia only has two seasons, the dry and rainy seasons. In the dry season, the climate is very hot. Therefore, workers are uncomfortable working with

DOI: 10.1201/9781003278368-11

full safety and health equipment, including additional equipment to prevent the spread of the coronavirus, such as face masks. The other problem is that most construction workers in Indonesia have low educational backgrounds. This condition is in line with the level of education of workers in Indonesia in general. According to the data that the Ministry of Manpower Republic of Indonesia published in 2020, 57.5% of 126.51 million of Indonesia's working-age population have a low educational background.

Moreover, this low educational background is not supported by adequate professional certification. The percentage of certified construction workers is still deficient. According to 2020 Statistics Indonesia, the number of construction workers in Indonesia has reached 8.3 million. Among them, only an estimated 666,000 have been certified. The low educational background and lack of professional certification have increased the workers' ignorance of working safely and healthily. This condition escalates the risk of work accidents at project sites, especially during the Covid-19 pandemic, which is very vulnerable to transmitting hazardous diseases.

Resolving Occupational Health and Safety (OHS) issues in construction, especially those related to the coronavirus, requires the role and commitment of various parties involved in construction projects, such as clients, contractors, and the government. Among all parties, the most significant role lies with the contractor, who is directly involved in project activities and a direct user of construction workers; therefore, the contractor is responsible for managing the workers and providing the proper facilities to support workers to work safely and healthily. In addition, the government also plays a significant role in encouraging and ensuring the implementation of OHS programs and in regulating healthy work practices during the coronavirus pandemic.

Although various regulations related to work safety in the construction sector both before and during the pandemic have been issued by the Indonesian government, a structured review that provides a clear picture of work safety arrangements in Indonesia before and during the pandemic has not been properly carried out. In addition, the important role of contractors in supporting the implementation of work safety programs in Indonesia during the pandemic has not been fully and thoroughly explored. Based on this gap, this chapter focuses on implementing the OHS program during the Covid-19 pandemic in Indonesia. To address this issue, first the Indonesian Government Regulations that related to OHS program and Covid-19 preventions will be explored and presented in a systematic way, and then the role of contractors in supporting the success of OHS program implementation will also be identified.

## The Covid-19 pandemic in the construction sector

The Covid-19 pandemic impacted all business sectors, including the construction sector. The impact on the construction sector became more significant because of its specific working environment. Construction projects include activities that cannot be run remotely. Several studies on the impact of the Covid-19 pandemic on the construction industry have been carried out on different topics and in countries worldwide. However, studies about the pandemic in the construction industry in Indonesia are quite limited.

Alenezi (2020) studied the delays in construction projects in Kuwait due to the Covid-19 pandemic. This study found escalation and inflation of construction material prices to be the leading cause of construction project delays during the pandemic. Another study related to project delay has been carried out in Indonesia by Parinduri and Parinduri (2020), but with a more general focus on the impact of the pandemic on the construction sector in Indonesia. This study found that the direct implications of the pandemic were delays in project time completion. The delays were caused by a supply chain that was not running very well, which impacted the supply of construction materials, equipment, and labor. Several projects had to be stopped, increasing project budgets and causing potential contract disputes. This condition has a multiplier effect on socio-economic aspects, such as termination of employment and enforcement of mobilization restrictions in various regions.

A study about the impact of the Covid-19 pandemic on construction contracts has been carried out in Indonesia by Larasati et al. (2021). This study found the significant effect of the pandemic on construction contracts was the project schedule. In addition, this study also found that implementing health protocols on the project site required assistance for people involved in project activities, additional costs, staff capacity improvement, and special equipment.

Gamil and Alhagar (2020) conducted a study identifying the impact of the pandemic on Malaysia's construction industry. This study found that most of the projects were suspended because of the pandemic and only a few continued, especially those related to medical facilities. In this situation, project planning and scheduling have been impacted significantly. Another effect is that all staff working on the project must be aware of the transmission of disease caused by coronavirus. Staff must work with full awareness and under strict supervision. This study also found that project suspension was the most significant impact, followed by job loss of labor, time overrun, and cost overrun.

Stiles et al. (2021) studied health and safety in construction in the UK. This study was concerned that the need for greater safety and flexibility within the construction sector was significant. More specifically, construction activities are expected to be carried out safely and be amenable to any changes, for example, local lockdown and work restrictions or future waves of conditions such as pandemics. This study makes four observations and then provides several recommendations based on those observations. The four recommendations were 1) how to manage coronavirus risk in construction; 2) broader implications of coronavirus for safety in construction; 3) the role of the organization; 4) the role of safety leadership. Several proposed recommendations focused on improving regulatory, policy, and safety control activities, including coronavirus control.

Based on the reality, coronavirus has significantly impacted various fields, including the construction sector. The OHS program is vital to apply in the construction industry because it comprises activities with considerable risk of accidents. Research related to OHS in construction, especially those related to the Covid-19 pandemic, is fundamental. Considering that research related to the impact of coronavirus on health and safety in the construction sector in Indonesia is still rare, it is crucial to conduct research to explore the OHS program in the construction sector.

**Methodology**

This study investigates the OHS program's implementation in Indonesia's construction projects during the Covid-19 pandemic. Due to the lack of relevant previous research in Indonesia, an exploratory approach was deemed necessary for this study. The qualitative method has been chosen to achieve the research aims and has been used to identify the provisions related to the OHS program on construction projects during the Covid-19 pandemic, as regulated by the Indonesian government. Furthermore, these methods were also used to explore the implementation of the OHS program on construction projects during the Covid-19 pandemic by contractors in Indonesia.

Data for this study's first aim was collected by reference to the laws issued by the Indonesian government that regulate the implementation of the OHS program in construction projects. The regulations were searched online using the following keywords: OHS, Pandemic, Covid-19, and Construction. Subsequently, an in-depth review of Indonesian Regulations relating to the implementation of the OHS program in construction was carried out. The analysis commenced by reading the regulations carefully, article by article, and then this was followed by the coding stage. In this stage, the article in the regulations governing the performance of the OHS program was collected. Finally, the idea of the regulation of the OHS program during the Covid-19 pandemic in Indonesia was depicted.

To achieve the second aim of this study, in-depth interviews have been carried out with five key persons who worked for contractors in Indonesia and have responsibility for the OHS program. By conducting an in-depth interview, detailed information could be obtained (Ling et al., 2022). The interviewees were chosen because they were intensively involved in planning, developing, and implementing OHS programs. Therefore, they are the most knowledgeable people about the policies and implementation of the OHS program on construction projects. In addition, the organizational criteria were also considered in order to select the right interviewees. The organizational criteria are related to the ownership and company size of the contractors. The contractors selected for this study were private and public-private contractors with equal-sized companies. The interviews with five interviewees were considered adequate because they had achieved data saturation, where no more new information was found. An in-depth interview was also conducted with an officer of the Social Insurance Administration Organization to complement the information obtained from contractors.

To obtain optimum results from the interviews, an interview guide was prepared and sent to the interviewees by email, prior to their interviews. The interview guideline consists of several questions, such as:

1. How is the OHS program being implemented in construction projects during the coronavirus pandemic?

2. How do the contractors determine and regulate the implementation of the OHS program in construction projects during the coronavirus pandemic?
3. How does the Indonesian government regulate the implementation of the OHS program in construction projects during the coronavirus pandemic?
4. What are the obstacles faced in carrying out the OHS program according to the health protocol during the coronavirus pandemic?

The way the questions were asked did not always follow the guidelines. They varied depending on the flow of the conversation. Additional questions were asked in cases where the interviewees mentioned issues that were important and relevant to the topic of the interview, and the interviewer found it beneficial to explore further. The interviewer controlled the conversations and made sure the focus stayed on the issue. The duration of each interview varied from 60 to 90 minutes. The discussions were fully audio-recorded with permission from the interviewees.

This study used less structured procedures and relied more on the researcher's interpretation in analyzing the data. The following processes were carried out to analyze the data from interviews to identify the implementation of the OHS program:

1. The analysis was started by listening to the interview recording carefully, which enabled the researchers to be familiar with the data and to capture initial ideas from the data.
2. It was followed by the coding stage. The first coding was done manually by sifting through the recording. Statements that indicated a potential pattern of OHS program implementation were written down manually. In this stage, the researchers tried to code as many phenomena as possible that emerged from the interviews.
3. Refining the coding process and re-collating the codes into appropriate themes was continuously undertaken to check whether or not the findings worked concerning the entire data set. Finally, the implementation of OHS program in Indonesia's construction project sites was identified.

**OHS regulation in Indonesia**

The Indonesian Government has issued several laws to regulate OHS in Indonesia, such as: the Law of the Republic of Indonesia Number 1 of 1970 (Republic of Indonesia, 1970), about Occupational Safety which underlies the implementation of OHS in Indonesia; the Law of the Republic of Indonesia Number 13 of 2003 (Republic of Indonesia, 2003) about employment; Government Regulation of the Republic of Indonesia Number 50 of 2012 (Republic of Indonesia, 2012), concerning the implementation of the OHS Management System (OHSMS).

All these regulations govern the OHS in general. However, construction projects have specific working conditions. Therefore, the rule that regulates OHS in the construction sector was needed. To fulfill this demand, the Indonesian government issued the Regulation of the Minister of Public Works and Public Housing

Number 05/PRT/M/2014 of 2014 (Ministry of Public Works and Public Housing of the Republic of Indonesia, 2014), concerning Guidelines for Construction OHSMS in the Public Work Sector. In this regulation, Construction OHS is defined as all activities to guarantee and protect workers' safety and health through occupational accidents and disease prevention efforts in construction work. Construction OHSMS of Public Works is defined as part of the contractor's management system to control safety and health risk on every construction job in the field of Public Works. In both definitions, construction work is a series of the whole or part of planning or constructing activities and supervision that covers buildings, mechanical and electrical installations, and other services to realize buildings or other physical facilities within a certain period. This regulation includes several issues in construction OHSMS, such as the implementation of construction OHSMS in public works, duties, responsibilities, and authorities; costs of implementing construction OHSMS in public works; and sanctions for not implementing the construction OHSMS.

In 2017, the Indonesian government issued Laws of the Republic of Indonesia Number 2 of 2017 about Construction Services (Republic of Indonesia, 2017). This law does not explicitly regulate OHS in construction, but in general, it contains provisions for OHS because it is an essential aspect of construction services. This law mandates that the implementation of construction services that are under the Standard of Security, Safety, Health, and Sustainability is the responsibility of the Central Government. The Standard of Security, Safety, Health, and Sustainability in this law is defined as technical guidelines for security, safety, health in the construction workplace, and social protection of workers, as well as local environmental management in the implementation of construction services. Provisions related to security, safety, health, and sustainability of construction are regulated explicitly in Chapter 6 of this law.

The government stipulated Government Regulation Number 14 of 2021 to update Government Regulation 22 of 2020. The update ensures the implementation of Law Number 2 of 2017 concerning construction services, including the role of each party involved. According to Article 84AK of Government Regulation Number 14 of 2021, OHSMS is regulated by the minister. Minister of Public Works and Public Housing Regulation Number 10 of 2021 concerning the Guidelines for Construction Safety Management Systems was stipulated to advocate the article. (Ministry of Public Works and Public Housing of the Republic of Indonesia, 2021). This regulation states that every user and provider of construction services must implement a Construction Safety Management System. Furthermore, this regulation covers three main chapters: 1) implementation of Construction Safety Management System; 2) components of the implementation of Construction Safety Management System; and 3) guidance and supervision.

After the Covid-19 pandemic in Indonesia, the Indonesian government was concerned about preventing the spread of coronavirus by managing community activities in several fields. For this purpose, the Ministry of Health of the Republic of Indonesia issued Decree of Minister of Health of the Republic of Indonesia

Number HK.01.07/MENKES/328/2020 of 2020 about Guidelines for Prevention and Control of Corona Virus Disease 2019 (Covid-19) in the Office and Industry Workplace to Support Business Continuity in Pandemic Situations (Ministry of Health of the Republic of Indonesia, 2020). This decree provides guidelines to be used as a reference for workplace managers/managers in government agencies, private companies, State-Owned Enterprises, and Provincial and District/City Health Offices. According to this decree, the Central Government, Provincial Governments, and Regency/Municipal Governments carry out guidance and supervision of implementing the guidelines under their respective authorities and may involve the community.

In particular, a protocol for coronavirus prevention in construction is regulated by Instruction of the Minister of Public Works and Public Housing Number 02/IN/M/2020 of 2020 concerning the Protocol to Prevent the Spread of Corona Virus Disease 2019 (COVID-19) in the Implementation of Construction Services (Ministry of Public Works and Public Housing of the Republic of Indonesia, 2020). This Instruction is part of the overall policy to achieve OHS in construction. Moreover, the safety of the public and environment at every stage of construction can be accomplished. This Instruction contains a mechanism regarding the protocol of coronavirus prevention in the implementation of construction services, which includes: 1) establishing a coronavirus prevention task force carried out by construction service users and providers; 2) providing coronavirus prevention facilities carried out by construction service providers; 3) educate everyone in the task force to protect themselves from coronavirus.

Various regulations related to OHS that the Indonesian government has issued from time to time show that the Indonesian government is concerned with the OHS program, including in the construction sector. However, according to Phuspa et al. (2019), implementing these regulations is still not optimal. Several reasons were found, such as lack of awareness to report occupational accidents, weak sanctions if contractors do not apply the regulations, lack of supervision, and low company commitment to implement the OHS program.

## OHS program in construction projects in Indonesia during the COVID-19 pandemic

Work activities in the construction industry involve many elements, such as workers, heavy equipment, and a large amount of material, which may lead to accidents (Asih and Latief, 2021). A safety program in the construction project is essential due to the higher risk of work accidents. In Indonesia, it is obligatory to have an OHSMS in place for large or high-risk enterprises. The law states that occupational health has to be considered not only to protect the health of all workers from workplace hazards but also to balance the productivity and the health and safety of workers (Buranatrevedh, 2015). According to Lingard and Rowlinson (2004), the OHS law guarantees that when workers experience a work-related accident or illness, they have the right to get compensation and undergo rehabilitation to resume their participation in the workforce and the community.

During the Covid-19 pandemic, the construction projects experienced even higher stakes. Ogunnusi et al. (2020) reported that the pandemic substantially affected construction projects. It was not only that the projects might be delayed, but also that the health and safety risks for the workers were escalated. The assessment of health and safety had to be conducted under integrated guidelines.

The construction industry in Indonesia is one of the government's focal points. When the Covid-19 pandemic hit the country, the construction industry had to continue working to achieve the targets. Larasati et al. (2021) stated that 80% of construction projects were still being operated during the pandemic. However, the construction industry demands the on-site involvement of every project member. In this case, every company working in the construction industry had to set a plan to accomplish the target without compromising the health and safety of the workers.

Thorough discussions were conducted with two state-owned companies and one private company working in the construction industry to understand the implementation of the OHS Program in Indonesia, especially during the Covid-19 pandemic. An interview with the officer of Badan Penyelenggara Jaminan Sosial (BPJS) or the Social Insurance Administration Organization, was conducted to find out the role of the public insurance organization in the case of the Covid-19 pandemic.

### Health protocol in construction project sites in Indonesia

Projects are the heart of every construction company. It means the survival of construction companies depends on the existence of projects. The Covid-19 pandemic increased concerns since the projects could be shut down once a cluster of Covid-19 had been confirmed. Preventive action had to be determined to neutralize the threats of Covid-19 to the construction projects. The main program for the prevention to minimize the Covid-19 risks to the projects was implementing health protocols in construction project sites.

According to the Decree of the Minister of Health of the Republic of Indonesia Number HK.01.07/MENKES/328/2020 of 2020, it was mandatory that every workplace had to carry out a health protocol during the Covid-19 pandemic. Contractors in Indonesia must commit to the regulation; therefore, they implement the health protocol in every construction project. They established a procedure that organized all the activities on the construction sites. The company evaluated the measures taken during the monthly project evaluation.

Considering all the facilities that were required for the preventive measures, every company reported that they needed to allocate an extra budget. This statement was in line with the results of Larasati et al. (2021), which stated that 62% of the respondents claimed that additional costs were required. The expenses went toward the procurement of washbowls, hand soap, masks, disinfectants, hand sanitizers, thermometer guns, nutrition supplements, and the Covid-19 antigen and Polymerase Chain Reaction (PCR) tests. For some projects, these additional costs might cause concern. The conclusion was that since implementing health protocols can interfere with project performance, stakeholders should consider these additional costs (Larasati et al., 2021).

The protocol implemented by the companies was not only for the workers on site but also for the staff in the back office. WFH and work from office (WFO) mechanisms had to be applied to adhere to the protocol. The WFH mode was intended to minimize the face-to-face sessions. The number of staff who had to WFH was 25% to 70%. When the pandemic was at its peak, 70% of the staff had to WFH. Consequently, meetings and any other communication were conducted online. Larasati et al. (2021) stated that 60% of their respondents found online coordination was effective and efficient. The rest of the respondents claimed that online coordination was ineffective due to lack of skilled personnel, limited facilities, and poor internet connections.

All interviewees confirmed that by implementing the health protocol, the cases of Covid could be minimized. The companies appreciated the government's involvement while implementing the rigid health protocol. They were not only forcing the companies to obey the rules but also very cooperative during the monitoring and evaluation phases. Several actions carried out by the contractors in Indonesia to support the implementation of health protocol have been found as follows.

### COVID-19 prevention task force

The company decided to form a task force to handle the issues related to Covid-19. The top management assigned a task force to focus on preventing Covid-19 cases on the construction site, especially to prevent the formation of a Covid-19 cluster. It was challenging to implement effective policies for dealing with the situation. On the other hand, the company must adhere to government policies that are brought in to deal with an emergency. It was not until the Decree of the Minister of Health of the Republic of Indonesia Number HK.01.07/MENKES/328/2020 of 2020 that the companies could decide on the measures that had to be taken. To fulfill the responsibility, the team focuses on the health screening of the workers every time they come to the construction site. Even a task force from one of the correspondent contractors carried out a regular safety patrol with the help of a military member to ensure that all the workers obeyed the protocol.

### The vaccination program

The vaccination program is one of the company policies to prevent the Covid-19 cases escalating and to minimize the risk. Several workers initially refused the vaccination program, and this issue became a constraint on implementing the policy. As a solution, the top management had to implement a strict rule where the workers who refused to be vaccinated would be penalized. By the time of the interview, around 98% of the workers had been vaccinated. In addition, the company provided food supplements for the workers to strengthen the workers' immune systems.

### Ensuring a hygienic working environment

The company had to ensure a clean area and good air quality to provide a hygienic workplace. The workplace had to include adequate washbowls and hand sanitizers. It was also a must to maintain physical distancing among workers in the workplace. In order to ensure a hygienic working environment, the health tracing program was conducted to ensure that there was no transmission of viruses. Every morning, each worker had to fill in a form, using an app that was developed by the top management. This tracing program included the monitoring of mobile staff. Every staff member traveling from another city had to take a few measures to guarantee that the viruses did not infect them. Another effort to ensure a hygienic working environment was a regular disinfecting program for several places on site, such as the workers' dormitory. The company also set up the workers' dormitory to support the protocol to fulfill the physical distancing pattern. Moreover, they renovated the bathroom in the dormitory. Before the pandemic, the dormitory had a traditional bathroom design that consisted of a tub and a plastic dipper. The workers had to use the bathroom in turns. To minimize the risk of Covid-19, the bathroom renovation involved changing the traditional design to a modern one with a shower. The company also provided a thorough assessment to ensure safe working conditions.

### Educating the workers

Worker education was crucial to prevent the spread of Covid-19. Education for the workers was carried out in several ways, such as conducting weekly safety talks and briefs that were arranged by the task force. The education focused on the dangers of Covid-19, the importance of vaccination programs, and the preventive action by carrying out the health protocol. Besides this formal and regular program to educate the workers, the task force also worked with the senior forepersons to inform the workers about the preventive measures the company had decided to conduct. In addition, the company provided a pocketbook containing all the health protocol information for every worker.

### Case handling

Even though the companies were able to minimize the cases by the rigid protocol, they were prepared for the worst scenario. The companies monitored the Covid-19 cases on the construction site by conducting regular meetings. During the meeting, the rate of the cases was discussed. This measure was able to confirm that the workers were in a healthy condition.

Every worker had to take the Covid-19 antigen test every two weeks to monitor the cases. The company took care of the workers who produced positive results. These workers had to be isolated from others, and the company supported them during the isolation period. Case handling at the second state-owned company was quite similar. The company provided a temporary shelter for the workers who needed to have an isolation period. This temporary shelter included the medicines required by the workers. The private company was also committed to helping their workers who were infected with coronavirus. For example, where necessary, they facilitated the workers being admitted to hospitals appointed by the government.

The scenario mentioned here proved that the companies working in the construction industry followed the guidelines enacted by the government. Detailed approaches might not be the same from one company to another, but they all adhered to the rules. These results confirmed the previous study by Larasati et al. (2021). According to the survey, 71% of the respondents declared that the health protocol had been implemented in the construction projects.

During the post-pandemic period, the worst-case scenario still needs to be considered. The implications of the results are that every construction site needs to be prepared with a temporary shelter, especially for those who are unwell. The temporary shelter should be centralized so that its control can be handled easily.

### *Role of the social insurance administration organization*

In managing the OHS of the workers in the construction industry in Indonesia, every company must cooperate with the BPJS. This organization ensures the workers are covered for every risk in the workplace that may endanger their health and safety. Regarding the Covid-19 pandemic, the BPJS is vital in hastening the vaccination program. However, since Covid-19 is deemed a pandemic, the responsibility is still in the government's hands. It means that the Social Insurance Administration Organization will not insure the Covid-19 cases in the workplaces during the pandemic. Once the status changes to an endemic disease, the BPJS is responsible for the infected patients.

### Conclusions

As a result of the regulations that provide Guidelines for Construction Safety Management Systems, the implementation of OHS during the pandemic has been easier to implement. A task force is formed with each person in charge of OHS in each construction project. No adjustments are needed in terms of organizational structure. Adjustments need to be made in the application of the protocol in accordance with prevention and treatment measures.

All existing stakeholders primarily determine the success of implementing the regulations that have been made. The compliance of construction workers in construction activities is one of the most influential things. Both the educational background of workers and the comfort of PPE affected worker compliance in implementing health protocols during the pandemic. The company seeks to improve employee compliance with various approaches, ranging from regulations that are accompanied by penalties to a more subtle approach by inviting workers to take part in determining their health.

Implementation of OHS within the construction industry during a pandemic has impacted project schedules and budgets. Although construction is one sector that could continue to run during the pandemic, due to restrictions on mobility, it will indirectly result in the supply chain being disrupted. PPE, vitamins and supplements, and other tools that need to be provided to meet health protocols and maintain workers' health result in additional costs that have not been considered in the budget.

A practical recommendation based on these results can be made. Since implementing health protocol increases the need for funding, the budgeting plan must be arranged carefully. At the beginning of the project, the budget planners have to include all the costs for implementing the health protocol. The practical significance that needs to be intensified is the education program. Since most workers come from lower educational backgrounds, boosting the education program will help the success of the OHS implementation in the post-pandemic period.

## References

Alenezi, T.A.N. (2020). The impact of Covid-19 on construction projects in Kuwait. *International Journal of Engineering Research and General Science*, 8(4), 6–9.

Asih, R., & Latief, Y. (2021). Evaluation of implementation within occupational health and safety management system based on Indonesia government regulation number 50 of 2012 and ISO 45001:2018 (Case Study: Company X). *In:* 2021.

Buranatrevedh, S. (2015). Occupational safety and health management among five ASEAN countries: Thailand, Indonesia, Malaysia, Philippines, and Singapore. *Journal of the Medical Association of Thailand*, 98(2), S64–S69.

Gamil, Y., & Alhagar, A. (2020). The impact of pandemic crisis on the survival of construction industry: A case of COVID-19. *Mediterranean Journal of Social Sciences*, 11(4), 122.

Larasati, D., et al. (2021). Impact of the pandemic COVID-19 on the implementation of construction contracts. *IOP Conference Series: Earth and Environmental Science*, 738(1), 12075.

Ling, F.Y., et al. (2022). Impact of COVID-19 pandemic on demand, output, and outcomes of construction projects in Singapore. *Journal of Management in Engineering*, 38(2), 04021097.

Lingard, H., & Rowlinson, S. (2004). *Occupational health and safety in construction project management*. Abingdon, UK: Routledge.

Ministry of Health of the Republic of Indonesia. (2020). Decree of Minister of Health of the Republic of Indonesia Number HK.01.07/MENKES/328/2020 of 2020 about Guidelines for Prevention and Control of Corona Virus Disease 2019 (Covid-19) in the Office and Industry Workplace to Support Business Continuity in Pandemic Situations.

Ministry of Public Works and Public Housing of the Republic of Indonesia. (2014). Regulation of the Minister of Public Works and Public Housing Number 05/PRT/M/2014 of 2014 concerning Guidelines for Construction OHSMS in the Public Work Sector.

Ministry of Public Works and Public Housing of the Republic of Indonesia. (2020). Instruction of the Minister of Public Works and Public Housing Number 02/IN/M/2020 of 2020 concerning the Protocol to Prevent the Spread of Corona Virus Disease 2019 (COVID-19) in the Implementation of Construction Services.

Ministry of Public Works and Public Housing of the Republic of Indonesia. (2021). Regulation of the Minister of Public Works and Public Housing Number 10 of 2021 concerning Guidelines for Construction Safety Management Systems.

Ogunnusi, M., et al. (2020). COVID-19 pandemic: The effects and prospects in the construction industry. *International Journal of Real Estate Studies*, 14(2), 120–128.

Parinduri, L., & Parinduri, T. (2020). Implementasi Manajemen Keselamatan Konstruksi dalam Pandemi Covid 19. *Buletin Utama Teknik*, 15(3), 222–228.

Phuspa, S., et al. (2019). Implications of Indonesian occupational safety and health management system award to the safety culture. In Z. Rusnalasari, et al. (eds.).

Republic of Indonesia. (1970). Law of the Republic of Indonesia Number 1 of 1970 on Occupational Safety.

Republic of Indonesia. (2003). Law of the Republic of Indonesia Number 13 of 2003 concerning Manpower.

Republic of Indonesia. (2012). Government Regulation of the Republic of Indonesia Number 50 of 2012 concerning Implementation of OHS Management System (OHSMS).

Republic of Indonesia. (2017). Laws of the Republic of Indonesia Number 2 of 2017 about Construction Services.

Stiles, S., Golightly, D., & Ryan, B. (2021). Impact of COVID-19 on health and safety in the construction sector. *Human Factors and Ergonomics in Manufacturing*, 31(4), 425–437.

## Section Two

# Impact of COVID-19 on occupational safety, health and well-being (OSHW)

# 11 Individual and organisational support mechanisms to foster career resilience during the COVID-19 pandemic

*Naomi Borg, Christina M. Scott-Young,*
*Nader Naderpajouh and Jessica Borg*

## Introduction

The 21st century work environment context is highly dynamic and complex, with employees expected to navigate multiple shocks and stressors that test their ability to adapt and survive, i.e., to be career-resilient. The global coronavirus (COVID-19) pandemic which emerged in late 2019 (Bushuyev et al., 2020) wrought havoc on some individuals' careers and on organisational performance. As a result, employees and organisations must constantly assess, re-organise, and adapt to the ongoing challenges imposed by COVID-19 (Hite and McDonald, 2020). The strain imposed by COVID-19 has impacted the project management (PM) profession as well. Prior to COVID-19, project management practitioners were already managing in a volatile, uncertain, complex, and ambiguous (VUCA) environment (Mack et al., 2016). The uncertainties and challenges caused by COVID-19 created an additional threat to their health and wellbeing and to their general career success (Seibert et al., 2016; Akkermans et al., 2020).

Career success is determined by an employee's capacity to not merely survive in complex, challenging, unpredictable, and turbulent work environments (Rossier et al., 2017), but to view associated threats, stressors, and shocks as potential opportunities for career growth. Without this optimistic lens, shocks like COVID-19 can "trigger deliberation about potential career transitions such as acquiring new skills, searching for a new job, changing occupations or retiring" (Seibert et al., 2016, p. 245). Career resilience, defined as "a person's resistance to career disruption in a less than optimal environment" (London, 1997, p. 621), is a self-regulatory capacity that plays a key role in adopting this optimistic lens (Waterman et al., 1994) that facilitates career success and continued employability (Bezuidenhout, 2011). Career resilience differs from an individual's personal resilience in that it is career-related and primarily concerned with the necessary capacities to assist in navigating career challenges to achieve sustainable career success. Conversely, individual resilience is defined as the "the positive psychological capacity to rebound, to 'bounce back' from adversity, uncertainty, conflict, failure, or even positive change, progress, and increased responsibility" (Luthans, 2002, p. 702). Hence, individual resilience is likely to be associated with the attainment of the more distal construct of career resilience, but this relationship has yet to be tested.

DOI: 10.1201/9781003278368-13

While the career success of PM practitioners relies heavily on their self-agency to manage their own careers, employers have much to gain from providing the necessary resources to foster their employees' career resilience to contribute to organisational resilience. Organisational resilience refers to the "measurable combination of characteristics, abilities, capacities or capabilities that allows an organisation to withstand known and unknown disturbances and still survive" (Ruiz-Martin et al., 2018, p. 21). As employees are the most valuable asset upon whom an organisation's resilience and success is dependent (Lynn, 2000), a career-resilient workforce is critical. Career-resilient employees deliver high levels of productivity and demonstrate strong organisational loyalty (Harari, 1995). Although the uncertain conditions of the global pandemic make it impossible for employers to offer certainty over job security, they can create appropriate support mechanisms to buffer the stress (Lazarus and Folkman, 1984) of this disruption. The provision of additional organisational support during sudden shocks like COVID-19 can nurture employees' health and wellbeing and bolster their resilience to withstand the difficult environment.

This chapter is based on an online survey administered during the first year of the pandemic to 148 Australian PM practitioners affiliated with two project management peak bodies (PMI and AIPM). Thematic analysis of free-text survey questions provided insights into their perceived levels of personal and career resilience during the early stage of COVID-19 and the type of organisational support they received. Drawing on the Job Demands and Resources (JD-R) theoretical perspective, this chapter identifies the job resources which organisations provided to assist their PM practitioners in overcoming the shocks and job demands they faced during the pandemic. The chapter also outlines organisational support mechanisms that can assist in fostering career-resilient PM practitioners.

## Literature review – perspectives and concepts

### *Career resilience in 21st century careers*

According to Cascio (2007, p. 552), "career resilience is an essential survival skill in the 21st century". The COVID-19 pandemic and its associated challenges underscore the importance for individuals to develop career resilience as a capability to overcome the pressures, demands, and dynamism associated with such volatile contexts (Daniels and Radel, 2018). Furthermore, the recent shift towards the boundaryless and protean career paradigm (Akkermans and Kubasch, 2017) has required employees to take more responsibility for their own careers and to exercise greater initiative in acquiring new skillsets and knowledge to progress their career development (Akkermans et al., 2018). However, employers must also provide necessary career support resources or risk losing their valuable talent to their competitors (Brundage and Koziel, 2010). An organisation's ability to effectively manage their human capital depends on their capacity to understand and meet their employees' career needs and their requirements for career development (Greenhaus et al., 2010). Both employees and employers have a vested interest in creating career resilience, even more so as the world continues to experience the challenges of the COVID-19 pandemic.

*Career shocks and stressors in the PM profession*

Throughout their careers, project professionals experience a number of transitions. Many of these changes are unexpected, limiting the extent to which employees can proactively prepare for and respond to sudden events or "shocks" (Seibert et al., 2013; Akkermans et al., 2018). A career shock has been defined as "a distinct and impactful event that triggers deliberation about potential career transitions such as acquiring new skills, searching for a new job, changing occupations or retiring" (Seibert et al., 2016, p. 245) and can have either a positive or negative impact on their career. According to researchers, career success is dependent on the thought processes and responses initiated by these shocks, which have the potential to alter an individual's career trajectory for better or for worse (Seibert et al., 2013; De Vos and Van der Heijden, 2015). The project environment has its own unique set of shocks and challenges that contribute to PM practitioners' stress (Darling and Whitty, 2019), including poorly defined project goals, scope changes, project risks, tight deadlines, and poor work-life balance (Patil, 2016).

*JD-R theory*

This research utilises the Job Demands and Resources (JD-R) theory (Bakker and Demerouti, 2014) to frame the investigation of the personal factors and contextual factors influencing the career resilience of PM practitioners. There have been numerous theories used to explore career development; for example, social learning theory (Savickas, 2005), happenstance theory (Bright et al., 2005), and person/environment fit (Super, 1975). As this research is concerned with understanding the job resources provided to PM practitioners to manage job demands during COVID-19, the JD-R theory, used frequently by other construction researchers to study stress (e.g., Bowen et al., 2017), has been selected as the most suitable. The JD-R theory considers the job demands faced as well as the job resources available to PM practitioners and how they take action to utilise these resources and demands in response to arising challenges. Hence, this research investigates the strategies applied by career-resilient PM practitioners to craft sustainable careers. By using the JD-R theoretical lens, this research seeks to understand the job resources PM practitioners require to respond to COVID-19-related job demands in a career-resilient manner, as well as the required level of support needed from their organisations to assist in building and maintaining their career resiliency.

## Methodological approach

*Survey*

An online Qualtrics survey was used to enable "the collection of data from a sizeable population, allowing easy comparison" (Saunders et al., 2015, p. 181). Survey research is typically utilised "to answer questions that have been raised, to solve problem that have been posed or observed, to assess needs and set goals . . . and generally, to describe what exists, in what amount, and in what context" (Isaac and Michael, 1997, p. 136). This aligns with the study's aim to obtain information from a reasonable population of PM practitioners to allow comparisons to be made regarding their levels of personal and career resilience and the support mechanisms provided by their organisations. An online survey approach was selected based on its flexibility and timely administration benefits (Evans and Mathur, 2005), since at the time most PM practitioners were working from home under state government restrictions.

Open-ended free-text questions were used to elicit in-depth self-perceptions and sharing of respondents' experiences (Saunders et al., 2015) in a safe, anonymous, and protected environment (Zull, 2016). While open-ended survey questions are used less frequently than quantitative questions, they are useful for gathering contextual data in the respondents' own words without limiting their answers to predefined categories (Pallant, 2020). This provides an avenue for respondents' salient concerns to be voiced (Foddy, 1993). As there is a dearth of research on PM practitioners' career resilience and the level of organisational support that they received during COVID-19, open-ended questions allowed new insights to emerge from the data (Zull, 2016).

The survey questions were pilot tested with 10 respondents consisting of fellow researchers and practising PMs in the construction industry. These respondents had gained expertise through working or researching in the field of PM. Based on their feedback, only one minor change was made to the question order, with some of the demographic questions moved to the end of the survey so participants could engage more quickly with the questions relating to the effects of COVID-19 on their work experience.

### Sample and data collection

A stratified sampling procedure was used which divided the PM population based on their affiliation with the two Australian peak project professional associations. The Project Management Institute (PMI) was selected as the sample as it is the world's "leading not-for-profit professional membership association for the project management profession" (PMI, 2019). The Australian Institute of Project Management (AIPM) was selected since it represents different industry sectors from PMI. After pilot testing, the survey link was advertised through these professional bodies' LinkedIn forums. Volunteers completed the survey between July and October 2020, when Australian organisations were undergoing disruption, changes, and transitions in the early COVID-19 context.

### Data analysis

Content analysis of the qualitative text was used based on its ability to explore the "content with references to the meanings, contexts and intentions contained in messages" (Prasad, 2008, p. 1). As a research technique, content analysis utilises objectivity, systematic analysis, and valid inference procedures to understand content and contextual meaning from text-based data (Cavanagh, 1997; Prasad, 2008). As this study is concerned with understanding the meaning, formation, and degree of career resilience of PM practitioners, its focus on the context and interpretation and exploration of their lived experience lent itself to the conventional content analysis approach (CCA). As the questions had no pre-determined answers or categories associated with them, it was expected that their open-ended nature would elicit diverse responses. The CCA approach allows codes to emerge directly from the participants' responses as opposed to preconceived categories derived from existing literature (Hsieh and Shannon, 2005) as well as assisting in grouping these responses in accordance with appropriate themes. This allows the analysis to "stay true to the text" (Bengtsson, 2016, p. 8), in order to capture complexities of shared experiences and accounts. This is particularly important for this study, as there is limited research on the career resilience of PM practitioners in the COVID-19 workplace. In order to make a worthwhile contribution to understanding their level of career resilience and their support mechanisms that organisations provided, it is critical that findings are directly derived from the PM practitioners themselves.

## Results and discussion

### *Sample characteristics*

The majority of the sample PM practitioners worked as project managers or project team members on construction projects. Just over one-quarter (27%) worked in commercial construction, with 14% working on road and rail construction projects, 11% on school construction, and 14% on construction projects in the health sector, while a smaller proportion worked in different sectors, including IT, defence, agriculture, oil and gas, telecommunications, and government. Respondents mostly worked client-side (79%) while the remainder worked contractor-side. Participants ranged across all ages up to 61 years and over. Forty-five percent of the sample was under the age of 40 years. The largest group were aged between 31–40 years (28.4%), followed by those aged 51–60 years (27%), with PMs in the 18–30 and 41–50 age groups making up 18.9% each of the sample. There was only a small proportion of respondents aged 61 years or older (8.8%), which can be expected due to this age group being in the process of retiring from the profession. Males made up 69% of the respondents, reflecting the gender imbalance in the PM profession in Australia (AIPM, 2021).

### *Emerging themes*

#### *Perceived career resilience during the early stage of COVID-19*

**Key Finding:** Career-resilient PM practitioners responded through strategies of drawing on learnt experiences, maintaining a positive mindset, and undertaking job crafting and adaptation in the face of change.

The majority (61%) of PM practitioners reported high levels of career resilience, with most (70.8%) believing that they would emerge from the pandemic with an enhanced level of career resilience. Most had initiated a series of personal strategies and practices that improved their career resilience during the early stage of the pandemic shock. These strategies included i.) developing adaptability through new ways of working, ii.) enhanced balance between work and personal life, iii.) the adoption of a positive mindset, and iv.) a focus on the importance of continual training and development. The remaining PM practitioners reported either i.) no change in their level of career resilience, or ii.) a reduction in their career resilience as a result of feeling overwhelmed by anxiety and uncertainty due to the changes unfolding in their workplace and community. In comparison to those who reported an increase in career resilience, those who experienced reduced career resilience appear to have fallen victim to the shock of COVID-19. They viewed the pandemic as a threat to their career, rather than a potential opportunity to enhance their capacities and challenge themselves to come out of the shock stronger than before. A smaller proportion of respondents reported they expected no change to their levels of career resilience based on i.) having already developed a good level of career resilience and adaptive capacity as a result of working in dynamic project environments, and ii.) having already established a capacity to be resilient through experiencing past challenges. There was a shared conception between respondents in this category that COVID-19 was yet another period of the type of changes to which they were accustomed from working in fast-paced and changing project environments. Supporting quotes for these themes are provided in Table 11.1.

*Perceived organisational support during the early stages of COVID-19*

**Key Finding:** PM employers can assist in developing PM practitioners' career resilience through providing support resources such as: training and development interventions for professional growth; encouraging connections between colleagues and subordinates; and providing support directed at ensuring mental health and wellbeing.

In order to ascertain the level of support that respondents felt, respondents were asked whether they believed that their organisations were supportive during the early stage of the pandemic, and what measures were put in place to assist with their career resilience during the pandemic. There were 68.9% of respondents who commended their organisations for the initiatives they provided, which included i) managerial support, ii) job security, iii) working from home support mechanisms, iv) training and development opportunities, and v) enhanced communication. Conversely, 31.1% reported a lack of perceived support from their organisations during COVID-19. Perceived shortfalls in organisational support in Australia were comprised of i) a lack of management proactivity and foresight, ii) a lack of training in remote working technologies, and iii) a lack of managerial support. A few respondents considered that they bore individual responsibility and agency for developing their own career resilience. Some also believed it was their own individual responsibility to reach out and request support. However, since only a few respondents believed that individuals are solely responsible for their own career resilience, the findings suggest that employers are expected to play a role in the development and

*Table 11.1* Perceived career resilience during early COVID-19 and personal coping strategies.

### Enhanced Career Resilience

- **Increased adaptability**
  - *"The different ways of working remotely with no physical interaction with work colleagues proved to be productive and effective." (Participant 41)*
  - *"I now have better technology skills and resources to work remotely" (Participant 28)*
- **Positive mindset to embrace change**
  - *"There are so many ups and downs and we need to stay positive to continue our current workload and for our families and clients" (Participant 34)*
  - *"There will be challenges and there will be opportunities—you need to embrace both" (Participant 48)*
- **Focus on continual development**
  - *"Challenges faced only add to my skillset, and although it may be a setback for now, in the long run, I believe I will be better for it" (Participant 47)*
  - *"Everything else will be put in a subjective viewpoint and be less stressful and easier to manage in perspective once this has passed" (Participant 27)*
- **Better work-life balance**
  - *"In the scheme of things, these are things that should come ahead of work and I think having a better appreciation of what will assist me in separating my personal life from my work life and not letting the pressures of one affect the other" (Participant 5)*
  - *"From a personal health perspective mindset, this is an improvement" (Participant 12)*

### Lower Career Resilience

- **Stress from uncertain conditions**
  - *"I believe I will come out with greater job insecurity" (Participant 10)*
  - *"Less work and a greater pool of applicants…loss of income or high uncertainty…impetus for change is limited" (Participant 7)*

### No Change

- **Already developed level of career resilience**
  - *"I am already resilient enough" (Participant 13)*
  - *"I already have a high degree of resilience" (Participant 42)*
- **Drew on past experience**
  - *"After 27 years of project management in multiple organisations…I already have a reasonable degree of career resilience" (Participant 44)*
  - *"I already have career resilience, having worked across industries and sectors in public and private organisations" (Participant 36)*

*Table 11.2* Perceived organisational support during the early stage of COVID-19.

**Organisational support**

- **Managerial support & job security**
  - "To move out of their comfort zones" (Participant 41)
  - "No full-time staff would be made redundant" (Participant 8)
- **Work-from-home support mechanisms**
  - "A small work-from-home allowance to set up an office" (Participant 23)
  - "Technology was in place for all" (Participant 28)
- **Training & development opportunities**
  - "[My organisation] continued to promote people" (Participant 5)
  - "Encouraging us to look at online trainings and launching a newly upgraded learning management tool" (Participant 45)
- **Enhanced communications**
  - "[My organisation was] proactive with their communication" (Participant 24)
  - "Distribution of key information [a measure put in place by organisation to assist with career resilience during COVID-19]" (Participant 10)

**Lack of Organisational support**

- **No action/measures**
  - "Organisation did not have a clear documented policy for the pandemic in general" (Participant 1)
  - "No direct measures; more of a "continue with what you are doing and let us know what you might need" (Participant 27)
- **Lack of managerial support**
  - "WFH support has not been as good as it should have been, especially for IT and office setup" (Participant 26)
  - "They [management] did not check in to see whether we had the right equipment etc. (even basic things like headphones)" (Participant 5)
- **Lack of training support**
  - "During difficult times, things like training can be put to the side, as they're not considered a priority. So, training and development won't happen for a while" (Participant 26)
  - "Impediment to career resilience is that availability for training has been cut" (Participant 17)
- **Lack of proactivity & foresight**
  - "There was a great deal of panic and fear and they offloaded all their contractors with one week's notice" (Participant 6)
  - "[During COVID-19 I was] made redundant without any warning or notice" (Participant 7)

**Shared responsibility**

- "I don't feel there is much more they can do...individuals now need to take responsibility and ownership of how they work" (Participant 31)
- "Career resilience is my job to do" (Participant 20)

support of their employees' career resilience. It should be noted that these observations should be interpreted in the context of Australia, with relatively higher level of support during the pandemic. To provide more context, supporting quotes for these themes are provided in Table 11.2.

The results reveal that while a large proportion of organisations in Australia provided support resources which contributed to the development of their employees' career resilience, there were some that did not. Consistent with JD-R theory, most PM practitioners indicated that their organisations had provided supportive tools such as extra training and development initiatives, feedback mechanisms, supportive management interactions, and initiatives aimed at ensuring mental health and wellbeing to assist with the management of their COVID-19-related job demands. However, while most organisations seemed to be providing tools to achieving career resilience, extra effort was required to create "the open environment, and opportunities for assessing and developing the skills" (Waterman et al., 1994, p. 88). Some respondents indicated that their workload prevented them from making use of these resources. Almost a third of respondents reported their organisation did not offer any support to facilitate their PM practitioners' career resilience during the early stage of the pandemic.

## Implications for practice and research

### *Practical implications for organisations*

When sudden shocks like COVID-19 cause an imbalance between job demands and job resources, organisations need to offer resources to their PM practitioners directed at developing and boosting their career resilience. The findings of this study support the view that the development of career resilience requires the combined efforts of both employees and their employers (CAC, 2019). It was promising to see that a large proportion of organisations were actively fulfilling their role in providing support resources aimed at encouraging the development of career-resilient PM practitioners who were well-equipped to manage sudden shocks and stressful job demands. However, the findings show that there is still room for improvement in terms of the level of support resources provided during times of shock, as well as providing employees with adequate time and opportunity to utilise them.

This study suggests that in order to support the development of career resilience in their PM workforce, organisations should provide support resources such as training and mentoring opportunities, fostering closer connections between colleagues and subordinates, and providing initiatives targeted at enhancing mental health and wellbeing. In addition to providing these resource opportunities, organisations should work with their employees to strategise how individuals can take advantage of these support mechanisms if they are to maximise the benefits which accrue to both their PM practitioners' individual careers and their organisation's success. By supporting interventions such as mentoring, support, and feedback channels (London, 1993; Chiaburu et al., 2006), organisations can create an environment that enables the lessons learnt by experienced project managers to be shared between employees, which will assist in the management of stress through enhanced coping skills (Peterson et al., 2011).

### Limitations of the study

There are some limitations to this study which should be considered when interpreting the findings. The method of data collection via an online survey did not provide the opportunity to probe or clarify respondents' responses (Evans and Mathur, 2005). However, some research (e.g., Miles and Huberman, 1994; Foddy, 1993) shows that the anonymity of a survey can be advantageous to avoid interviewer effects and to increase the likelihood of obtaining honest and uncensored information on the participants' experiences. A further limitation to the study is associated with the time horizon and location in which the study was undertaken. This study was not longitudinal and is limited to the Australian context. However, its cross-sectional nature aligns with the aim of exploring the career resilience and experiences of PM practitioners at a particular point in time, i.e., during the COVID-19 pandemic. A longitudinal design would take into account that career resilience can alter in response to contextual changes over time, while other contexts can provide more nuances to implications in different conditions such as lower level of support. Further, the adoption of a single theory (JD-R) limits the explanation of the findings to this particular lens.

### Implications for future research

It is hoped that this study will stimulate further research on career resilience, a capability which is essential for enabling individuals to maintain their careers in the volatile 21st century. There is a need for more research into the relationship between career resilience and PM practitioners' health and wellbeing during the inevitable shocks, stresses, and challenges encountered in their project work environments. It is recommended that future research adopts alternative theoretical lenses like social learning theory (Savickas, 2005), happenstance theory (Bright et al., 2005), and person/environment fit (Super, 1975). Studies can also use a longitudinal design to capture and explore the longer-term effects of the pandemic and its aftermath on the careers of PM practitioners. Further research could identify, measure, and monitor organisational support mechanisms to assess the relative effectiveness of different initiatives. More attention to the research area of career resilience will assist in understanding the necessary actions and strategies required by PM practitioners and their organisations to survive in a dynamic work context while maintaining a positive and sustainable career trajectory.

### Conclusions

The purpose of this chapter was to understand the impact that the shocks and stressors associated with the emergence of the COVID-19 pandemic presented to the wellbeing of PM practitioners. The JD-R theory was used to highlight that both

PM practitioners and their organisations have a role in ensuring that necessary support mechanisms and job resources are in place to help them cope with challenging job demands. PM practitioners who reported high degrees of personal resilience (a capacity associated with maintaining wellbeing in the face of adversity) perceived that this resulted from their maintaining a positive mindset, having access to support networks, and ensuring they had good work-life balance. They viewed that their own personal efforts were bolstered by key support initiatives provided by their organisation during the early stage of the pandemic. Our findings show that organisations can develop and support the career resilience of their workforce by providing an intensified focus on health and wellbeing initiatives, maintaining connections and communications between work teams, providing training and development opportunities for PM practitioners to enhance their job resources, and ensuring they feel secure in their jobs. Therefore, organisations play a critical role in nurturing a career-resilient and adaptable workforce – a key success factor in challenging circumstances like the COVID-19 work environment. This analysis of the lived experience of PM practitioners contributes new knowledge on how career resilience was fostered in the context of the project management profession during the early stage of the pandemic. Practical recommendations have been provided for PM practitioners and their organisations to assist them in maintaining a positive state of health and wellbeing and strong levels of career resilience in the event of future shocks or challenges.

## References

AIPM (Australian Institute of Project Management). (2021). The diversity challenge: AIPM gender equity report 2021. *AIPM Website*. Available at https://f.hub spotusercontent10.net/hubfs/7399164/AIPM%20Gender%20Equity%20in%20 the%20Workplace%202021%20V5.pdf?hsCtaTracking=c5a5b998-1393-4da8-9ad4-0d79667ab3df%7C64c970b7-d3df-4335-949d-a135c063595d (Accessed 30 July 2022).

Akkermans, J., & Kubasch, S. (2017). Trending topics in careers: A review and future research agenda. *Career Development International*, 22(6), 586–627.

Akkermans, J., Richardson, J., & Kraimer, M.L. (2020). The COVID-19 crisis as a career shock: Implications for careers and vocational behaviour. *Journal of Vocational Behaviour*, 119, 103–134.

Akkermans, J., Seibert, S.E., & Mol, S.T. (2018). Tales of the unexpected: Integrating career shocks in the contemporary career's literature. *SA Journal of Industrial Psychology*, 44, 1503.

Bakker, A.B., & Demerouti, E. (2014). *Job demands: Resources theory in wellbeing*. Hoboken, NJ: John Wiley & Sons Ltd.

Bengtsson, M. (2016). How to plan and perform a qualitative study using content analysis. *NursingPlus Open*, 2, 8–14.

Bezuidenhout, M. (2011). *The development and evaluation of a measure of graduate employability in the context of the new world of work*. Unpublished master's dissertation, University of Pretoria, Pretoria.

Bowen, P., Govender, G., Edwards, E., & Cattell, K. (2017). Work-related contact, work: Family conflict, psychological distress and sleep problems experienced by construction professionals: An integrated explanatory model. *Construction Management and Economics*, 36(3), 153–174.

Bright, J.E.H., Pryor, R.G.L., & Harpham, L. (2005). The role of chance events in career decision making. *Journal of Vocational Behavior*, 66, 561–576.

Brundage, H., & Koziel, M. (2010). Retaining top talent. *Journal of Accountancy*, 38–44.

Bushuyev, S., Bushuiev, D., & Bushuieva, V. (2020). Project management during infodemic of the COVID-19 pandemic. *Innovative Technologies and Scientific Solutions for Industries*, 2(12), 13–21.

Career Action Centre. (2019). *Career action centre*. Available at www.careeractioncentre.com.au/.

Cascio, W. (2007). Trends, paradoxes, and some directions for research in career studies. In *Handbook of career studies* (pp. 549–557). Los Angeles: SAGE Publications.

Cavanagh, S. (1997). Content analysis: Concepts, methods and applications. *Nurse Researcher*, 4(3), 5–16.

Chiaburu, D.S., Baker, V.L., & Pitariu, A.H. (2006). Beyond being proactive: What (else) matters for career self-management behaviors? *Career Development International*, 11(7), 619–632.

Daniels, C., & Radel, K. (2018). Career resilience in 21st century Australian labour markets, [conference presentation]. 29th Annual Conference of the Australian and New Zealand Academy of Management, New Zealand. Available at https://www.anzam.org/wp-content/uploads/pdf-manager/2639_205.PDF (Accessed 17 June 2020).

Darling, E.J., & Whitty, S.J. (2019). A model of projects as a source of stress at work: A case for scenario-based education and training. *International Journal of Managing Projects in Business*, 1753–8378.

De Vos, A., & Van der Heijden, B.I.J.M. (2015). *Handbook of research on sustainable careers*. Cheltenham: Edward Elgar Publishing.

Evans, J.R., & Mathur, A. (2005). The value of online surveys. *Internet Research*, 15(2), 195–219.

Foddy, M., & Crundall, I. (1993). A field study of social comparison processes in ability evaluation. *British Journal of Social Psychology*, 32, 287–305.

Greenhaus, J.H., Callanan, G.A., & Godshalk, V.M. (2010). *Career management* (4th ed.). London: Sage.

Harari, O. (1995). The new job security. *Your Management Review*, 84(9), 29–31.

Hite, L.M., & McDonald, K.S. (2020). Careers after COVID-19: Challenges and changes. *Human Resource Development International*, 23(4), 427–437.

Hsieh, H.F., & Shannon, S.E. (2005). Three approaches to qualitative content analysis. *Qualitative Health Research*, 15(9), 1277–1288.

Isaac, S., & Michael, W.B. (1997). *Handbook in research and evaluation: A collection of principles, methods, and strategies useful in the planning, design, and evaluation of studies in education and the behavioral sciences*. (3rd ed.). San Diego: Educational and Industrial Testing Services.

Lazarus, R., & Folkman, S. (1984). *Stress, appraisal and coping*. New York: Springer.

London, M. (1993). Relationships between career motivation, empowerment and support for career development. *Journal of Occupational and Organizational Psychology*, 66, 55–69.

London, M. (1997). Overcoming career barriers: A model of cognitive and emotional processes for realistic appraisal and constructive coping. *Journal of Career Development*, 24(1), 25–38.

Luthans, F. (2002). The need for and meaning of positive organisational behavior. *Journal of Organisational Behavior: The International Journal of Industrial, Occupational and Organisational Psychology and Behavior*, 23(6), 695–706.

Lynn, B.E. (2000). Intellectual capital. *Ivey Business Journal*, 64(13), 48–51.

Mack, O., Khare, A., Kramer, A., & Burgartz, T. (2016). *Managing in a VUCA world*. Switzerland: Springer International Publishing.

Miles, M.B., & Huberman, A.M. (1994). *Qualitative data analysis: An expanded sourcebook*. Thousand Oaks, CA: Sage Publications Inc.

Pallant, J., & Manual, S.S. (2020). *A step-by-step guide to data analysis using SPSS*. Berkshire, UK: McGraw-Hill Education.

Patil, G.V. (2016). Project management challenges. *Journal of Multidisciplinary Engineering Science and Technology*, 3(11), 6019–6024.

Peterson, B.D., Pirritano, M., Block, J.M., & Schmidt, L. (2011). Marital benefit and coping strategies in men and women undergoing unsuccessful fertility treatments over a 5-year period. *Fertility and Sterility*, 95(5), 1759–1763.

Project Management Institute (PMI). (2019). The future of work leading the way with PMTQ. *Project Management Institute Website*. Available at https://www.pmi.org/-/media/pmi/documents/public/pdf/learning/thought-leadership/pulse/pulse-of-the-profession-2019.pdf?sc_lang_temp=en (Accessed 11 December 2021).

Rossier, J., Ginevra, M.C., Bollmann, G., & Nota, L. (2017). The importance of career adaptability, career resilience, and employability in designing a successful life. In K. Maree (ed.), *Psychology of career adaptability, employability and resilience* (pp. 65–82). Champagne: Springer.

Ruize-Martin, C., Lopez-Paredes, A., & Wainer, G. (2018). What we know and do not know about organizational resilience. *International Journal of Production Management and Engineering*, 6(1), 11–28.

Saunders, M.N.K, Lewis, P., Thornhill, A., & Bristow, A. (2015). Understanding research philosophy and approaches to theory development. In M.N.K. Saunders, P. Lewis, & A. Thornhill (eds.), *Research methods for business students* (8th ed.). Harlow: Pearson Education.

Savickas, M.L. (2005). The theory and practice of career construction. In S.D. Brown & R.W. Lent (eds.), *Career development and counselling: Putting theory and research to work*. Hoboken, NJ: Wiley.

Seibert, S.E., Kraimer, M.L., & Heslin, P.A. (2016). Developing career resilience and adaptability. *Organizational Dynamics*, 45, 245–257.

Seibert, S.E., Kraimer, M.L., Holton, B.C., & Pierotti, A.J. (2013). Even the best laid plans sometimes go askew: Career self-management processes, career shocks, and the decision to pursue graduate education. *Journal of Applied Psychology*, 98(1), 169–182.

Super, D.E. (1975). Career education and career guidance for the life span and for life roles. *Journal of Career Education*, 2(2), 27–42.

Waterman, R.H., Waterman, J.A., & Betsy, C.A. (1994). Towards a career resilient workforce. *Harvard Business Review*, 87–95.

Zull, C. (2016). *Open-ended questions (version 2.0)*. Mannheim: GESIS-Leibniz-Institut für Sozialwissenschaften.

# 12 Assessing how pandemic lockdown upended construction work creed in Free State and Limpopo, South Africa

*Rose Matete and Fidelis Emuze*

## Introduction

Notably, the outbreak of the COVID-19 pandemic in March 2020 found a vulnerable South African economy. And as a result, the COVID-19 pandemic deepened the economic crisis (Republic of South Africa [RSA], 2020). Some measures introduced at the time faced resistance (Assaad and El-adaway, 2021). Even though the lockdown may be an essential strategy to break the chain of transmission, in response to the pandemic, the closure of businesses resulting from the inability to work safely without risk of exposure to the coronavirus was welcomed. For instance, clients and contractors must implement designs that enable social distancing and regular disinfecting facilities (Raliile, et al., 2021). Stiles, et al. (2020) argue that the implications of COVID-19 on construction are twofold. On the one hand, work was halted or changed, and new projects were paused while construction practices came to terms with new ways of working. On the other hand, sites have had to adjust to social distancing, implementing new hygiene and personal protective equipment (PPE) measures, and accommodating a greater level of working from home for roles that are not essential to front-line work (Aigbavboa et al., 2021; Alsharef et al., 2021; Ataei et al., 2021).

Bou Hatoum, et al.(2021) argued that while construction workers are the heartbeat of every construction project, there has been little discussion on workers' perception of the pandemic and the effectiveness of the newly established safety measures. This chapter reports on a study that assesses how the sudden lockdown restrictions upended work creed (rules) from the view of PiC.

## Research method

This chapter shows how COVID-19-related restrictions changed occupational health and safety (OHS) rules followed by people in construction (PiC). This has been done through qualitative data collection in the Free State and Limpopo, South Africa. Participants of the study had to answer questions that assessed the impact of the lockdown rule on H&S procedures, which ranged from the implications for hazard identification and risk assessment in construction sites, the implementation of H&S plan, H&S induction of workers, periodic safety audits, and

DOI: 10.1201/9781003278368-14

implementation of the compulsory medical fitness, examination, and testing of construction workers.

This section explains the procedure and methods used in collecting, organising, analysing, and synthesising the data. The study explored how the sudden lockdown restrictions upended work creed (rules) about the OHS of PiC. A qualitative approach was used, and primary data were collected through a semi-structured interview schedule (Creswell, 2014). The sample stratum included stakeholders who are professionals in the employ of state organs, consulting firms, and registered contractors in two South African provinces, the Free State and Limpopo. The 25 participants were identified through convenient sampling recruited in the Free State and Limpopo provinces through a professional working relationship with the principal investigator (PI). The PI called all the respondents to schedule telephonic interviews, and appointments were scheduled with each respondent. Informed consent was discussed in detail at the beginning of each interview, which included an emphasis on confidentiality and the significance of the study. After securing approval, telephonic interviews commenced. The interview protocols were sent through email for participants to familiarise themselves with the content and context. The PI conducted all telephonic interviews. Eighteen (18) interview textual data were analysed. Nine images were obtained from one research participant at a construction site in Giyani, Limpopo; the advantage of using visual materials is that people easily relate to ideas because they are so pervasive in our society. Pictures of the site were taken in June 2020.

Data were stored in the computer in audio recordings, portable document format (pdf) notes, and Microsoft Word for transcribed scripts (Kumar, 2014). All data were assigned codes to protect the identity of the participants. The method of analysis adopted in this study was deductive, and manual coding was used to manage the data. The data consisted of over 9½ hours of audio, which documented more than 165 hours of interviews, 152 pages of transcriptions, field notes, and nine pictures shared by one of the participants. Three participants were re-contacted to address some omissions and inadvertent failures to record certain information. Data screening was done manually to ensure that data were accurate and complete, and the PI performed the data analysis.

## Results and discussion

### *Demographic information*

Table 12.1 presents the demographic information of the participants involved in project planning, supervision, monitoring and reporting, building designs, construction management, administration, acquiring of contracts when awarded, scaling of resources, recruitment of experienced staff, and mobilisation of resources. The H&S practitioners are involved in compiling weekly and monthly reports, conducting toolbox talks, risk assessments (RA), safe work procedures (SOPs),

*Table 12.1* Demographic information.

| Profession | Employer | Position |
| --- | --- | --- |
| Architect (1) | Consulting firm (1) | Architectural technologist (1) |
| Quantity surveyor (1) | Consulting firm (1) | Junior quantity surveyor (1) |
| Civil engineer (3) | State Department/ Construction company (3) | Control works inspector/ Contracts manager/ Administrator (3) |
| Electrical engineer (2) | Construction company/state-owned enterprise (2) | General manager maintenance/ director/project manager (2) |
| Project manager (3) | State-owned enterprise/ construction company (3) | Construction manager/General supervisor (3) |
| Procurement Manager (1) | Construction company (1) | Bid office manager (1) |
| Construction (H&S) practitioner (5) | Consulting firm/construction company (5) | H&S officer/director/regional HSE specialist Limpopo (5) |
| Contractor (2) | Construction company (2) | Managing director/director (2) |

planning job observations, reviewing H&S/excavation and fall protection plans, and monitoring and reviewing task-specific RA. Additionally, they perform daily personal protective equipment (PPE) inspections, vehicle inspections, site inspections, and upkeep of H&S registers and COVID-19 screening registers. They also conduct site H&S audits, site inspections, induction training, and administration; prepare H&S files, oversee H&S compliance on construction sites and advise contractors on matters of compliance with the South African Occupational Health and Safety Act, 85. 1993.

The textual data from the interviews are presented in subheadings.

### The impact on hazard identification and risk assessment in construction sites

Participants experienced an impact as most projects were put on hold. They had to review their hazard, identification, and risk assessment (HIRA), and workers had to be trained to identify and protect themselves against the virus. State officials would vacate offices to allow workers time to complete their work. However, when they tested positive they locked up offices, which required contractors to wait for them to unlock offices, which caused some delays in their programmes. Others continued to have continuous risk assessments to identify and assess risks; there were high stress levels, and some workers lost their jobs. H&S officers were trained on the COVID-19 HIRA. H&S plans now cover COVID-19. Additionally, they experienced the placement of sanitation stations in multiple areas and improved H&S management systems for COVID-19. Those who disagree have not experienced an impact because they conduct HIRA daily and continue to check their risk assessment.

**The impact on the implementation of the H&S plan on construction sites**

Most participants (89%) experienced an impact because previous H&S plans never included COVID-19 and they had to review their plans to cover COVID-19 protocols, for implementation and introduction of the mandatory mask-up, use of sanitisers, placing of security personnel at access points, and COVID-19 signage. H&S officers had to ensure everyone on site followed the rules and instructions; contractors were forced to implement their plans and ensure that sanitisers and PPE were adequately procured (Figures 12.1 and 12.2). Other participants expressed that many contractors continued with work without amendments to their H&S plans. Additional requirements had to be implemented immediately; implementation of H&S plans is now costly, and clients had to allocate supplemental budgets to comply with COVID-19 requirements. COVID-19 protocols have overtaken the H&S plan as people now talk more about the COVID-19 pandemic.

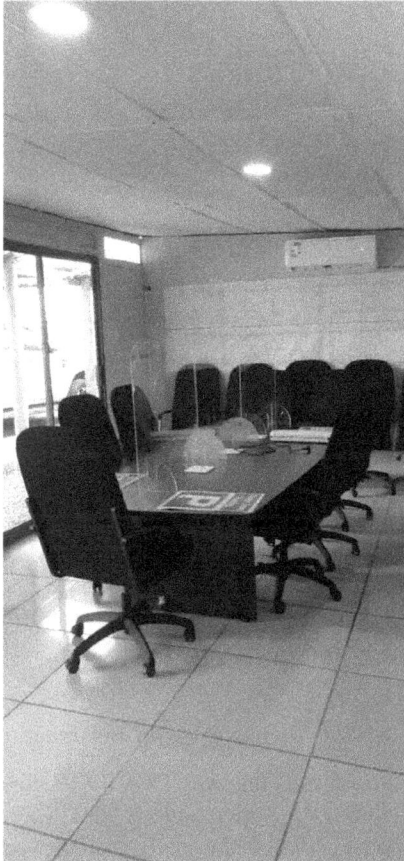

*Figure 12.1* COVID-19 screening in the boardroom.

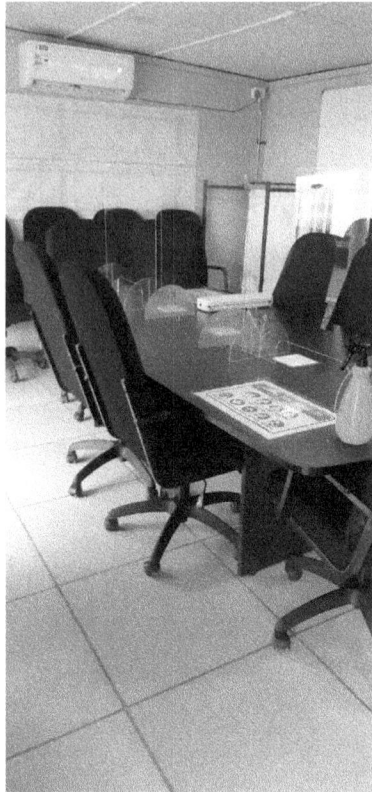

*Figure 12.2* Sanitiser and signage in the boardroom.

### The increased rate of absenteeism among workers in construction

Participants experience absenteeism after people have been vaccinated and after testing positive for COVID-19. Workers submit false sickness claims and fake other illnesses. Absenteeism becomes a major challenge as workers abscond from work claiming that they were exposed to COVID-19. Some participants mentioned that they had not experienced absenteeism due to COVID-19; in fact, they are of the view that workers wouldn't be absent unnecessarily and risk being laid off as a result because they rely on their salaries for survival.

### The impact on the bi-weekly toolbox talks on construction sites

Participants had to design topics in line with COVID-19, amend their previous topics, and maintain social distancing during toolbox talks. They experienced extended working hours due to toolbox talks. Additionally, their bi-weekly toolbox talks were changed to weekly. COVID-19 pandemic has become a topic on its own as COVID-19 statistics had to be obtained daily and communicated during the toolbox talks.

## The impact on H&S induction of workers on construction sites

Participants experienced the inability to conduct site-based induction. For instance, general workers on construction sites worked without being inducted. Online inductions were undertaken, which excluded most contractors and only management, and their head office-based workers accessed the training while community-based workers could not. They also included COVID-19 protocols and risks of COVID-19, emphasised the need for social distancing, use of sanitisers, wearing of cloth masks, and workers' interaction among themselves in every induction. Employers increased their efforts for H&S induction, and regular induction was conducted. COVID-19 protocols were incorporated into induction training programmes and compliance was strictly monitored by clients.

## The impact on routine daily safety inspections on construction sites

Participants agree that routine safety inspections were impacted because current daily checks include COVID-19 screening, which is positive. Workers disinfect their hand tools, and workers and H&S representatives conduct inspections before workers perform their site activities. Additionally, inspections improved, and daily safety inspections included checking up on the use of cloth masks, washing hands, provision of paper towels in toilets, and regular hygiene inspections. They further mention that checklists were used to monitor compliance. Some participants argue that in some construction sites, workers were just working without adhering to COVID-19 rules.

## The impact on the periodic safety audits on construction sites

Participants have experienced an impact since the audits have to cover COVID-19 prevention or control measures, including COVID-19 screening and sanitation stations. They had to provide for COVID-19 protocols and compliance. Participants also agreed that the audits were happening monthly to ensure compliance. Participants also stated more time is spent now than before during site safety audits. Some participants argue that audits were not happening on most construction sites since everybody just wanted to complete their work while their minds were preoccupied with the deaths. They went further to state that audits are not done accordingly since the lockdown rules came into effect.

## The impact on compulsory medical fitness of construction workers

Participants agreed that the medicals were done to ensure workers are set to return to work, and this ensures that those who are found not to be safe had to be quarantined at a formal facility. This caused a nightmare because of all the procedures that happened before people could start work. There has also been a positive impact considering that when employers would want to bring workers to their sites, their COVID-19 statuses would have been confirmed in due time. Others mention that they conduct continuous medical examinations to ensure that the certificates of medical fitness are updated. Compulsory medical fitness, inspection, and testing of a worker could be undertaken to cover essential COVID-19 screening to confirm their statuses. And this has an impact on the financial position of contractors in terms of loss of production time. Some participants argue that isolation that happens when people are awaiting their results from being suspected of having COVID-19 has an impact on production as workers must stay at home. Additionally, contractors didn't have complete access to people they could employ while starting up projects. Work schedules were extended as H&S severe measures had to be implemented to ensure everything is under control and workers obey the rules and follow instructions due to document processing.

### The impact on the provision and use of PPE on construction sites

Participants experienced a negative impact because of increased costs from additional procurement of clothes, masks, buying more PPE than before the pandemic, and lack of finances. They also experienced increased costs because of the requirements on the safe disposal of surgical masks. They mentioned that subcontractors struggle to provide PPE as they depend on supplies from their main contractors, they face some challenges from their workers who don't use the items issued to them as required, and they are also affected by budgets which have been a problem because they never made sufficient allocations while tendering. The positive impact has been that workers now have additional PPE. Participants noted that there have been some challenges when it comes to the mandatory use of cloth masks in construction, because workers are familiar with the wearing of safety boots and overalls and not the cloth masks, as they have been expected to do. There have been some positive impacts as workers used to exchange PPE on sites, and this practice has ended. They had to increase items such as safety gloves and overalls even in summer and provide cloth masks simultaneously with face shields for extra protection. It has been a priority for contractors to ensure they provide PPE for workers to be easily identified at their construction sites. Additionally, monitoring compliance through safety inspections and periodic audits has benefited workers. Lastly, even though contractors are compelled to provide additional PPE, clients now face the challenge of allocating additional funds for PPE provision.

### The impact on the provision and use of workers' rest areas on construction sites

Participants experienced an impact because workers had to be trained in social distancing and daily monitoring of the areas for the number of people inside, and to check the extent to which sites can prevent the spread of COVID-19. They must put more chairs in their rest areas and in areas where sharing spaces was no longer allowed due to social distancing. In most of the construction sites, rest areas provided were too small and workers couldn't sit and eat the same way they did before the pandemic started. Secondly, those who didn't have large enough areas to accommodate all their workers had to allow workers to rest outside, as they felt it was safer that way. In some sites, they had to provide additional rest areas. Some contractors were forced to reduce their workforce to comply with the lockdown rule. Additionally, they experienced an impact from the government that recommended that people shouldn't share and use eating utensils which used to be kept in their eating areas, and as a result, each person had to carry their equipment with them daily to work, which was also used to avoid reuse without cleaning up after multiple users.

### The impact on the provision and use of hand-washing facilities on construction sites

Most of the participants (83%) experienced an impact because water, hand sanitisers, and hand wash soaps are available unlike before the pandemic. Workers are also constantly cleaning their hands, so contractors needed to go an extra mile in the provision of the facilities, which has a financial impact. Figure 12.3 presents facilities provided on-site. Additionally, a positive impact on workers is that compliance has been consistent. Some participants have experienced additional facilities, which are even more accessible to workers.

### The rule resulting in amendments to the H&S policies

The majority of the participants (72%) agreed that they experienced amendments to the H&S policies to accommodate new H&S rules, address masking up, face shields, sanitisers, and social distancing to incorporate COVID-19 measures, issues of employees testing positive, the handling of incident claims to the Department of Employment and Labour (DEL), and to improve COVID-19 PPE policies in their existing one and to communicate the policy to their employees. The DEL also provided additional training for nurses, employees were no longer exchanging cars,

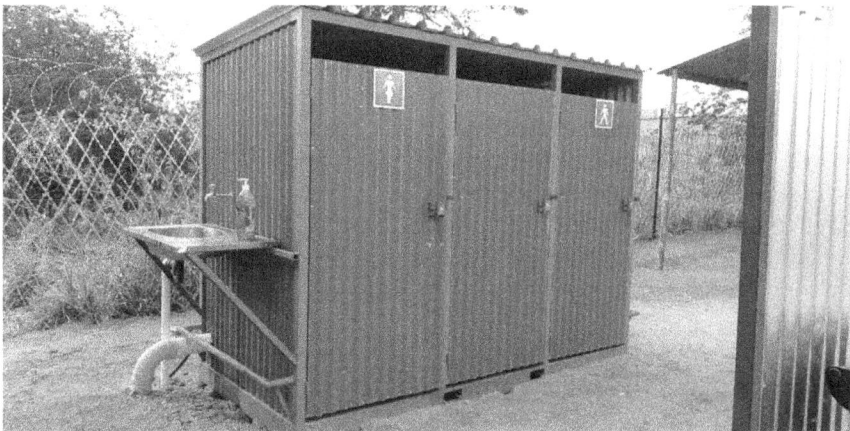

*Figure 12.3* Provision of toilet/hand wash facilities.

and they had to implement a one-worker/one-car policy, which could be additional costs to the clients and contractors.

### The impact on the transportation of workers to the construction sites

Most participants (78%) experienced an impact due to travel permits that were issued during alert level 5, increased trips on transporting workers to their sites, limiting the number of workers taken by their vehicles, which affected production time, sanitisation of transport vehicles, and increased costs associated with social distancing in buses or construction vehicles as social distancing resulted in more trips to their sites. Additionally, modes of transport became difficult as normal transport was not freely available, which resulted in some workers coming to work late.

### Impact of on social distancing on construction site productivity

Participants experience social distancing in eating areas, working areas, toolbox talks, during induction training, and when entering construction sites. They also mention that social distancing has negatively impacted the performance of activities and work programs. Communication on construction sites has also been negatively impacted; contractors are unable to meet their targets, and this has resulted in delay of project completion periods. However, some argued that it ensured workers adhered to social distancing practices. Workers who have been vaccinated have developed a tendency not to mask up or observe social distancing protocols. Some workers continue to work closely in small spaces, such as in truck-mounted buckets. They also mention that some workers feel unpleasant about being closer to other workers.

### The impact of sanitising measures on construction sites

Participants experienced an impact as workers continue to sanitise the same way it has been implemented nationally. Additionally, sanitising confers increased hygiene levels for workers as they don't experience a lot of infections among themselves. They mention that there is continuous use of sanitisers on sites. Participants who disagree argue that workers overuse sanitisers, and this is seen to reduce productivity on sites. Additionally, it has a negative impact on production time as hand tools need to be disinfected before and after use. The rule on sanitisers still needs to be implemented correctly, as they are being utilised without consistency.

### The impact of mask-up measures on construction sites

Participants experienced strict wearing of masks throughout their shift, and this benefits workers as fewer infections are being recorded. H&S officers and safety representatives enforce and closely monitor the use of masks without compromise.

Workers regularly wear their masks, and everyone who enters their gates also wears masks. They have COVID-19 awareness signage, and they implement a no-mask/no-entry policy at all gates and site offices. Additionally, masks were worn by workers working in dusty areas, but now masking up is compulsory. They mention that workers can't cope with mask-up, especially when they are bending and climbing up ladders; they complain that it gets hard for them to breathe, which negatively impacts productivity. It was noted that some employers also fail to adequately provide masks, and some workers only wear their masks when H&S officers approach them.

### The impact of isolation measures on construction sites

Participants initially experienced perfect practice of isolation; however, isolation was no longer in practice. They experienced workers who faked their illnesses while they were sent to isolation under false pretence. Again, people confused isolation with quarantine, as they were seen isolating for longer periods. They also mention that recommended isolation periods of 10–14 days hampered production. They experienced a negative financial impact on workers who were isolated as construction implements a no-work/no-pay policy, which also negatively affects all stakeholders as it results in a lack of site activities. Furthermore, workers became anxious when colleagues were isolated. Some participants have not experienced any impact because they don't have close contact activities, while other companies kept their positive COVID-19 cases secret without implementing isolation.

### The impact of vaccination measures on construction sites

Participants mention that a lot of people have volunteered to take the vaccine, and many continue to request time off duty to get the vaccination. Contractors are currently encouraging workers to obtain vaccine certificates. Others argue that vaccination has not been influenced by the rule and that vaccination doesn't affect construction sites negatively. They also mention that some workers are afraid that vaccines will result in their vulnerability to some sicknesses which can result in loss of their income. They also expressed those conspiracies to cause mixed feelings and panic among workers; as a result, implementation is quite slow from the lack of knowledge and information among workers. Some contractors have experienced between 30–50% vaccination rates among workers. They expressed that people's belief systems and the media influence their decision on vaccinations. They further mention that propaganda significantly drives negativity, and mandatory vaccination is likely to increase the rates once implemented, while workers will be fighting to keep their jobs.

### Conclusions

The primary purpose of this chapter is to assess how the sudden lockdown restrictions upended work creed (rules) in relation to the OHS of PiC. The newly established changes to the rule resulted in amendments to the H&S practices, implementation of social distancing, sanitisers, mask-up measures, isolation, and vaccination. Routine site safety inspections and audits included COVID-19 screening for the identification of positive cases. Workers can no longer start any activities without the disinfection of hand tools and work equipment. Vehicles must be sanitised before workers can be transported to sites. Compulsory medical fitness, examination, and testing associated with COVID-19 have resulted in project delays. Workers misused isolation as they fake sicknesses while claiming to be either sick or being persons under investigation. This has cost implications to the clients and contractors. Limiting the number of workers accessing rest areas, toilets, and hand wash facilities delayed work activities.

As presented in Figure 12.1, the themes developed from literature indicate that, due to the lockdown rule, construction is bearing huge losses due to unexpected delays and suspended operations for the sake of workers' OHS. Findings revealed that most contractors amended their HIRA and H&S plans to cover COVID-19 before they could resume their construction site activities, and monitoring of H&S compliance by stakeholders has increased through routine site inspections and periodic H&S audits. Induction training of workers and toolbox talks were ramped up. Contractors and clients experience increased costs resulting from the implementation of their policies and H&S plans, which have resulted from mandatory mask-up, use of sanitisers, and PPE. Furthermore, the H&S measures that have been introduced have been a blessing in disguise when it comes to the prevention and control of risks on construction sites since the PiC has seen improved levels of protection through stricter enforcement by authorities. Even though some of the PiC may feel that there has not been much change in certain matters of H&S compliance, a lot has been gained by the industry, and direct benefits have been experienced.

## Acknowledgement

We would like to express our special thanks to all the participants of this study. Their participation in this wonderful project of a chapter in a book on *"Construction Safety, Health and Well-being in the COVID-19 Era"* is of great value to our industry. We would like to say that Occupational Safety and Health is a shared responsibility. Lastly, we would like to thank our families for their support and encouragement as we finalised this project in a limited time.

## References

Aigbavboa, C.O., Aghimien, D.O., Thwala, W.D., & Ngozwana, M.N. (2021). Unprepared industry meet pandemic: COVID-19 and the South Africa construction industry. *Journal of Engineering, Design and Technology*, 20(1), 183–200.
Alsharef, A., Banerjee, S., Uddin, S.M.J., Albert, A., & Jaselskis, E. (2021). Early impacts of the COVID-19 pandemic on the United States construction industry. *International Journal of Environmental Research and Public Health*, 18(4), 1559–1579.

Assaad, R., & El-adaway, I.H. (2021). Guidelines for responding to COVID-19 pandemic: Best practices, impacts, and future research directions. *Journal of Management in Engineering*, 37(3), 1–17.

Ataei, H., Becker, D., Hellenbrand, J.R., Mehany, M.S.H.M., Mitchell, T.E., & Ponte, D.M. (2021). *COVID-19 pandemic impacts on construction projects*. Reston, VA: ASCE.

Bou Hatoum, M., Faisal, A., Nassereddine, H., & Sarvari, H. (2021). Analysis of COVID-19 concerns raised by the construction workforce and development of mitigation practices. *Frontiers in Built Environment*, 7(688495), 1–15. doi: 10.3389/fbuil.2021.688495.

Creswell, J.W. (2014). *Research design: Qualitative, quantitative, and mixed methods approach* (4th ed.). Thousand Oaks, CA: SAGE Publications, Inc.

Kumar, R. (2014). *Research methodology: A step by step guide for beginners* (4th ed.). Los Angeles: SAGE Publications Ltd.

Raliile, M.T., Haupt, T.C., & Akinlolu, M. (2021). Rethinking construction health and safety legislation compliance: Lessons learnt from COVID-19. Proceedings of the Joint CIB W099 & W123 Annual International Conference 2021: Good Health, Changes & Innovations for Improved Wellbeing in Construction, 9th–10th September, Glasgow (on-line), UK, pp. 337–346.

Stiles, S., Golightly, D., & Ryan, B. (2020). Impact of COVID-19 on health and safety in the construction sector. *Human Factors and Ergonomics in Manufacturing & Service Industries*, 31(4), 425–437.

Republic of South Africa (RSA). (2020). *The South African economic reconstruction and recovery plan*. Pretoria: South African Government.

# 13 COVID-19 pandemic

## A case study of mental health of migrant construction workers at TTDI Sentralis, Selangor, Malaysia

*Mohd Amizan Mohamed @ Arifin,
Nur Izzati Sofia Shuhaimi, Syahirah Intan
Mohd Sheffie and Nazirah Mohd Apandi*

## 1.0 Introduction

The COVID-19 pandemic has impacted the lives of billions of people throughout the world (Pandey et al., 2021). The Malaysian Government introduced the MCO and total lockdown and applied it to the Prevention and Control of Infectious Diseases Act 1988 and the Police Act 1967. Throughout the years of 2020 and 2021, several phases of the MCO have been implemented across the country. Consequently, the construction sector was one of the sectors that was greatly affected as all work got halted immediately owing to the implementation of the MCO. As mentioned in The Straits Times (2020), the Senior Minister of Works, Datuk Seri Fadillah Yusof, suggests that Malaysia's construction industry had lost RM18.5 billion in the first three phases of the country's lockdown while complying with the order aimed at preventing the spread of the coronavirus. With the MCO being implemented, which has caused most non-essential industries to be on hold, the public has been significantly affected by work-related stress, alongside adapting to the new norms while also complying with the new boundaries set by the government (Pandey et al., 2021).

According to (Wahab, 2020) research, Malaysia is home to around two million migrant workers. Migrant construction workers in Malaysia are known for living in cramped accommodations, which made it hard for them to practice social distancing, and even exposed them to vulnerabilities of the life-threatening COVID-19 virus. In fact, as a result, many of them were infected with COVID-19. Research by Tan et al. (2020) reveals that out of 14,187 migrant construction workers who were screened for COVID-19, 676 of them tested positive. Foreign workers were reported to account for 11.8% of Malaysia's confirmed cases.

Due to the extended duration of the MCO, many migrant workers may have suffered from psychological effects such as stress, sadness, and anxiety. The COVID-19 pandemic may have resulted in most workers losing part or even all of their income (Mathiaparanam, 2020). Despite still being employed, workers in most industries are forced to comply with reduced hours and salary cutbacks (International Labour Organization (2020): Poor mental health can affect productivity,

DOI: 10.1201/9781003278368-15

performance, physical health, safety, and well-being in the workplace (Nwaogu et al., 2020). According to Wahab (2020), most migrant construction workers primarily live in *kongsi* houses with an average of 80 people. Therefore, they were suspected of being more likely to contract COVID-19 because of their cramped living conditions.

The state of one's mental health should not be taken lightly at any point in time. Even before COVID-19 hit the world, the number of workers in the industry who experienced work-related stress, depression, or anxiety increased by 0.7% in 2019, compared to 0.6% in 2018 (Relojo-Howell, 2020). Since these workers have no easy access to mental healthcare, they might not even notice that they have the symptoms of mental illnesses. Insufficient studies focus on the mental health of migrant construction workers in Malaysia. Therefore, this study investigated the effect of the COVID-19 pandemic on the mental health of migrant construction workers at TTDI Sentralis. Then, the relationship between mental health and perceived work productivity of migrant construction workers is highlighted in this manuscript on how to mitigate the effects of the COVID-19 pandemic on the mental health of migrant construction workers towards work productivity.

## 2.0 Perspectives and concepts

### a) *Effects of COVID-19 lockdown on migrant construction workers*

The pandemic has severely affected the construction industry, and all new constructions and projects have been halted until further notice (Zakaria and Singh, 2021). Beginning with the first phase of MCO and continuing through the third phase, the government has ordered most construction sites to close for around six weeks, except for important projects (Esa et al., 2020). Most construction companies temporarily stopped work, while employees were urged to work from home. However, migrant workers could not do their job from home. Not only that, but they were also detained in overcrowded detention centres, where thousands of people were afflicted by the pandemic and while there were blamed for spreading COVID-19 (The Star, 2020). According to Choudhari (2020), migrant workers are at a higher risk of developing severe, acute, and chronic mental health disorders due to the COVID-19 pandemic, which various multidimensional factors would cause. Multiple actions, all taken together, can result in suffering on various levels, including physical and socio-economic.

### b) *Migrants workers' mental health*

Workers in the construction industry are more likely to have accidents related to their jobs, including those that can affect both their physical and emotional health (Peng and Chan, 2020). Employees may tolerate poor mental health and well-being without recognising it (Turner and Lingard, 2020). Being away from home may affect migrant workers' mental health, psychological pressure, and homesickness (Htay et al., 2020; Shen et al., 1998). Previous research indicates that patients' mental health can be affected when a pandemic outbreak occurs (Shah et al., 2020). This includes anxiety symptoms, including feeling agitated, lacking aspiration and desire, and treatment and health result concerns (Hossain, Sultana et al., 2020; Hossain, Tasnim, et al., 2020). They develop anxiety and sadness due to limited resources and space. Being away from their families, losing friends and family members due to the pandemic, and a sense of vulnerability in caring for their family while working might contribute to mental illness (Mucci et al., 2020; Pamidimukkala and Kermanshachi, 2021). Job stress was associated with depressive symptoms via reduced self-esteem (Li et al., 2019). Thus, their ability to handle their job and support their family was crucial to their self-esteem. 25% of rural-urban migrants believed inadequate income caused work-related stress (Cui et al., 2012). Social exclusion, joblessness, budgetary limitations, and working from home while caring for children and other family members are among the stresses studied. Also, depression symptoms rose from 8.5% before the outbreak to 27.8% during the lockdown (Ettman et al., 2020).

### c)   *Factors affecting the mental health of migrant construction workers during COVID-19*

According to the government, construction industries may increase their working capacity to 100% from 60% if 80% to 100% of their staff are vaccinated (The Star, 2021). During the COVID-19 pandemic, workers must work longer, continuous shifts with increased workloads and shorter rest periods (ILO, 2020). Due to workforce shortages and self-isolation, workers may get stressed or anxious (Pamidimukkala and Kermanshachi, 2021). Alsharef et al. (2021) note that there was much concern about the virus spreading at construction sites. Workers must share workspaces, amenities, and toilet facilities. Workers must take extreme precautions to prevent viral transmission. Alsharef et al. (2021) claimed that workers were worried about exposure to COVID-19 at work and about implementing and enforcing unrealistic safety safeguards on construction sites. Since most male migrant workers do not live with their families, their loneliness might lead to mental health conditions, including depression (Zhou et al., 2020). Losing loved ones during the pandemic and feeling helpless to care for family members' health while living abroad may exacerbate stress (Choudhari, 2020). According to Karim et al. (2020), migrant workers and their dependents are socially and economically disadvantaged due to COVID-19.

### d)   *Work productivity of migrant construction workers*

While seeking to lower the dangers of the spread of COVID-19 among construction workers by reducing the number of employees and their interactions, it is logical to predict decreased worker productivity (Araya, 2021). There is no research regarding the effects of COVID-19 on the work productivity of migrant construction workers. However, studies have reported that having adjustments in working schedules which includes rotating shifts, night shifts, as well as other forms of working schedules during the COVID-19 pandemic, has significant impacts on the absence of workers and turnover rates, as well as the productivity of construction workers (Bavel et al., 2020; Pamidimukkala and Kermanshachi, 2021). Sato et al. (2020) note that workers with mental health issues are more likely to be under-productive, whereas research by Johari and Jha (2020) indicates that productivity declines as workers' motivation deteriorates. Other mental health issues, such as anxiety disorders, have been linked to poor performance and sick days from work (Burton et al., 2008).

*e)* *Mitigation of the effects of lockdown on the mental health of migrant construction workers*

Construction companies may lessen the mental health consequences of the COVID-19 lockdown in numerous ways. Publicly complimenting or thanking workers in front of managers and co-workers may increase productivity, according to Johari and Jha (2020). Outdoor exercise helps people mingle with others, socialise, and improve their health. In preventing and managing cardiovascular diseases, exercise training improves the quality of life, mortality, disability, and co-morbidity (Anselmi et al., 2021). Employers can also give migrant construction employees extra time off if they have mental health issues. Lastly, attending counselling is another technique to handle mental health issues, such as cognitive behavioural therapy.

## 3.0   Research methods

This study focused on the migrant construction workers at a construction site in Seksyen 13, Shah Alam, Malaysia, TTDI Sentralis, with 55 respondents. This study focused on the impact of the COVID-19 lockdown in Malaysia on the mental health of migrant construction workers and their work productivity. The scope of mental health focused on anxiety, depression, and stress. This study was conducted quantitatively through a survey using Google Forms and offline questionnaires. Data analysis for this methodology was extracted into Microsoft Excel and analysed by SPSS software utilising descriptive statistics. The details of the research methodology are discussed based on Figure 13.1.

## 4.0   Results and discussion

### 4.1   *Factors affecting the mental health of the migrant construction workers*

The highest rate of the factor affecting the mental health of migrant construction workers is five, which is strongly agreed upon. According to Choudhari (2020), migrant workers are at higher risk of developing severe, acute, and chronic mental health disorders due to the COVID-19 pandemic, which various multidimensional factors would cause. The factors affecting the mental health of migrant construction workers were listed from the previous literature review as guidance for the

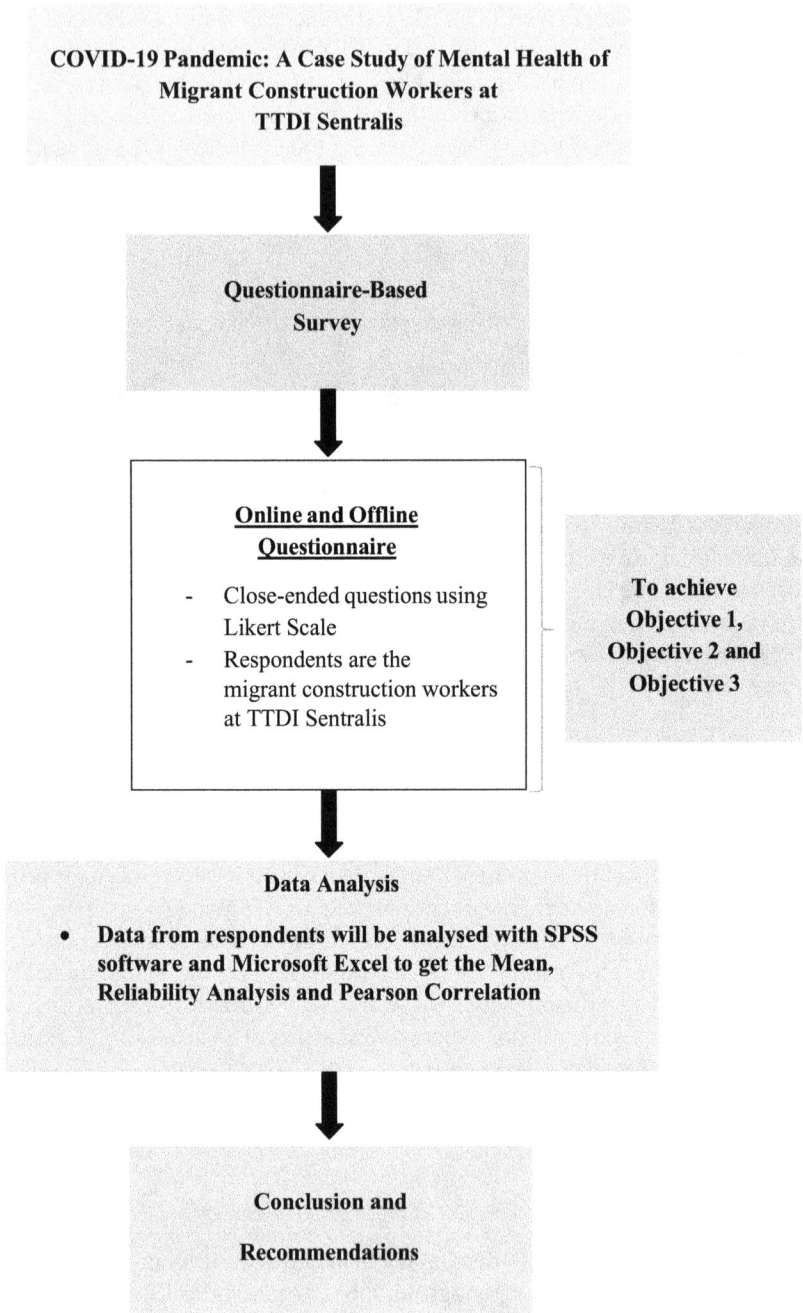

*Figure 13.1* Research design and method.

researcher and for the respondents to rate and validate whether they affected them during the COVID-19 pandemic.

Figure 13.2 shows several factors that affect the mental health of migrant construction workers at TTDI Sentralis the most. It has been found that they are worried about the financial difficulties experienced by the COVID-19 pandemic. Many migrant workers did not live with their family members, and their ability to do their job well and financially support their families was an essential source of their self-esteem (Li et al., 2019). They may face negative consequences such as unemployment, short working hours, isolation, poor living conditions, social discrimination, and mental stress resulting from the lockdown, while their dependents at home face financial difficulties due to limited or reduced cash flow from their working relatives. The socio-economic slump may impact their mental health due to job loss and financial constraints (Christodoulou and Christodoulou, 2013). Figure 13.2 shows the response to financial worries during the COVID-19 pandemic.

Migrant construction workers were also concerned about losing their job at TTDI Sentralis during the MCO's implementation in Malaysia since they were the first to lose their job, as shown in Figure 13.3. They were also the first to be denied government assistance and forced to live in cramped, unhygienic conditions. For instance, Bangladeshis who have migrated to other countries for work face negative consequences such as joblessness, shorter working periods, seclusion, poor living conditions, social ostracism, and mental stress (Karim et al., 2020).

Another factor is that these workers also felt helpless for not being able to help their families during the lockdown. Separation from their families, the death of friends and family members because of the pandemic, and a sense of helplessness

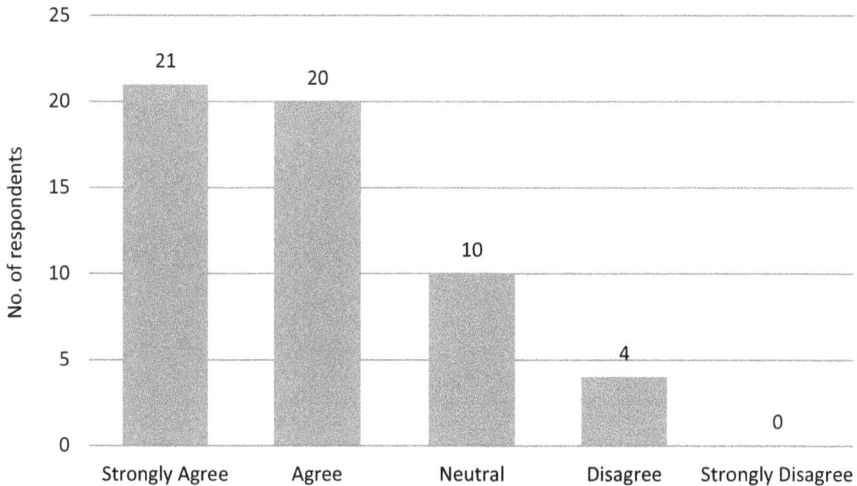

*Figure 13.2* Response to financial worries during the COVID-19 pandemic.

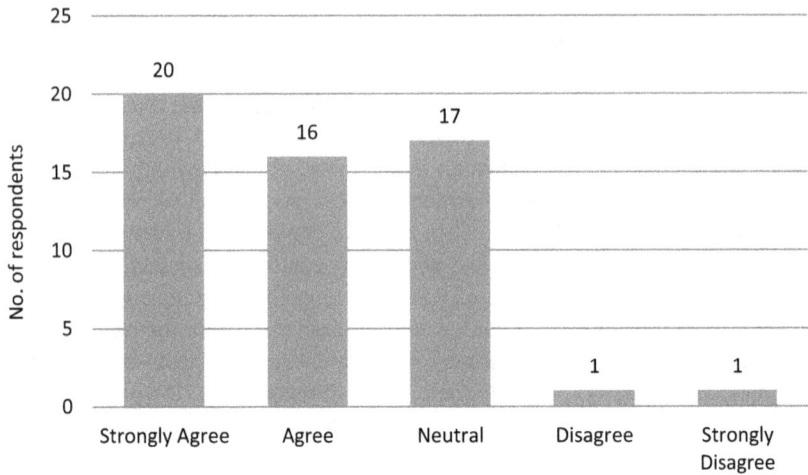

*Figure 13.3* Response to fear of unemployment during the COVID-19 pandemic.

*Table 13.1* Mean value of each of the questions asked in the survey.

| Items | N | Mean | Rank |
| --- | --- | --- | --- |
| I am worried about my financial difficulties during the COVID-19 pandemic | 55 | 4.0545 | 1 |
| I am scared of losing my job with my current construction company during the COVID-19 pandemic | 55 | 3.9636 | 2 |
| I feel helpless for not being able to help my family during the lockdown | 55 | 3.9273 | 3 |
| I am sad, scared, and anxious about the deaths of my family members and friends | 55 | 3.8182 | 4 |
| I feel anxious about being infected with COVID-19 | 55 | 3.7818 | 5 |
| Staying away from home makes me feel homesick | 55 | 3.7273 | 6 |
| I feel lonely because I live far away from my family | 55 | 3.6545 | 7 |
| Isolations make me feel lonely and anxious | 55 | 2.9636 | 8 |
| I suffer from physical pain due to too much work | 55 | 2.8364 | 9 |
| I feel restless when working during the COVID-19 pandemic | 55 | 2.7091 | 10 |
| I feel my heart rate increased rapidly while working at the construction site during the COVID-19 pandemic | 55 | 2.6364 | 11 |
| I feel shortness of breath while working at the construction site during the COVID-19 pandemic | 55 | 2.5455 | 12 |
| I have difficulty maintaining my sleep due to working at the construction site during the COVID-19 pandemic | 55 | 2.4000 | 13 |

in catering to their family's needs while working all contribute to developing the mental condition mentioned (Mucci et al., 2020; Pamidimukkala and Kermanshachi, 2021). It can be said that the top three factors that affect the mental health of migrant construction workers are (i) being worried about their financial difficulties, (ii) feeling scared of losing their job, and (iii) feeling helpless about not being able to help their families during the lockdown, as highlighted in Table 13.1.

*Table 13.2* Pearson correlation for the relationship between mental health and perceived work productivity of migrant construction workers.

|  |  | Mental health | Perceived work productivity |
|---|---|---|---|
| Mental Health | Pearson Correlation | 1 | .591 |
|  | Sig. (2-tailed) |  | .000 |
|  | N | 55 | 55 |
| Perceived Work Productivity | Pearson Correlation | .591 | 1 |
|  | Sig. (2-tailed) | .000 |  |
|  | N | 55 | 55 |

### 4.2   The relationship between mental health and perceived work productivity of migrant construction workers at the construction site

For this objective, Pearson correlation has determined the relationship between the mental health and perceived work productivity of migrant construction workers, as shown in Table 13.2. It is expected that this research would hypothesise a positive relationship between the mental health of migrant construction workers and their perceived work productivity.

To accomplish this study, Pearson correlation has investigated the connection between the mental health of migrant construction workers and their perceived levels of workplace efficiency.

It is anticipated that the hypothesis that emerges from this research suggests a positive association between the mental health of migrant construction workers and their reported work productivity levels. Pearson correlation was run to determine the relationship between mental health and the perceived work productivity of migrant construction workers. This test was used to test the relationship between them because there is one continuous and one categorical variable in this study. Based on Table 13.1, the Pearson correlation was obtained for analysis. The relationship between mental health and the perceived work productivity of migrant construction workers was 0.591. Therefore, this shows that the strength of a linear relationship is fair based on the data (Chan, 2005).

Figure 13.4 shows the scatter plot graph for the relationship between mental health and the perceived work productivity of migrant construction workers at the construction site. The two variables have a positive correlation. Based on the graph, all the points fall near the straight line, which indicates that the variables are assumed to be generally distributed in the population. As the score for mental health increases, the score for perceived work productivity also increases. Based on the survey, it can be said that respondents with a higher total score in Section B indicate a more significant mental health issue. Meanwhile, a higher score in Section C indicates low perceived work productivity. Therefore, the hypothesis of the mental health of migrant construction workers and their perceived work productivity is the same as predicted, which is a positive relationship between mental health and perceived work productivity.

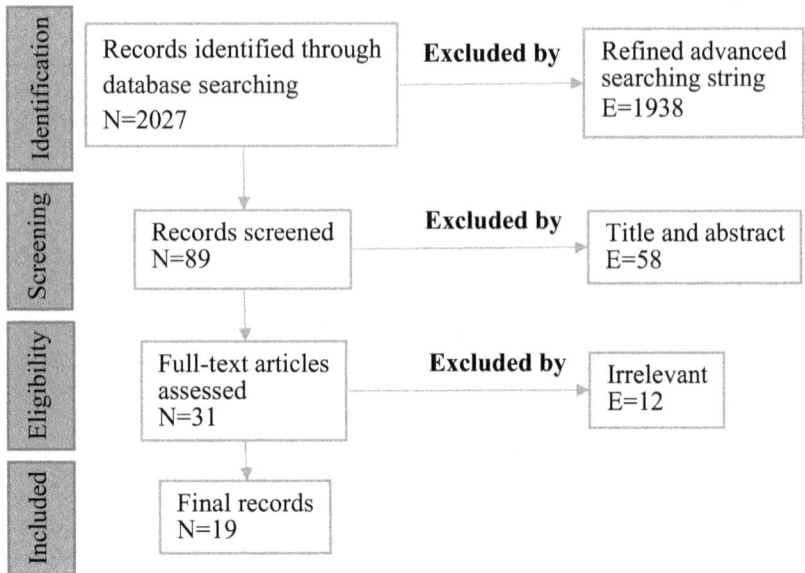

```
Identification   Records identified through     Excluded by     Refined advanced
                 database searching          ───────────────►   searching string
                 N=2027                                          E=1938

Screening        Records screened               Excluded by     Title and abstract
                 N=89                        ───────────────►   E=58

Eligibility      Full-text articles             Excluded by     Irrelevant
                 assessed                    ───────────────►   E=12
                 N=31

Included         Final records
                 N=19
```

*Figure 13.4* The scatter plot graph for the relationship between mental health and perceived work productivity of migrant construction workers at the construction site.

*Table 13.3* Mean value for the second objective.

| Items | N | Mean | Rank |
|---|---|---|---|
| Unpredictable and extreme weather conditions have made me less motivated | 55 | 3.3091 | 1 |
| I feel burnout | 55 | 2.8727 | 2 |
| I feel underproductive | 55 | 2.7273 | 3 |
| I do not enjoy my job | 55 | 2.6909 | 4 |
| I feel less motivated | 55 | 2.6727 | 5 |
| I am not satisfied with my job | 55 | 2.5273 | 6 |
| I procrastinate a lot | 55 | 1.8909 | 7 |
| I often take emergency leaves/days off | 55 | 1.8182 | 8 |
| Valid N (listwise) | 55 | | |

The data about the perceived work productivity of migrant construction
workers were listed based on a previous literature review. This data shows the
respondents' reaction to the statement that mental health significantly affects
work productivity. According to the survey results in Table 13.3, the respondents stated feeling less motivated due to unpredictable and extreme weather conditions. These findings agree with what Johari and Jha (2020) have said: the
respondents work at the exact location, their task is very domain-specific, and

they face several dangers, including unpredictable and extreme weather conditions. Feeling burnout is ranked as the second-highest. Lack of work-life quality is linked to more significant stress, anxiety, and burnout caused by work pressures, leading to a significant drop in job performance and company expenses (Leitão et al., 2021). Lastly, the third-highest statement ranked by the respondents is feeling underproductive. It is said that workers with mental health concerns are more likely to be underproductive (Sato et al., 2020). Job burnout is associated with absenteeism, decreased productivity, loyalty to the organisation, motivation, contentment, and poor physical and mental health. Therefore, it can be said that the second objective is to understand the relationship between mental health and the perceived work productivity of migrant construction workers at the construction site.

### 4.3 Suggestions on how to mitigate the effects of the COVID-19 pandemic on the mental health of migrant construction workers

This section presents the third objective of this research, which is to suggest how to mitigate the effects of the COVID-19 pandemic on the mental health of migrant construction workers. These suggestions include boosting morale, regular exercise, extra days off, and counselling. According to the statistics, some effort should be made to reduce the negative impact of the COVID-19 epidemic on the mental health of migrant construction workers. A few approaches can be taken to reduce the adverse effects of some factors on the mental health of migrant construction workers. The respondents in this study agreed that a good environment could help them boost their morale during work. According to Johari and Jha (2020), public compliments or expressions of appreciation in front of on-site meetings of supervisors and co-workers contribute significantly to higher productivity. Motivated employees are more likely to be content with their job and stay with the organisation for an extended time.

The second-highest rank for mitigating the effect is that they also agreed that the company should provide a leave of absence when they feel sick or tired. Rest is essential for maintaining excellent mental health, improving focus and memory, strengthening the immune system, and reducing stress. The third-highest ranking is that they feel motivated if their boss praises their work. Following the findings of Johari and Jha (2020), it has been found that instances in which workers are publicly commended or shown gratitude in front of gatherings of supervisors and co-workers on-site contribute considerably to higher productivity. In conclusion, the third objective is achieved.

### 5.0 Implications for practice and research

This study can suggest several recommendations to help migrant workers with severe mental health issues. Future researchers could build on it and look at the impact of the COVID-19 pandemic on migrant workers' mental health at other construction sites, different regions, or even in Malaysia itself. This would allow us

*Table 13.4* Mean value for the third objective.

| Items | N | Mean | Rank |
|---|---|---|---|
| Having a good environment can help me to boost my morale during work | 55 | 3.6909 | 1 |
| My company should provide a leave of absence when I feel sick or tired | 55 | 3.6727 | 2 |
| I feel motivated if my boss praises my work | 55 | 3.6364 | 3 |
| Exercising may improve my health condition | 55 | 3.3818 | 4 |
| Exercising before work may improve my mood and motivation to work | 55 | 3.2909 | 5 |
| Counselling may help me in coping with mental health issues | 55 | 2.8000 | 6 |
| My company should provide counselling sessions for mental health issues during the COVID-19 pandemic | 55 | 2.6909 | 7 |
| Valid N (listwise) | 55 | | |

to analyse the impact of the COVID-19 pandemic on the mental health of migrant workers with a bigger sample size. Future studies can concentrate on a specific mental health issue, such as migrant workers' post-traumatic stress disorder. In addition, future researchers can use quantitative research to perform the survey and obtain reliable answers and data from migrant workers.

## 6.0   Conclusions

Furthermore, this study also found that several factors have a significant impact on the migrant workers at TTDI Sentralis, such as financial difficulties, being scared of losing one's job, feeling helpless because of not being able to help their family throughout the lockdown, and feeling sad, scared, and anxious from the deaths of their family members and friends. Even though their mental health is affected by other variables, they are found not to be concerned about their inability to adopt social distancing adequately. It has also been found that they do not mind sharing facilities. It is also fortunate that they did not consider suicide while working on the construction sites during the COVID-19 outbreak. The second objective is to understand the relationship between mental health and the perceived work productivity of migrant construction workers at the construction sites. It is reasonable to expect a drop in worker productivity, especially when they have had many issues. Based on the questionnaire and data collected, the mental health and perceived work productivity score are high. Therefore, it can be concluded that the greater the mental health issues, the lower the work productivity. The findings showed that mental health and work productivity are positively correlated. Thus, the hypothesis is accepted. The final goal is to make recommendations for reducing the impact of the COVID-19 pandemic on migrant construction workers' mental health. Several recommendations have been made to alleviate the consequences of the COVID-19 pandemic on mental health. The respondents agreed that having a good environment, providing leave, and regular exercise can help them cope with the mental health impacts of the COVID-19 pandemic. However, many respondents disagree with the idea of a counselling session. Therefore, it can be said that this section is crucial in ensuring that this company collaborates to assist and enhance the mental health of its migrant workers.

## References

Alsharef, A., Banerjee, S., Uddin, S.M.J., Albert, A., & Jaselskis, E. (2021). Early impacts of the COVID-19 pandemic on the United States construction industry. *International Journal of Environmental Research and Public Health*, 18(4), 1–21. https://doi.org/10.3390/ijerph18041559.

Anselmi, F., Cavigli, L., Pagliaro, A., Valente, S., Valentini, F., Cameli, M., Focardi, M., Mochi, N., Dendale, P., Hansen, D., Bonifazi, M., Halle, M., & D'Ascenzi, F. (2021). The importance of ventilatory thresholds to define aerobic exercise intensity in cardiac patients and healthy subjects. *Scandinavian Journal of Medicine and Science in Sports*, 31(9), 1796–1808. https://doi.org/10.1111/sms.14007.

Araya, F. (2021). Modelling the spread of COVID-19 on construction workers: An agent-based approach. *Safety Science*, 133(September 2020), 105022. https://doi.org/10.1016/j.ssci.2020.105022.

Bavel, J.J.V., Baicker, K., Boggio, P.S., Capraro, V., Cichocka, A., Cikara, M., Crockett, M.J., Crum, A.J., Douglas, K.M., Druckman, J.N., Drury, J., Dube, O., Ellemers, N., Finkel, E.J., Fowler, J.H., Gelfand, M., Han, S., Haslam, S.A., Jetten, J., . . . Willer, R. (2020). Using social and behavioural science to support COVID-19 pandemic response. *Nature Human Behaviour*, 4(5), 460–471. https://doi.org/10.1038/s41562-020-0884-z.

Burton, W.N., Schultz, A.B., Chen, C.Y., & Edington, D.W. (2008). The association of worker productivity and mental health: A literature review. *International Journal of Workplace Health Management*, 1(2), 78–94. https://doi.org/10.1108/17538350810893883.

Chan, Y.H. (2005). Biostatistics 304: Cluster analysis. *Singapore Medical Journal*, 46(4), 153–160.

Choudhari, R. (2020). COVID-19 pandemic: Mental health challenges of internal migrant workers of India. *Asian Journal of Psychiatry*, 54(May), 102254. https://doi.org/10.1016/j.ajp.2020.102254.

Christodoulou, N.G., & Christodoulou, G.N. (2013). Financial crises: Impact on mental health and suggested responses. *Psychotherapy and Psychosomatics*, 82(5), 279–284. https://doi.org/10.1159/000351268.

Cui, X., Rockett, I.R.H., Yang, T., & Cao, R. (2012). Work stress, life stress, and smoking among rural-urban migrant workers in China. *BMC Public Health*, 12(1), 1. https://doi.org/10.1186/1471-2458-12-979.

Esa, M.B., Ibrahim, F.S.B., & Kamal, E.B.M. (2020). Covid-19 pandemic lockdown: The consequences towards project success in the Malaysian construction industry. *Advances in Science, Technology and Engineering Systems*, 5(5), 973–983. https://doi.org/10.25046/aj0505119.

Ettman, C.K., Abdalla, S.M., Cohen, G.H., Sampson, L., Vivier, P.M., & Galea, S. (2020). Prevalence of depression symptoms in US adults before and during the COVID-19 pandemic. *JAMA Network Open*, 3(9). https://doi.org/10.1001/jamanetworkopen.2020.19686.

Hossain, M.M., Sultana, A., & Purohit, N. (2020, July). Mental health outcomes of quarantine and isolation for infection prevention: A systematic umbrella review of the global evidence. *SSRN Electronic Journal*. https://doi.org/10.2139/ssrn.3561265.

Hossain, M.M., Tasnim, S., Sultana, A., Faizah, F., Mazumder, H., Zou, L., McKyer, E.L.J., Ahmed, H.U., & Ma, P. (2020). Epidemiology of mental health problems in COVID-19: A review. *F1000Research [revista en Internet] 2018 [acceso 10 de diciembre de 2020]*, 9, 1–16.

Htay, M.N.N., Latt, S.S., Maung, K.S., Myint, W.W., & Moe, S. (2020). Mental well-being and its associated factors among Myanmar migrant workers in penang, Malaysia. *Asia-Pacific Journal of Public Health*, 32(6–7), 320–327. https://doi.org/10.1177/1010539520940199.

ILO. (2020). *Managing work-related psychosocial risks during the COVID-19.* Available at www.ilo.org/wcmsp5/groups/public/-ed_protect/-protrav/-safework/documents/instructionalmaterial/wcms_748638.pdf.

Johari, S., & Jha, K.N. (2020). Impact of work motivation on construction labor productivity. *Journal of Management in Engineering*, 36(5), 04020052. https://doi.org/10.1061/(ASCE)me.1943-5479.0000824.

Karim, M.R., Islam, M.T., & Talukder, B. (2020). COVID-19's impacts on migrant workers from Bangladesh: In search of policy intervention. *World Development*, 136, 105123. https://doi.org/10.1016/j.worlddev.2020.105123.

Leitão, J., Pereira, D., & Gonçalves, Â. (2021). Quality of work life and contribution to productivity: Assessing the moderator effects of burnout syndrome. *International Journal of Environmental Research and Public Health*, 18(5), 1–20. https://doi.org/10.3390/ijerph18052425.

Li, Q., Chi, P., Hall, B.J., Wu, Q., & Du, H. (2019). Job stress and depressive symptoms among migrant workers in Macau: A moderated mediation model of self-esteem and perceived social support. *Psych Journal*, 8(3), 307–317. https://doi.org/10.1002/pchj.298.

Mucci, N., Traversini, V., Giorgi, G., Tommasi, E., De Sio, S., & Arcangeli, G. (2020). Migrant workers and psychological health: A systematic review. *Sustainability (Switzerland)*, 12(1), 1–28. https://doi.org/10.3390/SU12010120.

Nwaogu, J.M., Chan, A.P.C., Hon, C.K.H., & Darko, A. (2020). Review of global mental health research in the construction industry: A science mapping approach. *Engineering, Construction and Architectural Management*, 27(2), 385–410. https://doi.org/10.1108/ECAM-02-2019-0114.

Pamidimukkala, A., & Kermanshachi, S. (2021). Impact of Covid-19 on field and office workforce in the construction industry. *Project Leadership and Society*, 2, 100018. https://doi.org/10.1016/j.plas.2021.100018.

Pandey, K., Thurman, M., Johnson, S.D., Acharya, A., Johnston, M., Klug, E.A., Olwenyi, O.A., Rajaiah, R., & Byrareddy, S.N. (2021). Mental health issues during and after COVID-19 vaccine era. *Brain Research Bulletin*, 176(May), 161–173. https://doi.org/10.1016/j.brainresbull.2021.08.012.

Peng, L., & Chan, A.H. (2020). Adjusting work conditions to meet the declined health and functional capacity of older construction workers in Hong Kong. *Safety Science*, 127, 104711.

Relojo-Howell, D. (2020). Mental health and the everyday construction worker _ Free Malaysia Today (FMT). *Free Malaysia Today*. Available at www.freemalaysiatoday.com/category/leisure/2020/02/04/mental-health-and-the-everyday-construction-worker/.

Sato, K., Kuroda, S., & Owan, H. (2020). Mental health effects of long work hours, night and weekend work, and short rest periods. *Social Science and Medicine*, 246(December 2019), 112774. https://doi.org/10.1016/j.socscimed.2019.112774.

Shah, K., Kamrai, D., Mekala, H., Mann, B., Desai, K., & Patel, R.S. (2020). Focus on mental health during the coronavirus (COVID-19) pandemic: Applying learnings from the past outbreaks. *Cureus*, 12(3).

Shen, Q., Lu, Y.W., Hu, C.Y., Deng, X.M., Gao, H., Huang, X.Q., & Niu, E.H. (1998). A preliminary study of the mental health of young migrant workers in Shenzhen. *Psychiatry and Clinical Neurosciences*, 52(SUPPL.). https://doi.org/10.1111/j.1440-1819.1998.tb03272.x.

The Star. (2020). The unnoticed, unsung heroes during this time of the pandemic. *The Star*. Available at www.thestar.com.my/opinion/letters/2020/12/19/the-unnoticed-unsung-heroes-during-this-time-of-pandemic.

The Star. (2021). The construction sector could fully reopen by October. *The Star*. Available at www.thestar.com.my/business/business-news/2021/09/09/construction-sector-could-fully-reopen-by-october.

The Straits Times. (2020). Malaysia's construction industry records $6b losses in the first three lockdown phases, SE Asia news and top stories: The Straits Times. *The Straits Times*. Available at www.straitstimes.com/asia/se-asia/malaysias-construction-industry-records-s6-bil-losses-in-first-three-lockdown-phases.

Tan, T.T., Noor, N.M., & Khalidi, J.R. (2020, June). Covid-19: We must protect foreign workers. *Khazanah Research Institute*, 1–36. Available at www.KRInstitute.org.

Turner, M., & Lingard, H. (2020). Examining the interaction between bodily pain and mental health of construction workers. *Construction Management and Economics*, (11), 1009–1023. https://doi.org/10.1080/01446193.2020.1791920.

Wahab, A. (2020). The outbreak of Covid-19 in Malaysia: Pushing migrant workers at the margin. *Social Sciences and Humanities Open*, 2(1), 100073. https://doi.org/10.1016/j.ssaho.2020.100073.

Zakaria, S.A.S., & Singh, A.K.M. (2021). Impacts of Covid-19 outbreak on civil engineering activities in the Malaysian construction industry: A review. *Jurnal Kejuruteraan*, 33(3), 477–485.

Zhou, X., Snoswell, C.L., Harding, L.E., Bambling, M., Edirippulige, S., Bai, X., and Smith, A.C. (2020). The role of telehealth in reducing the mental health burden from COVID-19. *Telemedicine and E-Health*, 26(4), 377–379. https://doi.org/10.1089/tmj.2020.0068.

# 14 COVID-19 and the Ghanaian construction industry

## Current state of impact and mitigation measures

*Kofi Agyekum, Emmanuel Adinyira,
Anita Odame Adade-Boateng, Patrick Manu and
Victoria Maame Afriyie Kumah*

### Introduction

Following the discovery of a new virus in the Wuhan Region of China, later identified by the World Health Organisation (WHO) as SARS-CoV-2 (a new type of coronavirus) and subsequently declared a public health emergency, several sectors have been impacted. One such sector which was hard hit by the pandemic is the construction sector. The activities of the construction industry are inevitable in nations across the world. Although the construction industry is known for its massive contribution to the gross domestic product (GDP) of various countries, it is prone to health and safety issues. Hence, various stakeholders become concerned anytime there are public health emergencies like the COVID-19 pandemic. In the views of Chigara and Moyo (2022), since the sector is already vulnerable to other risks, the outbreak of COVID-19 aggravates health and safety issues.

With the spread of the virus worldwide, most construction-related matters continue to change, with its effect felt among contracting parties and their agreed terms of contracts (Salami et al., 2022). The Ghanaian construction industry is noted for developing infrastructure like dams, bridges, townships, and offices, among others. It constitutes about 10% of the workforce in Ghana and contributes 30% to the Ghanaian GDP (Agyekum et al., 2022). This makes it a major contributor to the Ghanaian economy. Like the construction industries in other countries, the Ghanaian construction industry is known for accident occurrences that lead to fatalities (Simpeh and Amoah, 2022; Agyekum et al., 2018). In addition to the known factors that contribute to poor construction health and safety in the Ghanaian construction industry (e.g., focus on profit, insufficient supervision, poor health and safety training, and inadequate health and safety management (Danso et al., 2022; Adinyira et al., 2020), the COVID-19 pandemic has become a key health issue to reckon with.

The impact of the pandemic on the construction industry worldwide is well reported. Stride et al. (2021) hinted at the exceptional changes which the pandemic has brought to many construction companies in the United Kingdom. Rehman et al. (2022) also revealed that in the construction industry in the United Arab

DOI: 10.1201/9781003278368-16

Emirates (UAE), the impact of the pandemic resulted in schedule delays, disrupted cashflows, delayed permits, approval, and inspections. In Nigeria, Olatunde et al. (2022) studied the impact of the pandemic on indigenous construction firms and revealed that time overrun, loss of profit, and dispute creation were among the impacts. In Ghana, a study by Amoah et al. (2021), revealed that the pandemic has affected small construction firms in terms of their cashflows, inability to secure contracts, and inability to effectively manage their sites. In a similar study, Agyekum et al. (2022) studied the impact of the pandemic on three selected large construction firms in Ghana and revealed that the impact is revealed in the following areas: decreased work rate, delays in payment, and an increased cost of materials arising from border closure.

Currently, only two scientific studies (Agyekum et al., 2022; Amoah et al., 2021) have been conducted and published with regard to the impact of COVID-19 on the Ghanaian construction industry. For the few studies carried out in Ghana, it is evident that responses were received from few respondents, making it quite difficult to generalise the findings among the larger construction industry. For instance, in the study of Agyekum et al. (2022), the qualitative approach was used to select nine (9) interviewees from three different construction companies. Also, in the study of Amoah et al. (2021), the qualitative approach was used to solicit the views of thirty (30) interviewees in small construction firms in Ghana. With the shortcomings identified in this approach as employed in the various papers, there is a need to seek the broader views of industry professionals on the impacts of the pandemic on the industry. With the gradual recovery of the construction industry from the impacts of the pandemic, the questions worth asking at this point are: what is the current state of impact of COVID-19 on the Ghanaian construction industry? What mitigation measures are currently practiced to control the spread of the virus in the Ghanaian construction industry? To address these questions, this chapter examines the current state of the Ghanaian construction industry in the midst of the COVID-19 pandemic. It identifies the impacts of the pandemic on the construction industry, and the mitigation measures practiced to control the spread of the virus in the construction industry.

## Construction health and safety management in Ghana and during COVID-19

Ghana has enacted and ratified several statutes and regulations aimed at safeguarding the health and safety of workers in various sectors. Unfortunately, these regulations are rarely enforced, and this makes workers prone to many kinds of injuries and at times deaths. In the view of Boadu et al. (2021), the laxity in enforcing occupational health and safety regulations plays a key role in poor health and safety performance in the Ghanaian construction industry. One could not disagree with Boadu et al. (2021) when there is no single occupational health and safety regulation directed at the construction industry in Ghana. As an industry that is labor-intensive with temporary working environments, there are several conditions that expose workers to various health and safety risks (Agyekum et al., 2018).

Notwithstanding this, there are several regulations that deal with safety issues that occur in numerous industries across Ghana (Annan et al., 2015). They include: The Mining and Minerals Regulations 1970 LI 665; The Workman's Compensation Law 1987; The Ghana Health Services and Teaching Hospital Act 2003 (ACT 651); The Radiation Protection Instrument LI 1559 of 1993, an amendment of the Ghana Atomic Energy Act 204 of 1963, and The EPA Act 1994 (ACT 490) (Annan et al., 2015). Enshrined in some sections of these Acts are issues that pertain to health and safety in the construction industry. Despite the institutionalisation of these important frameworks in Ghana, compliance with the requirements of these Acts leaves much to be desired (Agyekum et al., 2018).

Now more than ever there is a need for occupational health and regulatory bodies in Ghana to modify the various Acts to capture unforeseen situations like the COVID-19 pandemic. On December 31, 2019, Wuhan, the Hubei province's capital in China, registered the first case of a novel pneumonia-like sickness with its origin unknown (Hui et al., 2020). This became popularly known as the 2019 n-CoV. 2019. n-CoV as a name illustrates the fact that the virus was novel and was discovered in 2019. The virus is spread by close contact between people: in the form of respiratory droplets, aerosols, or through contact with respiratory surfaces (Jones et al., 2022). This implies that the virus can easily spread on construction projects, irrespective of outdoor activities. With the spread of the virus still paramount in several parts of the world, the woes of the construction industry are far from over. There is a need for the enforcement of construction companies within this part of Sub-Saharan Africa to be on guard to implement most of the health and safety measures documented in approved guidelines to safeguard their activities.

### Impact of COVID-19 on the construction industry and mitigation measures

The construction industry has not been spared the brunt of COVID-19, with impacts ranging from mild to severe across the globe. In a global study undertaken by Ogunnusi et al. (2020), it was revealed that low business turnover, delays in construction payment and output, difficulties working from home, and job losses were some negative impacts of the pandemic on the industry. In a critical analysis of the impact of the pandemic on Architecture, Engineering and Construction (AEC) organisations in Malaysia, King et al. (2022), revealed that reduced construction productivity, reduced foreign investment in the construction industry, reduced demand for construction-related works, disruption in the supply chain, and reduced number of public projects were key impacts. In Zimbabwe, Chigara et al. (2022) examined the factors that affected the delivery of optimum health and safety in the construction industry following the pandemic. Their study categorised the factors into nine broad components to include change and innovation-related factors, monitoring and enforcement-related factors, production-related factors, access to information and health service-related factors, on-site facilities and welfare-related factors, risk assessment and mitigation-related factors, job security and funding-related factors, cost-related factors, and COVID-19 risk perception related factors.

In Jordan, Alhusban et al. (2022) examined how the pandemic would change the future of architectural design and revealed that the design of building components has the potential to be heavily impacted in response to future pandemics. In the United Arab Emirates (UAE), Rehman et al. (2022) studied the impact of the pandemic on construction project performance. The impacts were identified to include schedule delays, disrupted cashflows, delayed permits, approvals and inspections, travel restrictions, material and equipment shortages, among others (Rehman et al., 2022). Indigenous contractors in Nigeria were not spared by COVID-19. A recent study by Olatunde et al. (2022) revealed that such contractors faced time overrun, loss of profit, dispute creation, disruption in supply of labour, and additional cost of locally sourced materials, among others. Most of these impacts were also confirmed by Oladimeji (2022), who later examined the influence of COVID-19 on local construction firms' viability in Nigeria. In Ghana, a survey of a few D1 building construction firms revealed the impacts of the pandemic on such firms included decrease in work rate, delays in payments, and increase in the cost of materials arising from border closure (Agyekum et al., 2022).

In the wake of the pandemic, organisations like the World Health Organisation (WHO) and the Centres for Disease Control (CDC) developed some guidelines to assist in curbing the spread of the virus in various organisations. Portions of those guidelines were extracted by individual sectors and modified to suit the conditions of their organisations. Some of the proposed measures included social/physical distancing, screening, using personal protective equipment, sanitization, and proper hygiene and housekeeping, among others (WHO, 2020).

## Methodology

This study sought to examine the current state of impact of COVID-19 on the Ghanaian construction industry and identified measures put in place to mitigate its spread. A quantitative (survey) research strategy was adopted for this study. Creswell (2009) indicated that this approach is suitable where a study captures and explores relationships between factors and where a study seeks to ascertain a generic view of a phenomenon being studied. The adoption of the quantitative survey approach, therefore, ensured that the experience and views of the respondents were adequately captured.

### Population and sample size

The unit of analysis from which the primary data was collected were construction project managers, health and safety officers, and directors of D1, D2, and D3 building construction firms across Ghana. In Ghana, building construction firms are registered according to the categories criteria set out by the Ministry of Water Resources, Works, and Housing (MWRWH). There are four categories of company classifications: D (building), K (civil engineering), E (electrical works), and G (plumbing works) (Agyekum et al., 2018). Within these categories, there are four financial sub-classifications in the order of Classes 1 (>500,000 USD),

2 (200,000–500,000 USD), 3 (75,000–200,000 USD), and 4 (>75,000 USD) (Agye-kum et al., 2018). The limits of the companies based on their assets, plant and equip-ment, labour holdings, etc., are determined by these financial sub-classifications. Class 1 has the highest resource base, and decreases through Classes 2, 3, and 4 in that order (Agyekum et al., 2018). In this study, D1, D2, and D3 building construction firms that are reachable across Ghana were considered. It must be acknowledged that the inclusion of a contractor's name in the MWRWH register is not compulsory in Ghana (Agyekum et al., 2018). This means that it is difficult to obtain an accurate list of such firms. Owing to this problem, readily available construction firms were located using purposive sampling, and by referrals using the snowball method, other firms were contacted for the study. In all, a total of 223 construction firms were reached.

### Data collection

Data for the study were collected through a questionnaire survey. Closed-ended questions were posed and respondents were limited to choosing between several given options from the provided Likert response scale of 1 to 5. The questions were designed to be as simple and unambiguous as possible. The confidentiality of responses by participants was taken into consideration in order to enable them to answer the questions sincerely and confidently as much as possible.

The literature review supported the development of the survey questionnaire. The questionnaire consisted of three main sections. The first section sought back-ground information of the respondents. This included the class of firm they worked with, their profession, and their experience in the construction industry. The second section required the respondents to score on the Likert scale of 1 to 5 (where 1= Not severe, 2 = Less severe, 3 = Moderately severe, 4 = Severe, and 5 = Very severe) the severity of selected impacts of COVID-19 on their firms. The third section further required the respondents to score on the Likert scale of 1 to 5 the level of importance (where 1 = Not important, 2 = Less important, 3 = Moderately impor-tant, 4 = important, 5 = Highly important) they attached to some measures put in place by their firms to control the spread of the virus. The 5 – point rating scale was chosen for the last two sections of the questionnaire because it provides unambigu-ous results that are easy to interpret (Agyekum et al., 2022). The questionnaires were distributed and retrieved online as part of the adherence to COVID-19 safety. The data for this study were collected within three weeks, from October 5 to Octo-ber 26, 2021, the period when most construction firms were resuming work after the nationwide lockdown in Ghana.

Out of the total number (223) of questionnaires returned, Directors constituted 20% (n = 45), Health and Safety Officers constituted 36% (n = 80), and Construc-tion Managers constituted 44% (n = 98). In terms of the respondents' educational backgrounds, 46% (n = 103) possessed master's degrees, 45% (n = 100) bachelor's degrees, and 9% (n = 20) had Higher National Diploma degrees. The working experience revealed most of the respondents (80%, n = 178) had between 5 to 25+ years of experience. Twenty percent (20%, n = 45) had less than five years of working experience. Concerning the types of companies the respondents worked in, 22% (n = 50) were with D1, 44% (n = 98) were with D2, and 34% (n = 75) were with D3 building construction companies. This demographic data reveals that the respondents were well-experienced in the construction industry and had the requisite knowledge to provide the feedback needed.

*Data analyses*

The data gathered were analysed using the Statistical Package for Social Sciences (SPSS) Version 26. The tools selected for the analysis were the Shapiro-Wilk test, mean score ranking, and the Kruskal-Wallis test. A normality test was first carried out to determine the nature of the data obtained using the Shapiro-Wilk test. This test is suitable when the data sample size is less than 2000 (Ghasemi and Zahediasl, 2012). The significant values obtained for both the impacts and measures were less than 0.05, indicating that the data gathered were non-parametric in nature. The reliability of the research instrument was further determined using Cronbach's Alpha test. The values obtained for the impact and measures were 0.912 and 0.815 respectively. This indicates that the instrument was reliable. Following these tests, the mean score ranking was used to rank the impacts and measures for the various groups of respondents.

The mean score ranking is a typical quantitative analytical method that has been widely used in previous studies for ranking the relative significance of factors pertaining to given scenarios. Hence, in this study, the mean values of responses from the respondents were used to obtain the severity of the impacts as well as the relative importance of the mitigation measures. The higher the mean value (greater than or equal to 3.0), the more severe the impact and the more important the mitigation measure. The Kruskal-Wallis Test was used to test the formulated hypotheses as follows: There is no statistically significant difference in the ranking of the assessed impacts and measures by the respondents; there is no statistically significant difference in the views of the respondents regarding the impacts and measures. According to Eze et al. (2021), the Kruskal-Wallis Test is suitable when the perceptions of at least three groups of respondents are to be determined.

## Results

*Impacts of COVID-19 on the Ghanaian construction industry*

Table 14.1 summarises the survey results of the impacts of the COVID-19 pandemic on the Ghanaian construction industry. The three respondents' group views regarding the individual impacts showed different mean scores across the various factors. For the respondent group that fell under the D1 building construction firm, the results show that the severity of the impact ranged from 4.00 to 3.56. For the D2 building construction firms, it ranged from 4.12 to 3.70, and for the D3 building construction firms, it ranged from 4.89 to 3.61.

Respondents from the D1 building construction firms ranked effects on conditions of contract [$\bar{X}$ = 4.00, SD = 0.969] as the most severe impact while suspension of projects [$\bar{X}$ = 3.56, SD = 1.072] was ranked as the least. Also, for the D2 building construction firms, respondents ranked interruption of planning and scheduling [.., SD = 1.008] as the most severe, while job loss and workforce shortage [$\bar{X}$ = 3.70, SD = 1.086] was ranked as the least. For the D3 building construction firms, respondents ranked anxiety leading to the poor mental health of workers [$\bar{X}$ = 4.89, SD = 0.311] as the most severe, while the uncertainty of survival of construction firms [$\bar{X}$ = 3.61, SD = 0.490] was ranked as the least.

The results of the Kruskal-Wallis H-test revealed that seven out of the twelve impacts have significant *p-values* below 0.05, indicating that those variables were rated differently by the respondents. Those impacts include: Uncertainty of survival of construction firms; Scarcity and hikes in the prices of materials and equipment; Increase in the cost of materials; Workers have become more conscious of their health and surroundings; Anxiety leading to the poor mental health of workers; Interruption of planning and scheduling; and Job loss and workforce shortage. The significant *p*-values (i.e., $p < 0.05$) obtained for these seven variables mean the null hypotheses for those variables must be rejected. On the other hand, the five remaining impacts, i.e., Lack of firms' working capital, Delay in project delivery leading to cost overruns, Effects on conditions of contracts, Effects on operations due to social distancing, and Suspension of projects, obtained significant *p*-values greater than 0.05. This means that there exists no statistically significant difference in the views of the respondents regarding these five impacts. Hence, the opinions of the respondents converge on these five impacts.

Notwithstanding this revelation, all twelve impacts were ranked higher with mean scores greater than the mean value of 3.0. Overall, the factors *anxiety leading to the poor mental health of workers* [$\bar{X}$ = 4.30, SD = 0.975], *interruption of planning and scheduling* [$\bar{X}$ = 4.20, SD=0.948], and *scarcity of materials and equipment* [$\bar{X}$ = 4.17, SD = 1.031], were ranked by all the respondents from the three different classes of construction firms as the three key impacts of COVID-19 on the Ghanaian construction industry.

One of the key impacts identified by the respondents was anxiety leading to poor mental health of workers. This finding agrees with that of Agyekum et al. (2022) and Brown (2022). In their study, Agyekum et al. (2022) revealed that workers in class D1 building construction firms in Ghana reported of severe cases of anxiety in the midst of the COVID-19 pandemic. Brown (2022) also postulated that the symptoms of anxiety and depression among construction workers have worsened during the COVID-19 pandemic. Work is good for mental health, but a negative working environment can lead to physical and mental health problems. The presence of informal and undeclared work arrangements poses threats to the global construction workforce through the creation of gaps in social security protection for workers (International Labour Organisation, 2019). The constellation of differential exposures of the construction sector depicts a high-risk public health situation in many countries preceding the COVID-19 pandemic (King and Lamontagne, 2022). In view of this, many construction firms have responded to the COVID-19 pandemic by boosting the mental health of their employees. King and Lamontagne (2022) report that these actions have become necessary because of the high rate of suicide and mental health issues that have risen in the construction industry in the wake of the COVID-19 pandemic. This impact identified is serious because the interruption to projects caused by the pandemic is likely to have caused anxiety about continuity of work/employment, especially among the smaller companies, i.e., D3 (see Table 14.1) and income for the respondents and the site workers they oversee (Bourne et al., 2021).

The respondents ranked interruption of planning and scheduling as the second most severe impact of COVID-19 on the construction industry in Ghana. This finding agrees with that reported in the literature (see Agyekum et al., 2022; Gamil and Alhagar, 2020). In the wake of the pandemic, it is inevitable that construction schedules will be impacted due to supply chain disruption, reduced workforce, material shortages, new safety protocols, reduced productivity, and other snowball effects (Jain, 2021). Understandably, owners are worried about the impact on their schedule and how that might translate to a potential increase in project costs and contractual issues (Jain, 2021).

The third key impact of the pandemic on the Ghanaian building industry was identified as the scarcity of materials and equipment. The COVID-19 pandemic disrupted most supply chains around the world and reduced or halted most international commercial activities related to the supply of construction materials and equipment. This caused major delays in projects. In the view of Husien et al. (2021), the COVID-19 crisis caused disruption to most of the materials supply transactions, and equipment rental companies have complained of major problems due to the remaining defective equipment at the sites. This finding agrees well with the literature (Agyekum et al., 2022; Husien et al., 2021). In the study of Agyekum et al. (2022), professionals working with class D1 building construction firms revealed that the supply of building equipment and renting equipment all came to a halt because of the COVID-19 pandemic.

### Measures to mitigate the spread of COVID-19 in the Ghanaian construction industry

Table 14.2 summarises the survey results of the measures employed to mitigate the spread of COVID-19 in the Ghanaian construction industry. The three respondents' group views regarding the individual measures showed different mean scores across the various factors. For the respondent group that fell under the D1 building construction firm, the results show that the importance of the measures ranged from 4.14 to 3.86. For the D2 building construction firms, it ranged from 4.13 to 3.57, and for the D3 building construction firms, it ranged from 4.60 to 3.95.

Respondents from the D1 building construction firms ranked proper hygiene and housekeeping [$\bar{X} = 4.14$, SD = 0.935] as the most important measure while cautiousness in handling delivery of materials/equipment [$\bar{X} = 3.86$, SD = 1.021] was ranked as the least. Also, for the D2 building construction firms, respondents ranked creating awareness and sharing information [$\bar{X} = 4.13$, SD = 1.017]

Table 14.1 Impact of COVID-19 on the firms.

| Impact | D1 Construction Firm | | | D2 Construction Firm | | | D3 Construction Firm | | | Overall | | | K-W | |
|---|---|---|---|---|---|---|---|---|---|---|---|---|---|---|
| | $\bar{X}$ | S.D | R | $\bar{X}$ | S.D | R | $\bar{X}$ | S.D | R | $\bar{X}$ | S.D | R | $X^2$ | P-Value |
| Uncertainty of survival of construction firms | 3.70 | 1.129 | 10 | 3.81 | 1.128 | 10 | 3.61 | .490 | 12 | 3.72 | .961 | 12 | 6.531 | .038 |
| Lack of firms working capital | 3.86 | 1.069 | 5 | 4.02 | .995 | 4 | 3.99 | .780 | 9 | 3.97 | .944 | 8 | 1.212 | .545 |
| Scarcity of materials and equipment | 3.78 | 1.112 | 7 | 3.91 | 1.113 | 7 | 4.79 | .412 | 2 | 4.17 | 1.031 | 3 | 50.399 | .000 |
| Increase in the cost of materials | 3.72 | 1.161 | 9 | 3.74 | 1.187 | 11 | 4.60 | .493 | 3 | 4.03 | 1.078 | 5 | 30.273 | .000 |
| Workers have become more conscious of their health and surroundings | 3.64 | 1.120 | 11 | 3.83 | 1.046 | 8 | 4.49 | .503 | 4 | 4.01 | .982 | 6 | 28.282 | .000 |
| Delay in project delivery leading to cost overruns | 3.86 | .990 | 4 | 3.98 | .930 | 5 | 4.11 | .709 | 8 | 4.00 | .878 | 7 | 1.061 | .588 |
| Effects on conditions of contracts | 4.00 | .969 | 1 | 4.05 | 1.009 | 2 | 4.19 | .896 | 7 | 4.09 | .962 | 4 | 1.728 | .422 |
| Effects on operations due to social distancing | 3.84 | 1.095 | 6 | 3.93 | 1.077 | 6 | 3.71 | 1.024 | 11 | 3.83 | 1.063 | 10 | 3.551 | .169 |
| Anxiety leading to the poor mental health of workers | 3.96 | 1.068 | 3 | 4.02 | 1.055 | 3 | 4.89 | .311 | 1 | 4.30 | .975 | 1 | 55.221 | .000 |
| Interruption of planning and scheduling | 4.00 | .990 | 2 | 4.12 | 1.008 | 1 | 4.43 | .791 | 5 | 4.20 | .948 | 2 | 7.816 | .020 |
| Suspension of projects | 3.56 | 1.072 | 12 | 3.82 | 1.078 | 9 | 3.85 | .881 | 10 | 3.77 | 1.016 | 11 | 2.235 | .327 |
| Job loss and workforce shortage | 3.74 | 1.175 | 8 | 3.70 | 1.086 | 12 | 4.29 | .632 | 6 | 3.91 | 1.014 | 9 | 13.285 | .001 |

$X^2$: Chi-Square; K-W: Kruskal-Wallis Test

$\bar{X}$: Mean Score; S.D: Standard Deviation; R: Ranking; Cronbach's Alpha: .912

as the most important, while cautiousness in handling the delivery of materials/ equipment [$\bar{X} = 3.57$, SD = 1.071] was ranked as the least. For the D3 building construction firms, respondents ranked creating awareness and sharing information [$\bar{X} = 4.60$, SD = 0.678] as the most important, while putting in place policies/ guidelines [$\bar{X} = 3.51$, SD = 1.032] was ranked as the least.

The results of the Kruskal-Wallis H-test revealed that five out of the eight measures have significant *p*-values below 0.05, indicating that those variables were rated differently by the respondents. Those measures include: creating awareness and sharing information; putting in place policies/guidelines; proper hygiene and housekeeping; social distancing; and cautiousness in handling the delivery of materials/equipment. The significant *p*-values (i.e., $p < 0.05$) obtained for these five variables mean the null hypotheses for those variables must be rejected. On the other hand, the three remaining measures, i.e., Use of Personal Protective Equipment (PPE); Regular screening of workers; and Restricting site access (dealing with visitors)/Security obtained significant *p*-values greater than 0.05. This means that there exists no statistically significant difference in the views of the respondents regarding these three measures. Hence, the opinions of the respondents converge at these three.

Notwithstanding this revelation, all eight measures were ranked higher with mean scores greater than the mean value of 3.0. Overall, the factors creating awareness and sharing information [$\bar{X} = 4.26$, SD = 0.947], proper hygiene and housekeeping [$\bar{X} = 4.24$, SD = 1.001], and regular screening of workers [$\bar{X} = 4.13$, SD = 0.918], were ranked by all the respondents from the three different classes of construction firms as the three key measures put in place to control COVID-19 on construction sites in Ghana.

The first measure identified by the respondents as key in mitigating the spread of the virus is by creating the needed awareness and sharing information. Education and awareness creation help to improve safety regulations in the construction industry (Umeokafor et al., 2020). Therefore, it is important that the employer tries to create the necessary awareness of what the virus is, how it spreads, and ways in which employees can protect themselves. In the views of Simpeh and Amoah (2020), some of the ways to enhance COVID-19 awareness creation include loud hailer to remind workers to wash their hands frequently, COVID-19 posters/ signboards, COVID-19 induction, regular toolbox talks awareness sessions and training, among others.

Regular screening of workers was the second measure considered as important in mitigating COVID-19 in the Ghanaian construction industry. Regular screening of workers is important to track those infected with the virus to control its spread. The employer must be able to conduct symptom screening of all workers and determine if any of the workers shows symptoms of COVID-19. The need to conduct regular screening of employees is well reported. In the views of Simpeh and Amoah (2022), this activity could be successful if the needed gadgets (e.g., thermometer), and facilities (e.g., screening rooms, isolation areas, etc.) are provided. In an earlier study in South Africa, it was reported that though most construction

Table 14.2 Measures to control the spread of COVID-19.

| Measures | D1 Construction Firm | | | D2 Construction Firm | | | D3 Construction Firm | | | Overall | | | | K-W | |
|---|---|---|---|---|---|---|---|---|---|---|---|---|---|---|---|
| | $\bar{X}$ | S.D | R | $\bar{X}$ | S.D | R | $\bar{X}$ | S.D | R | $\bar{X}$ | S.D | R | $X^2$ | $X^2$ | P-Value |
| Use of Personal Protective Equipment (PPE) | 4.00 | .866 | 5 | 3.83 | 1.000 | 7 | 3.96 | .951 | 6 | 3.91 | .954 | 6 | 1.187 | 1.187 | .552 |
| Creating awareness and sharing information (induction, training, orientation, toolbox, posters, meetings, safety briefing) | 4.00 | 1.021 | 6 | 4.13 | 1.017 | 1 | 4.60 | .678 | 1 | 4.26 | .947 | 1 | 16.632 | 16.632 | .000 |
| Putting in place general policies/ guidelines | 4.04 | 1.020 | 4 | 3.97 | .984 | 5 | 3.51 | 1.032 | 8 | 3.83 | 1.030 | 7 | 13.572 | 13.572 | .001 |
| Regular screening of workers | 4.10 | .895 | 2 | 4.10 | .931 | 2 | 4.19 | .926 | 4 | 4.13 | .918 | 3 | .524 | .524 | .769 |
| Proper hygiene and housekeeping | 4.14 | .935 | 1 | 4.04 | 1.039 | 4 | 4.56 | .919 | 2 | 4.24 | 1.001 | 2 | 20.806 | 20.806 | .000 |
| Social distancing | 3.98 | .924 | 7 | 3.97 | 1.005 | 6 | 4.35 | .707 | 3 | 4.10 | .910 | 4 | 7.353 | 7.353 | .025 |
| Restricting site access (dealing with visitors)/Security | 4.10 | .963 | 3 | 4.10 | .995 | 3 | 3.99 | .993 | 5 | 4.06 | .984 | 5 | .959 | .959 | .619 |
| Cautiousness in handling the delivery of materials/equipment | 3.86 | 1.021 | 8 | 3.57 | 1.071 | 8 | 3.95 | 1.173 | 7 | 3.76 | 1.105 | 8 | 7.179 | 7.179 | .028 |

$X^2$: Chi-Square; K-W: Kruskal-Wallis Test

$\bar{X}$: Mean Score; S.D: Standard Deviation; R: Ranking

*Cronbach's Alpha:* .815

companies have facilities and gadgets in place to enforce screening, there are still some construction firms without such facilities (Simpeh and Amoah, 2020).

The third measure considered significant in the Ghanaian construction industry is proper hygiene and housekeeping. Construction site hygiene encourages good housekeeping and helps to avoid cross-contamination to safeguard the health and safety of everyone. This measure is recommended by the World Health Organization (2020) as key to preventing the spread of the virus. Measures like providing wipes, alcohol-based sanitisers, and hand rubs, among others can help to control the spread (Simpeh and Amoah, 2020). Hatoum et al. (2021) recommends common contact surfaces like tables, chairs, doorknobs, handrails, and lift buttons among others to be sanitised regularly.

## Discussion of key findings

Although all the impacts and measures identified in this study were severe and important according to respondents from the three different classes of construction firms, the implications of this study are discussed around the three impacts and mitigation measures respectively. A recap of the findings on the current impact of COVID-19 on construction firms in Ghana revealed that anxiety leading to the poor mental health of workers, interruption of planning and scheduling, and scarcity of materials and equipment were the key impacts.

The construction industry is associated with mental health issues partly due to the high pressure and the physically demanding nature of work, long hours, the transient and unpredictable nature of work, and the macho culture existing in some parts, among others. The lockdowns, social distancing, and other related restrictions associated with the COVID-19 pandemic have greatly impacted all sectors. Growing mental health concerns exist in the construction industry because it ranks second-highest in suicide rates among major industries (Peterson et al., 2016). With the inclusion of the stress and anxiety associated with the COVID-19 pandemic, the rate of these mental health issues may increase. For the respondents of this study to indicate that the pandemic has a great impact on their health means if appropriate measures are not put in place there is a tendency for these professionals to suffer mental health issues. Therefore, this revelation places the Ghanaian construction industry in the spotlight to quickly make changes in their policies and practices and raise the needed awareness to control the anxieties that have arisen due to the COVID-19 pandemic. As part of the measures, a safe space for conversation could be created, mental health benefits and resources could also be created, educating oneself and the entire team, and offering mental health first aid training, among others, could all be instituted to minimise the anxiety.

The identification of interruptions of planning and scheduling as a key impact offers the contractors the ability to evaluate and quantify idle times, incurred costs, and schedule delays caused by the pandemic. This will enable the contractors to assess the current conditions and update project schedules to reflect new late-start and late-finish dates of activities with the updated dates for project completion (Critelli et al., 2020). The supply chain disruptions globally have made it difficult for manufacturers and distributors to replace or replenish their inventory and equipment or machinery (PricewaterhouseCoopers Limited, 2020). The identification of scarcity of materials and equipment as a potential impact of the COVID-19 pandemic offers players in the construction, logistics, and supply chain industries the opportunity to deploy innovative measures that could improve inventory management and distribution. This will help to engage in strategic partnerships with players and intermediaries across the value chain to deal with or control this impact.

Furthermore, the identification of the specific measures like awareness creation, proper hygiene and housekeeping, regular screening of workers, social distancing and the like present the industry with efficient and effective strategies that have been tried and tested through the trying times. With the proper enforcement of some of these measures, there is the potential for the construction industry to fully recover from the majority of the adverse impacts. Some of these measures could be developed in the form of operational policies exclusive to the construction industry setting of Ghana and could be adopted by all classes of construction firms in Ghana.

## Conclusion

The COVID-19 pandemic has affected almost every aspect of the construction industry in Ghana. This chapter examined the current state of the Ghanaian construction industry amid the COVID-19 pandemic. It identified the impacts of the pandemic on various aspects of the Ghanaian construction industry, and the mitigation measures practiced to control the spread of the virus in the industry. It is evident from this study that the construction industry has been severely impacted. Key impacts are anxiety leading to the poor mental health of workers, interruption of planning and scheduling, scarcity of materials and equipment, effects on conditions of contracts, and an increase in the cost of materials. The measures that have been employed by the construction firms to control the spread of the virus were identified to include awareness creation, proper hygiene and housekeeping, regular screening of workers, social distancing, use of Personal Protective Equipment (PPE), putting in place general policies/guidelines, and cautiousness in handling the delivery of materials/equipment.

The implications of the findings could both be theoretical and practical. Theoretically, the findings contribute to the state-of-the-art by providing an overview of the impact of COVID-19 on construction companies of different classes and characteristics. Practically, the findings could inform policymakers in developing more effective pandemic responses for the current COVID-19 pandemic and future pandemics.

Some key limitations of this study were identified. This study only considered the impact of COVID-19 on general issues of construction. However, it must be acknowledged that it would have been better if the impact on specific issues like finance, health and safety, and sustainability had been determined to better position the study in the context of the current situation. This creates the need for further studies to delve deeper into this issue. Another limitation is that the simple tests conducted in this study did not uncover the interrelationships, causal relationships, etc. among the factors and measurements considered in the study. Future research could consider using robust analyses like the Structural Equation Modelling (SEM), Fuzzy-based algorithms, network analyses, etc. to uncover such relationships.

## References

Adinyira, E., Manu, P., Agyekum, K., Mahamadu, A.-M., & Olomolaiye, P.O. (2020). Violent behavior on construction sites: Structural Equation Modelling of its impact on unsafe behavior using partial least squares. *Engineering, Construction and Architectural Management*, 27(10), 3363–3393.

Agyekum, K., Kukah, A.S., & Amudjie, J. (2022). The impact of COVID-19 on the construction industry in Ghana. *Journal of Engineering, Design and Technology*, 20(1), 222–244.

Agyekum, K., Simons, B., & Botchway, S.Y. (2018). Factors influencing the performance of safety programmes in the Ghanaian construction industry. *Acta Structilia*, 25(2), 39–68.

Alhusban, A.A., Alhusban, S.A., & Alhusban, M.A. (2022). How the COVID-19 pandemic would change the future of architectural design. *Journal of Engineering, Design and Technology*, 20(1), 339–357.

Amoah, C., Bamfo-Agyei, E., & Simpeh, F. (2021). The COVID-19 pandemic: The woes of small construction firms in Ghana. *Smart and Sustainable Built Environment*. doi: 10.1108/SASBE-02-2021-0025.

Annan, J.S., Addai, E.K., & Tulashie, S.K. (2015). A call for action to improve occupational health and safety in Ghana and a critical look at the existing legal requirement and legislation. *Safety and Health at Work*, 6(2), 146–150.

Boadu, E.F., Wang, C.C., & Sunindijo, R.Y. (2021). Challenges for occupational health and safety enforcement in the construction industry in Ghana. *Construction Economics and Building*, 21(1), 1–21.

Bourne, N.K., Balmforth, H., Beers, H., Cao, R., Cheung, C., Clarke, S., Collinge, W., Cooper, G., Corbett, E., Hartwig, A., Johnson, S., Kirkham, R., Li, L., Ling, D., Liu, C., Manu, P., Van Tongeren, M., Weightman, A., Yuan, P., & Yunusa-Kaltungo, A. (2021). Keeping the UK building safely: A scoping study: Prepared for the PROTECT COVID-19 National Core Study on transmission and environment. *University of Manchester*. Available at https://documents.manchester.ac.uk/display.aspx?DocID=56698.

Brown, S. (2022). Construction worker mental health during the COVID-19 pandemic. *Data Bulletin*. Available at www.cpwr.com/wp-content/uploads/DataBulletin-January2022.pdf (Accessed 16 March 22).

Chigara, B., & Moyo, T. (2022). Factors affecting the delivery of optimum health and safety on construction projects during the COVID-19 pandemic in Zimbabwe. *Journal of Engineering, Design and Technology*, 20(1), 24–46.

Creswell, J.W. (2009). *Research design: Qualitative, quantitative, and mixed method s approaches* (3rd ed.). Thousand Oaks, CA: Sage Publications, Inc.

Critelli, J., Jbara, K., & Sahota, R. (2020). *Impacts of COVID-19 on construction projects*. Available at www.protiviti.com/US-en/insights/covid-19-impact-construction-projects (Accessed 5 April 2022).

Danso, F.O., Adinyira, E., Manu, P., Agyekum, K., Ahadzie, D.K., & Badu, E. (2022). The mediating influence of local cultures on the relationship between factors of safety risk perception and risk-taking behavioural intention of construction site workers. *Safety Science*, 145(2022), 105490.

Eze, E., Ugulu, R.A., Egwunatum, S.I., & Awodele, I.A. (2021). Green building materials products and service market in the construction industry. *Journal of Engineering, Project and Production Management*, 11(2), 89–101.

Gamil, Y., & Alhagar, A. (2020). The impact of pandemic crises on the survival of construction industry: A case of COVID-19. *Mediterranean Journal of Social Sciences*, 11(4), 122–128.

Ghasemi, A., & Zahediasl, S. (2012). Normality test for statistical analysis: A guide for non-statisticians. *International Journal of Endocrinol Metabolism*, 10(2), 486–489.

Hatoum, M.B., Faisal, A., Nassereddine, H., & Sarvari, H. (2021). Analysis of COVID-19 concerns raised by the construction workforce and development of mitigation practices. *Frontiers in Built Environment*, 11, 1–17.

Hui, D.S.I., Azhar, E., Madani, T.A., Ntoumi, F., Kock, R., Dar, O., & Zumla, A. (2020). The continuing 2019-nCoV epidemic threat of novel coronaviruses to global health: The latest 2019 novel coronavirus outbreak in Wuhan, China. *International Journal of Infectious Diseases*, 91, 264–266.

Husien, I.A., Borisovich, Z., & Naji, A.A. (2021). COVID-19: Key global impacts on the construction industry and proposed coping strategies. *E3S Web of Conferences*, 263, 05056.

International Labour Organisation. (2019). *Extending social security to construction workers [L'extension de la Sécurité Sociale aux Ouvriers du Bâtiment]*. Available at www.social-protection.org/gimi/Emodule.action?id=64 (Accessed 31 January 2021).

Jain, N. (2021). *Coping with COVID-19: Part II, impacts on schedule*. Available at www.mgac.com/blog/coping-with-covid-19-part-ii-impacts-on-schedule/ (Accessed 16 March 2021).

Jones, W., Gibb, A.G.F., & Chow, V. (2022). Adapting to COVID-19 on construction sites: What are the lessons for long term improvements in safety and worker effectiveness?. *Journal of Engineering, Design and Technology*, 20(1), 66–85.

King, S.S., Rahman, R.A., Fauzi, M.A., & Haron, A.T. (2022). Critical analysis of pandemic impact on AEC organisations: The COVID-19 case. *Journal of Engineering, Design and Technology*, 20(1), 358–383.

King, T., & Lamontagne, A.D. (2022). COVID-19 and suicide risk in the construction sector: Preparing for a perfect storm. *Scandinavian Journal of Public Health*, 49, 774–778.

Ogunnusi, M., Hamma-Adama, M., Salman, H., & Kouider, T. (2020). COVID-19 pandemic: The effects and prospects in the construction industry. *International Journal of Real Estate Studies*, 14(2), 120–128.

Oladimeji, O. (2022). Influence of COVID-19 pandemic on local construction firms' viability. *Journal of Engineering, Design and Technology*, 20(1), 201–221.

Olatunde, N.A., Awodele, I.A., & Adebayo, B.O. (2022). Impact of COVID-19 on indigenous contractors in a developing economy. *Journal of Engineering, Design and Technology*, 20(1), 267–280.

Peterson, C., Sussell, A., Li, J., Schumacher, P.K., Yeoman, K., & Stone, D.M. (2020). Suicide rates by industry and occupation: National violent death reporting system, 32 States, 2016. *MMWR Morb Mortal Wkly Rep*, 69, 57–62. http://dx.doi.org/10.15585/mmwr.mm6903a1.

PricewaterhouseCoopers Limited. (2020). *Impact of COVID-19 on the supply chain industry*. Available at www.pwc.com/ng/en/assets/pdf/impact-of-covid19-the-supply-chain-industry.pdf (Accessed 05 April 2022).

Rehman, M.S.U., Shafiq, M.T., & Afzal, M. (2022). Impact of CIVID-19 on project performance in the UAE construction industry. *Journal of Engineering, Design and Technology*, 20(1), 246–266.

Salami, B.A., Ajayi, S.O., & Oyegoke, A.S. (2022). Coping with the Covid-19 pandemic: An exploration of the strategies adopted by construction firms. *Journal of Engineering, Design and Technology*, 20(1), 159–182.

Simpeh, F., & Amoah, C. (2020). Assessment of measures instituted to curb the spread of COVID-19 on construction site. *International Journal of Construction Management*. doi: 10.1080/15623599.2021.1874678.

Simpeh, F., & Amoah, C. (2022). COVID-19 guidelines incorporated in the health and safety management polices of construction firms *Journal of Engineering, Design and Technology*, 20(1), 6–23.

Stride, M., Suresh, R., Suresh, S., & Egbu, C. (2021). The effects of COVID-19 pandemic on the UK construction industry and the process of future-proofing business. *Construction Innovation*. doi: 10.1108/CI-03-2021-0045.

Umeokafor, N., Evangelinos, K., & Windapo, A. (2020). Strategies for improving complex construction health and safety regulatory environments. *International Journal of Construction Management*. doi: 10.1080/15623599.2019.1707853. Advance online publication.

World Health Organization (WHO). (2020). *Q&A on coronaviruses (COVID-19)*. Available at www.who.int/emergencies/diseases/novel-coronavirus-2019/question-and-answers-hub/q-a-detail/q-acoronaviruses (Accessed 24 March 2022).

# 15 Developing resilient construction professionals in the COVID-19 era

## Examining architecture students' personality perspective

*Alime Sanlı and Pinar Irlayici Cakmak*

### Introduction

The COVID-19 pandemic, which was declared a global epidemic by the World Health Organization (WHO) at the end of March 2020, has greatly affected the world (World Health Organization, 2020; Chih et al., 2022). Since it first broke out in Wuhan, China in December 2019, the world has changed drastically in just one month due to this unprecedented pandemic (Ogunnusi et al., 2020). COVID-19, an infectious disease, spread violently all over the world, causing health problems and death (Gamil and Alhagar, 2020). This epidemic has significantly affected not only human health but also different sectors and the economy (Ogunnusi et al., 2020). The COVID-19 pandemic has created a complex system of stressors such as sudden changes, future uncertainties, and economic disruptions. The construction industry, one of the sectors most affected by the COVID-19 pandemic, faced many stress factors due to the pandemic (Gamil and Alhagar, 2020).

Construction professionals, who were exposed to intense stress even in the normal period before the pandemic, encountered new stress factors such as changes in the way they do business, uncertainties, remote working, and the risk of COVID-19 contamination during the pandemic process (Ogunnusi et al., 2020). In such a dynamic industry, construction project professionals need to cope with these stressors to survive, recover from the COVID-19 pandemic, and be prepared for future contingencies (Chih et al., 2022). Ramazani and Jergeas (2015) state that future professionals should be prepared to engage in the context of real-life projects, and the university has an important role in encouraging future construction project professionals to start a learning process that will continue throughout their careers.

Resilience, which is the ability to bounce back and adapt, is considered an important skill that enables individuals to cope with stress (Turner et al., 2019). Universities can offer assets and resources that create a learning environment that promotes resilience-building (Turner et al., 2019). This research focuses on architecture education as an important area for resilience development. Students' attitudes and behaviors toward stress during their education follow them in their professional careers (Groen et al., 2019). Thus, it is important to understand the coping strategies and supports needed to assist and develop student resilience (Holdsworth et al., 2019). Researches show that decision-making (Al-Dabbagh,

DOI: 10.1201/9781003278368-17

2020), problem-solving (Knight, 2007), self-management (Groen et al., 2019), bouncing back (Turner et al., 2016), maintaining a positive attitude (Turner and Simmons, 2020), and adaptability (Sirotiak and Sharma, 2019) skills improve resilience. Also, personality traits can be used to support resilience development and stress management (Vollrath, 2001).

Personality characteristics that have an important effect on the stress process affect the choice, reaction, and outcome of the stressful condition (Vollrath, 2001). The response to similar stressors differs due to personality types. Therefore, personality types should be taken into account in determining strategies for coping with stress (Dumitru and Cozman, 2012). In this study, the Enneagram model was chosen to determine personality types. The Enneagram model is considered a valuable tool for personal development by trainers and practitioners (Sutton et al., 2013). Enneagram personality types enable individuals to recognize themselves under stress and development conditions (Riso and Hudson, 2008) and give an idea of personality and potential qualities before experiencing an event (Oraz et al., 2016). This study aims to develop suggestions using the Enneagram model as a practical guide to explore the relationship between personality types and stress and resilience during the pandemic and to encourage resilience development of architecture students and develop resilient construction project professionals.

## Stress in architectural education during COVID-19 pandemic

With the outbreak of the COVID-19 pandemic, universities had to close their academic activities at the end of March 2020 (Allu-kangkum, 2021). Never before has the education system been disrupted to this magnitude. Many governments ordered most educational institutions to end face-to-face education and move to online teaching and virtual education almost overnight. This sudden and unprecedented distance learning has affected all educational institutions (Salama and Crosbie, 2020). Many architectural schools also shelved face-to-face education in less than three weeks and decided to switch to online (Salama and Crosbie, 2020). The adoption of online learning in architectural education was quite difficult due to inadequate preparation, infrastructure difficulties, and teachers' indifference to this change (Varma and Jafri, 2020).

Architecture students faced increased stress factors brought about by sudden changes with the outbreak of the pandemic (Salama and Crosbie, 2020). The social nature and physical environment of architectural education are critical to the learning environment, such as activities, nonverbal cues, and chance encounters (Varma and Jafri, 2020). Online education has made students feel lonely and inadequate, increasing their procrastination tendencies and anxieties about academic time uncertainties caused by the change (Milovanović, 2020; Varma and Jafri, 2020). Students who are suddenly disconnected from social life are very worried about when life will return to normal (Daniel, 2020). Addressing this sudden change in the history of architectural education and new and old stress factors is important (Salama and Crosbie, 2020).

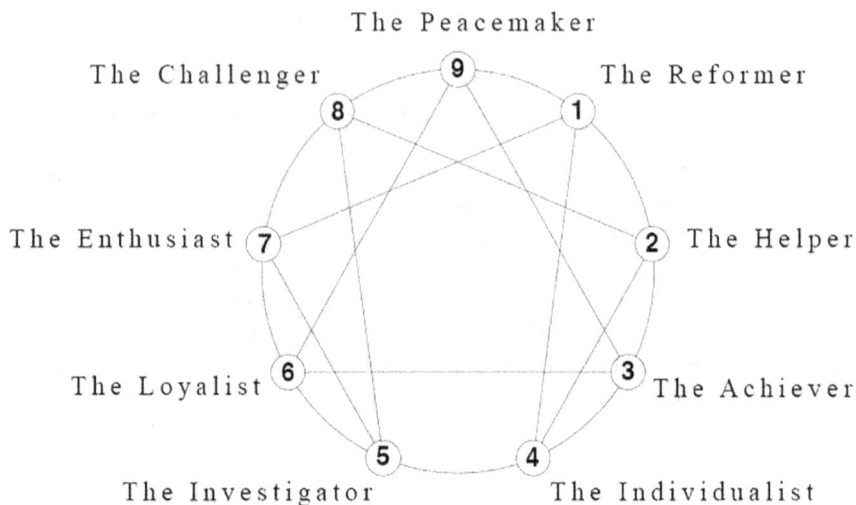

*Figure 15.1* The Enneagram.

## The Enneagram

The word "Enneagram" (pronounced "any-a-gram") consists of the Greek words "ennea," meaning "nine," and "gramma" or "grammos," meaning "written" or "point" (Riso and Hudson, 1999). In line with this word meaning, Enneagram is a geometric symbol as shown in Figure 15.1 with nine points representing the nine main personality types and dynamics of human nature (Palmer, 2010). These types are Type 1-The Reformer, Type 2-The Helper, Type 3-The Achiever, Type 4-The Individualist, Type 5-The Investigator, Type 6-The Loyalist, Type 7-The Enthusiast, Type 8-The Challenger, and Type 9-The Peacemaker (Riso and Hudson, 2008). Enneagram is a scientifically proven model that assumes that none of these nine personality types is superior to the other (Bland, 2010), and each type perceives the world differently (Riso and Hudson, 1999).

One of the potentially promising features of the Enneagram is that it describes the behavior and developmental levels of individuals in situations of stress and growth (Sutton et al., 2013). The Levels of Development provide a framework that shows the harmony of all the different traits of each personality type in a large whole (The Enneagram Institute, 2020). These levels of development are divided into three groups: healthy, average, and unhealthy. The movement toward health, up the Levels, is a sign of increased mental health and balance (Riso and Hudson, 2008).

## Methodology

In this part, hypotheses have been created to address the purpose of this study and to present the use of the Enneagram model as a practical guide. Hypotheses are developed by associating Enneagram personality types with resilience skills and stress factors. These hypotheses are put forward in two ways: null hypotheses (usually a statement of null effect) and alternative hypotheses (usually the opposite of a null hypothesis) (Dahiru, 2008).

An online web-based questionnaire survey method is selected to test the proposed hypotheses. The questionnaire consists of three sections. The first section contains personal information to identify the participant profile. In the second part, there are items determined through the literature to measure the stress factors and resilience skills of the participants during the pandemic era. The response to each item is measured on a five-point Likert scale. The third part consists of the Enneagram Type Indicator to determine the personality types of the participants. The designed questionnaire is tested through a pilot study. At first, the survey was planned to be conducted face-to-face to inform participants about Enneagram and to encourage them to answer the questionnaire. However, due to the pandemic, it was decided to provide this information online, and a video introducing Enneagram was prepared for the participants. The video and the final questionnaire were delivered to the participants via online access in December 2020, and a total of 96 usable surveys were returned by the end of February 2021.

Data were analyzed using the Statistical Package for Social Sciences (SPSS) for Windows™ Version 27. Before the statistical analysis of data, a reliability test was conducted to ascertain the reliability of the questionnaire survey (Sekaran and Bougie, 2016). The value of Cronbach's $\alpha$ coefficient must equal or exceed 70 percent to determine the reliability of the questionnaire (Cronbach and Shavelson, 2004). The values of Cronbach's $\alpha$ coefficient for the resilience scale were 0.814 in this study. Since this value was more than 0.7, the reliability of the questionnaire was established for further statistical analysis. The normality aspect was tested using the Shapiro – Wilk test, and it was found that the data was not normally distributed. Kruskal-Wallis H-test evaluates the differences between more than two independently sampled groups that are not normally distributed (McKight and Najab, 2010). Therefore, the non-parametric Kruskal-Wallis H-test was applied to test the significance of differences between Enneagram personality types, stress factors, and resilience skills. To provide further statistical insight into how each personality type pair is differentially related to stress and resilience, the post-hoc Dunn's statistical test corresponding to the pairwise comparison set was applied.

**Results and discussion**

Since the study aimed to examine the relationship between Enneagram personality types and stress and resilience during the pandemic and to offer suggestions for future construction project professionals to cope with stress and develop resilience, the profile of survey participants was determined to be architecture students. Among 96 participants, 29.2% of them are undergraduate students, 54.2% of them are graduate students, and 16.7% of them are doctoral students. According to the distribution of the Enneagram personality, among participants (n:96), 24% of them are Type One, 16.7% of them are Type Two, 7.3% of them are Type Three, 8.3% of them are Type Four, 9.4% of them are Type Five, 14.6% of them are Type Six, 4.2%

of them are Type Seven, 6.3% of them are Type Eight, and 9.4% of them are Type Nine. Before the statistical analysis of the data collected from the questionnaire study with 96 participants, the reliability test was performed and the reliability of the questionnaire for statistical analysis was ensured by finding Cronbach's α coefficient of 0.814. The data collected are analyzed using the Kruskal-Wallis H-test and post-hoc Dunn's statistical test to determine the significant differences between the variables. The results of this analysis are presented in Table 15.1, where statistically significant relationships were found between Enneagram personality types, resilience skills, and stress factors in the pandemic era.

In line with this evidence, the relationship between each personality type and stress factors and resilience skills is as follows:

Architecture students experience stress due to the sudden changes that occurred with the COVID-19 pandemic (Salama and Crosbie, 2020). The application of the Kruskal-Wallis H-test to the "sudden change" stress factor returned a p-value of 0.092, providing sufficient statistical evidence to reject the null hypothesis, concluding that this stress factor significantly differs across the examined personality types at a 10% significance level. The application of post-hoc Dunn's tests to the "sudden change" stress factor returned a p-value of 0.004, providing sufficient statistical evidence at a 95% confidence level to support the following conclusions: Sixes and Nines experience this stress factor more than Ones. At a 90% confidence level evidence is as follows: Sixes and Nines experience this stress factor more than Threes. In line with this statistical evidence, Sixes and Nines experience this stress factor more than Ones and Threes. Type Threes are goal- and achievement-oriented (Riso and Hudson, 2008) and may try to turn the change into opportunity and gain a competitive edge. Therefore, Threes may experience less stress due to the pandemic changes. Type Ones care about following rules and think that breaking the rules should be punished (Daniels and Price, 2004). Because of the mandatory rules that suddenly appeared due to the pandemic, Ones may look favorably at change. Type Sixes are planned, programmed, cautious, and prepared for potential future problems (Williams et al., 2008). Because of these sudden changes, Sixes can experience stress by having trouble making plans and anticipating possibilities. Type Nines love routines and do not want their peaceful environment to be disrupted by differences (Palmer, 2010). Nines may experience stress because the sudden changes disrupt their order and peaceful environment, and they feel unsafe. Therefore, Sixes and Nines should develop strategies to cope with the sudden changes during the COVID-19 pandemic. To cope with this stressor, instead of constantly thinking about the future, living in the moment and avoiding excessively anxious thoughts support Sixes' resilience development; Nines can cope with sudden change by stepping out of their comfort zone and being open to change (Daniels and Price, 2004; Riso and Hudson, 1999, 2008; Palmer, 2010; The Enneagram Institute, 2020).

Students' tendency to procrastinate has increased during the pandemic era (Milovanović, 2020). The application of the Kruskal-Wallis H-test to the "tendency to procrastinate" stress factor returned a p-value of 0.012, providing sufficient statistical evidence to reject the null hypothesis, concluding that this stress

Table 13.1 Kruskal – Wallis H-test and Post-hoc Dunn's statistical test results.

| Factors | sig. | Type 1 (T1) | Type 2 (T2) | Type 3 (T3) | Type 4 (T4) | Type 5 (T5) | Type 6 (T6) | Type 7 (T7) | Type 8 (T8) | Type 9 (T9) |
|---|---|---|---|---|---|---|---|---|---|---|
| Bouncing back | 0,023* | (T2) 0,054** (T4) 0,002* | (T1) 0,054** (T3) 0,064** (T9) 0,069** | (T2) 0,064** (T4) 0,004** (T6) 0,74** (T9) 0,05** | (T3) 0,004* (T5) 0,007* (T6) 0,086** (T7) 0,022* (T8) 0,011* (T9) 0,004* | (T4) 0,007* | (T4) 0,086** (T3) 0,74** | (T4) 0,022* | (T4) 0,011* | (T2) 0,069** (T4) 0,004* (T3) 0,05** |
| Decision-making | 0,006* | (T2) 0,007* (T4) 0,018* (T9) 0,034* | (T1) 0,007* (T3) 0,001* (T8) 0,073** | (T2) 0,001* (T4) 0,003* (T5) 0,017* (T7) 0,022* (T9) 0,005* | (T1) 0,018* (T3) 0,003* (T8) 0,077** | (T3) 0,017* | | (T3) 0,022* | (T2) 0,073** (T4) 0,077** | (T1) 0,034* (T3) 0,005* |
| Self-management | 0,002* | (T2) 0,02* (T4) 0,003* | (T1) 0,02* (T3) 0,001* (T8) 0,011* | (T2) 0,001* (T4) 0,00* | (T1) 0,003* (T3) 0,00* (T5) 0,077** (T8) 0,002* | (T4) 0,077** | | (T8) 0,086** | (T2) 0,011* (T4) 0,002* (T7) 0,086** | |
| Maintaining positive attitude | 0,057** | (T5) 0,005* | (T7) 0,09* (T8) 0,075** | | (T1) 0,005* (T5) 0,013* (T7) 0,01* (T8) 0,006* (T9) 0,077** | (T4) 0,013* | (T7) 0,088** (T8) 0,075** | (T2) 0,09* (T4) 0,01* (T6) 0,088** | (T2) 0,075** (T4) 0,006* (T6) 0,075** | (T4) 0,077** |
| Adaptability | 0,262 | | | | | | | | | |
| Problem-solving | 0,162 | | | | | | | | | |
| Sudden change | 0,092** | (T6) 0,004* (T9) 0,004* | | | | | (T1) 0,004* (T3) 0,074** | | | (T1) 0,004* (T3) 0,005* |
| Tendency to procrastinate | 0,012* | (T2) 0,005* (T4) 0,001* (T5) 0,054* (T6) 0,042* | (T1) 0,005* (T3) 0,062** (T8) 0,071** | (T2) 0,062** (T4) 0,01** | (T1) 0,001* (T3) 0,01** (T8) 0,012* (T9) 0,019* | (T1) 0,054** | (T1) 0,042* | | (T2) 0,071** (T4) 0,012* | (T4) 0,019* |
| Feeling inadequate | 0,037* | (T2) 0,001* (T4) 0,013* (T6) 0,07** | (T1) 0,001* (T8) 0,034* (T9) 0,01** | | (T1) 0,013* (T8) 0,064** (T9) 0,029* | | (T1) 0,07** | | (T2) 0,034* (T4) 0,064** | (T2) 0,01** (T4) 0,029* |
| Future anxiety | 0,628 | | | | | | | | | |
| Lack of social activity | 0,374 | | | | | | | | | |

* Results displaying statistical evidence of dissimilar performance at a 0.05 significance level.
** Results displaying statistical evidence of dissimilar performance at a 0.1 significance level but not at a 0.05 significance level.

factor significantly differs across the examined personality types at a 5% significance level. According to the results, Twos and Fours experience this stress factor
more than Ones, Threes, and Eights. Eights and Threes tend to act immediately
rather than procrastinate. Type Ones can postpone a project, task, or selection as a
strategy to avoid criticism and punishment for fear of making mistakes. However,
Ones' procrastination tendency is a relaxation option to get away from more stressful events. Type Fours tend to delay, waiting for the best moment to act. Type Twos
postpone their needs to satisfy the needs of others (Williams et al., 2008; Riso and
Hudson, 2008). The procrastination tendency of the Twos and Fours creates stress.
To cope with this stressor, Twos should go ahead and take action instead of running
away from their problems; Fours should take action by focusing on the moment
(Daniels and Price, 2004; Riso and Hudson, 2008; Palmer, 2010; The Enneagram
Institute, 2020).

Students may experience stress by feeling inadequate. Students studying architecture during the pandemic period think that they are inadequate compared to
those in the normal period (Daniel, 2020). The application of the Kruskal-Wallis
H-test to the "feeling inadequate" stress factor returned a p-value of 0.037, providing sufficient statistical evidence to reject the null hypothesis, concluding that this
stress factor significantly differs across the examined personality types at a 5%
significance level. According to the results, Twos, Fours, and Sixes experience this
stress factor more than Ones, Threes, and Eights. Type Ones, Threes, and Eights
are self-confident and believe they are self-sufficient. Twos tend to find themselves
and what they do inadequate. Fours can feel insecure, inadequate, and depressed
by comparing themselves to other people. The Sixes find themselves inadequate
and seek a guide. To cope with this stressor, Twos should believe that they are
self-sufficient. Fours should be at peace with themselves rather than criticizing
themselves. Sixes should believe in and trust themselves. (Daniels and Price, 2004;
Riso and Hudson, 2008; Palmer, 2010; The Enneagram Institute, 2020).

Bouncing back makes it easier to manage and adapt to stressors effectively and
develops resilience (Turner et al., 2016). The application of the Kruskal-Wallis
H-test to the "bouncing back" resilience skill returned a p-value of 0.023, providing sufficient statistical evidence to reject the null hypothesis, concluding that
this resilience skill significantly differs across the examined personality types at a
5% significance level. This skill is more prominent for Ones, Threes, Eights, and
Nines. Also, this skill is less prominent for Fours than others. Type Ones believe
that they can correct all the wrongs in the world on their own. Threes and Eights are
combative in the face of difficulties. Nines ignore discomfort to avoid stress factors. Fours tend to give up in the face of difficulties (Daniels and Price, 2004; Riso
and Hudson, 2008). Therefore, Fours should develop their bouncing-back skill to
develop their resilience. By turning to positive emotions and believing in themselves, Fours can bounce back from difficult times and build resilience (Daniels
and Price, 2004).

Decision-making plays an important role in students' lifestyle choices, life planning, purposeful life development, and goals in their professional and educational
careers. Decision-making skills should be developed against sudden events such as

COVID-19 (Al-Dabbagh, 2020). The application of the Kruskal-Wallis H-test to the "decision-making" resilience skill returned a p-value of 0.006, providing sufficient statistical evidence to reject the null hypothesis, concluding that this resilience skill significantly differs across the examined personality types at a 5% significance level. This skill is more prominent for Ones, Threes, and Eights than for Twos, Fours, and Nines. Type Ones are determined to do the right thing and stick to their principles. Type Threes are determined and do whatever it takes to achieve their goals. Type Eights are determined individuals and can make tough decisions (Riso and Hudson, 2008; The Enneagram Institute, 2020). Twos, Fours, and Nines are more indecisive because Twos and Nines often act according to the wishes of others, and Fours focus on shortcomings and constantly analyze their thoughts. Therefore, Twos, Fours, and Nines should develop their decision-making skills to improve their resilience and move forward in the direction of development. Developing their awareness and thinking proactively, critically, and creatively before reacting can improve their decision-making skills (Al-Dabbagh, 2020).

Self-management is the control of an individual over their behaviors, especially in pursuit of a particular goal (APA Dictionary of Psychology, 2020). Students' abilities in self-management may better equip them to cope with stressful situations and increase resilience (Groen et al., 2019). The application of the Kruskal-Wallis H-test to the "self-management" resilience skill returned a p-value of 0.002, providing sufficient statistical evidence to reject the null hypothesis, concluding that this resilience skill significantly differs across the examined personality types at a 5% significance level. This skill is more prominent for Ones, Threes, Fives, and Eights than Twos, Fours, and Sevens. Type Ones are organized, self-directed, and responsible individuals who make good use of time. Type Threes think that the time they don't use is wasted and will never come back. Threes want to do a lot in a short time and use their time efficiently. Type Fives are self-controlled and analyze before acting. Type Eights do not like to be controlled and want to maintain control of their lives themselves. Eights organize resources and try to use them in the best way possible. Twos disrupt their plans because they care about the wishes of others. Type Fours have trouble with self-management. Type Sevens are enthusiastic, easily out of control, and act impulsively (Daniels and Price, 2004; Williams et al., 2008; Palmer, 2010). Therefore, Twos, Fours, and Sevens should develop their self-management skills to improve their resilience and move forward in the direction of development. Individuals managing their behavior set personal standards, evaluate their performance in terms of these standards, and self-manage based on their self-assessments. Tactics such as self-observation, goal setting, and rehearsal can be used to practice self-directed behavior (Manz and Sims, 1980).

Maintaining a positive attitude is an aspect of resilience and makes it easier to deal with stress (Knight, 2007). The application of the Kruskal-Wallis H-test to the "maintaining a positive attitude" resilience skill returned a p-value of 0.057, providing sufficient statistical evidence to reject the null hypothesis, concluding that this resilience skill significantly differs across the examined personality types at a 10% significance level. This skill is less prominent for Fours and Sixes than others. Also, this tactic is more prominent for Sevens and Eights. Type Sevens are full of life, talking about good things instead of negativities. Type Eights believe they are strong enough to deal with all the challenges in the world. Type Fours tend to think about what is missing and tend toward negativity. Type Sixes are pessimistic and tend to think about negative possibilities (Daniels and Price, 2004; Riso and Hudson, 2008). Therefore, Fours and Sixes should develop their maintaining positive attitude skills to improve their resilience and move forward in the direction of development. The skill to adapt positively to stress and distress situations enables the student to progress, grow, and learn (Turner et al., 2019). Students can display a positive attitude with the tactics they choose while experiencing a stressful event (Groen et al., 2019). Developing tactics that maintain a positive attitude, such as the ability to keep a calm head in difficult times, can significantly reduce stress. These tactics which will increase the positive attitude, such as avoiding disappointments, not being overwhelmed, and putting the work to be done into perspective, are important to turn the negative choices made when dealing with stress into positive ones (Turner and Simmons, 2020).

### Implications for research

In this study, significant relationships were found between Enneagram personality types and resilience skills and stress factors. These relationships show that the personality traits of architecture students influence the effects and responses of this unexpected COVID-19 pandemic. The findings suggest that Enneagram

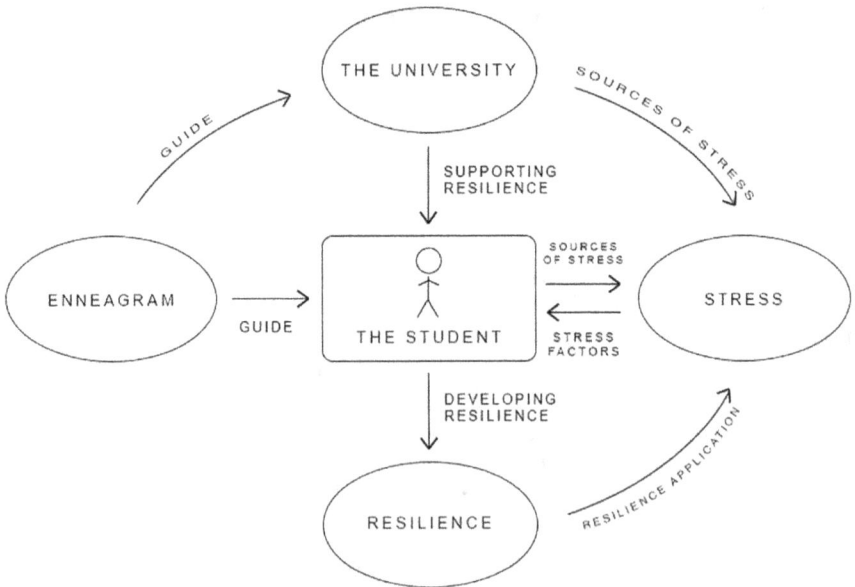

*Figure 15.2* The iterative process of resilience development in undergraduate architecture students.

personality types can be used to help future construction professionals prepare for situations like the pandemic and increase their resilience.

The ability of each type to explain their changing behaviors and potential for stress and relaxation can facilitate the use of the Enneagram model as a practical tool (Oraz et al., 2016). With the practical use of the Enneagram model, students can gain individual awareness, and advisors and mentors who do not have enough time to get to know students in the pandemic era can offer faster solutions to support students' development. Thus, students develop strategies for coping with stress and building resilience to advance toward development both in their academic life and in their careers. As illustrated in Figure 15.2, the Enneagram is an important tool as a practical guide to support the iterative resilience development process at the university and beyond.

This research supports previous studies that identified the positive role of promoting resilience development at university in preparing students for their careers (Holdsworth et al., 2019; Groen et al., 2019; Turner et al., 2019; Turner and Simmons, 2020). This is the first research to associate stress factors of architecture students and resilience skills with Enneagram personality types during the COVID-19 pandemic era. By addressing this gap, this research is highly contributing to the body of knowledge. This research is to identify the relationships between the stress of the pandemic on students from their perspective. Additionally, this research draws attention to the importance of focusing on the student's perspective to prepare future construction project professionals at the university for the demanding and stress-filled construction industry.

This study is limited to architecture students. In future research, the approach in this thesis research can be examined within the context of students in other disciplines who will be future construction industry professionals. Also, this approach can be projected beyond the university to construction industry professionals.

**Conclusions**

The construction industry has faced many stress factors with the outbreak of the COVID-19 pandemic. Future construction professionals need to be prepared for unexpected events such as pandemics, learn how to cope with stress factors, and be resilient. Personality characteristics affect stress and resilience. The university encourages future construction project professionals to initiate a development process that will continue throughout their careers. The purpose of this thesis research is to examine how to develop the resilience of future construction project professionals at the university by exploring the relationship between personality types and resilience and stress. Architecture undergraduate education is designated as the scope of this study. In this context, hypotheses were formed to understand the relationship between Enneagram personality types, resilience skills, and stress factors. The questionnaire method was chosen to test the hypotheses. The reliability of the data collected from 96 participants was established for further statistical analysis. Kruskal-Wallis H and post-hoc Dunn's statistical tests were performed to test the proposed hypotheses and identify significant differences between the variables. The analysis results provided sufficient statistical evidence to reject null hypotheses concluding that there is no relationship between the Enneagram personality types, stress factors, and resilience skills. Sudden change, tendency to procrastinate, feeling inadequate, stress factors and bouncing back, decision-making, self-management, and maintaining a positive attitude resilience skills are associated with personality types.

In conclusion, statistically significant correlations were found between Enneagram personality types and resilience and stress during the COVID-19 pandemic era. These findings are an important contribution to developing the resilience of future construction professionals (architecture students). This study provides the Enneagram as a practical guide to support the iterative process of building resilience in the university and beyond. Enneagram guides both students to increase their self-awareness and university advisors to understand and support students. Thus, future construction professionals who develop resilience and cope with stress by using the Enneagram as a guide can move in the direction of development beyond being prepared and surviving unexpected events such as COVID-19 pandemics.

## References

Al-Dabbagh, Z.S. (2020). The role of decision-maker in crisis management: A qualitative study using grounded theory (COVID-19 pandemic crisis as a model). *Journal of Public Affairs*, 20(4), e2186.

Allu-Kangkum, E.L. (2021). Covid-19 and sustainable architectural education: Challenges and perceptions on online learning. *Journal of Educational Research*, 6(2), 7–13.

APA (American Psychological Association). *Dictionary of psychology* [Online]. Available at https://dictionary.apa.org/ (Accessed 17 July 2020).

Bland, A.M. (2010). The Enneagram: A review of the empirical and transformational literature. *The Journal of Humanistic Counseling, Education and Development*, 49(1), 16–31.

Chih, Y.Y., Hsiao, C.Y.L., Zolghadr, A., & Naderpajouh, N. (2022). Resilience of organizations in the construction industry in the face of COVID-19 disturbances: Dynamic capabilities perspective. *Journal of Management in Engineering*, 38(2), 04022002.

Cronbach, L.J., & Shavelson, R.J. (2004). My current thoughts on coefficient alpha and successor procedures. *Educational and Psychological Measurement*, 64(3), 391–418.

Dahiru, T. (2008). P-value, a true test of statistical significance? A cautionary note. *Annals of Ibadan Postgraduate Medicine*, 6(1), 21–26.

Daniel, S.J. (2020). Education and the COVID-19 pandemic. *Prospects*, 49(1), 91–96.

Daniels, D.N., & Price, V.A. (2004). *Enneagram Kendini Bilme Sanatı*. Turkey: Kaknüs Yayınları.

Dumitru, V.M., & Cozman, D. (2012). The relationship between stress and personality factors. *Human and Veterinary Medicine*, 4(1), 34–39.

The Enneagram Institute. [Online]. Available at www.enneagraminstitute.com/ (Accessed 27 April 2020).

Gamil, Y., & Alhagar, A. (2020). The impact of pandemic crisis on the survival of construction industry: A case of COVID-19. *Mediterranean Journal of Social Sciences*, 11(4), 122–122.

Groen, C., Simmons, D.R., & Turner, M. (2019). Developing resilience: Experiencing and managing stress in a US undergraduate construction program. *Journal of Professional Issues in Engineering Education and Practice*, 145(2), 04019002.

Holdsworth, S., Turner, M., & Scott-Young, C.M. (2019). Developing the resilient learner: A resilience framework for universities. In *Transformations in tertiary education* (pp. 27–42). Singapore: Springer.

Knight, C. (2007). A resilience framework: Perspectives for educators. *Health Education*, 107(6), 543–555.

Manz, C.C., & Sims Jr, H.P. (1980). Self-management as a substitute for leadership: A social learning theory perspective. *Academy of Management Review*, 5(3), 361–367.

McKight, P.E., & Najab, J. (2010). Kruskal-wallis test. In *The corsini encyclopedia of psychology* (pp. 1–1). Wiley Online Library. Available at https://onlinelibrary.wiley.com/ (Accessed 20 July 2020).

Milovanović, A., Kostić, M., Zorić, A., Đorđević, A., Pešić, M., Bugarski, J., Todorović, D., Sokolović, N., & Josifovski, A. (2020). Transferring COVID-19 challenges into learning potentials: Online workshops in architectural education. *Sustainability*, 12(17), 7024.

Ogunnusi, M., Hamma-Adama, M., Salman, H., & Kouider, T. (2020). COVID-19 pandemic: The effects and prospects in the construction industry. *International Journal of Real Estate Studies*, 14(Special Issue 2).

Oraz, G., Günaydın, H.M., Giritli, H., & Tezel, E. (2016). Proje Yönetimi Performansı ve Kişilik Etkileşimleri. 4th International Project and Construction Management Conference, Eskişehir, Turkey (in Turkish).

Palmer, H. (2010). *Ruhun Aynası Ennegram'a Yansıyan İnsan Manzaraları*. İstanbul, Turkey: Kaknüs Yayınları (in Turkish).

Ramazani, J., & Jergeas, G. (2015). Project managers and the journey from good to great: The benefits of investment in project management training and education. *International Journal of Project Management*, 33(1), 41–52.

Riso, D.R., & Hudson, R. (1999). *The wisdom of the Enneagram: The complete guide to psychological and spiritual growth for the nine personality types* (Vol. 20). New York: Bantam Books.

Riso, D.R., & Hudson, R. (2008). *Enneagram ile Kişilik Analizi*. Turkey: Butik Yayınevi (in Turkish).

Salama, A.M., & Crosbie, M.J. (2020). Educating architects in a post-pandemic world. *Common\Edge* [Online]. Available at https://commonedge.org/educating-architects-in-a-post-pandemic-world/ (Accessed 9 October 2020).

Sekaran, U., & Bougie, R. (2016). *Research methods for business: A skill building approach*. New York: John Wiley & Sons.

Sirotiak, T., & Sharma, A. (2019). Problem-based learning for adaptability and management skills. *Journal of Professional Issues in Engineering Education and Practice*, 145(4), 04019008.

Sutton, A., Allinson, C., & Williams, H. (2013). Personality type and work-related outcomes: An exploratory application of the Enneagram model. *European Management Journal*, 31(3), 234–249.

Turner, M., Scott-Young, C.M., & Holdsworth, S. (2016). Bouncing back to move forward: Resilience of students in the built environment. *Association of Researchers in Construction Management*, 1, 589–598.

Turner, M., Scott-Young, C., & Holdsworth, S. (2019). Developing the resilient project professional: Examining the student experience. *International Journal of Managing Projects in Business*, 12(3), 716–729.

Turner, M., & Simmons, D.R. (2020). Taking a partnered approach to managing academic stress: An undergraduate study. *International Journal of Construction Education and Research*, 16(4), 251–269.

Varma, A., & Jafri, M.S. (2020). COVID-19 responsive teaching of undergraduate architecture programs in India: Learnings for post-pandemic education. *Archnet-IJAR: International Journal of Architectural Research*, 15(1), 189–202.

Vollrath, M. (2001). Personality and stress. *Scandinavian Journal of Psychology*, 42(4), 335–347.

Williams, K.C., Petrosky, A.R., & Hernandez, E.H. (2008). The Enneagram and its possibilities for student learning. *Journal of Business and Change Management*, 3, 63–93.

World Health Organization. (2020). *Director-General's opening remarks at the mission briefing on COVID-19*. Geneva, Switzerland: Tedros Adhanom Ghebreyesus.

# 16 Safety, health and wellbeing of construction workers in Nigeria – opportunities and challenges associated with the COVID-19 pandemic

*Haruna Musa Moda, Bello Mahmud Zailani, Mu'awiya Abubakar, Abdullahi Muhammad and Yahaya Makarfi Ibrahim*

## 1.0 The state of the Nigerian construction industry in the COVID-19 era

The unique characteristics of the construction industry make it among the economic sectors that were severely affected by the pandemic (Osuizugbo, 2021). Many significant activities in construction require physical presence and close interactions among different groups of workers. This was not possible during the pandemic due to restrictions imposed by government which brought about physical distancing between individuals, among other measures. Authorities were strongly advised by health experts to restrict movement and public gatherings, which led to shutdown of almost all construction sites and office activities. The nature of the construction business is such that not all activities can be performed in the "work from home" system adopted in Nigeria and many other parts of the world. However, certain activities such as designs, review meetings and other matters that do not require physical presence on site were carried out remotely. Despite these restrictions, some construction activities in critical sectors were not fully closed. This enabled such projects that were considered essential (e.g., construction of healthcare facilities) to be delivered on time.

Generally, the construction sector as a major contributor to the GDP of large and small economies suffered unprecedented consequences (Alsharef et al., 2021). On construction sites where works were critically managed and pushed to continue, there were serious reductions in productivity rates, leading to sharp delays and cost overruns. These challenges were faced not only in Nigeria but also in other countries. Almost all countries of the world have suffered the impact, with many of them falling into recession. This prompted several studies to investigate the impact of the pandemic on economic sectors across the globe to devise counter-strategies. For instance, Fernandes (2020) reported that the pandemic had the likelihood of causing a decrease in the gross domestic product (GDP) of countries by as much as 3–6%. Many countries witnessed a reduction in construction productivity, declining foreign investment and lower number of public projects. As Gamil and Alhagar (2020) concluded, the impact

DOI: 10.1201/9781003278368-18

of COVID-19 on the construction sector spanned issues of delays, cost over-runs and reduction in productivity. In addition, the high rate of labour turnover across small and medium businesses that lacked the ability to pay wages and salaries have been reported. The procurement of built assets and the construction industry at large have been affected by the full and partial stoppage of works which were majorly carried out with minimal competition and scrutiny (Ogunnusi et al., 2021). Other impacts include delays in payment and inflation in prices of materials arising from border closure and movement restrictions (Agyekum et al., 2021). These caused disruptions in the construction supply chain with attendant negative impacts on the construction companies in many countries (King et al., 2021). Similarly, project abandonment, claims and litigations arising from construction disputes were other financial impacts of the pandemic (Yusuf et al., 2021).

The industry was reported to have underperformed in 2020 with an average output falling by 7.7% in real terms. While a significant output drop of 31.8% year-on-year (YoY) was witnessed in the second quarter of 2020, it recovered in Q3 of 2020, with a 2.8% YoY growth (NBS, 2021). In a bid to restore economic growth and stability, although not as direct response to the pandemic, the government's "Economic Recovery and Growth Plan" (ERGP, 2017–2020) came in handy. The plan targeted a 7% real annual GDP growth by 2020 and specifically targeted the construction industry as one to leverage in terms of job creation, as huge resources have been earmarked for investment in the provision of infrastructure. Growth in construction output significantly improved in 2021 compared to the second quarter of 2020, when works were highly restricted. This was facilitated by the significant recovery in production levels. Overall, the industry is projected to grow at an average annual rate of 2.8% from 2022 to 2025, supported by the government's plans to invest in national infrastructure (NBS, 2021).

Ogunnusi et al. (2021) reported that the COVID-19 pandemic has resulted in efforts by various stakeholders towards the improvement of workplace health and safety protocols in construction compared to the pre-pandemic era. Construction organisations in Nigeria were reported to have integrated aspects of the global COVID-19 guidelines into their respective organisational policies, especially after the restrictions (Simpeh et al., 2021). Also, there was rapid adoption of the opportunity to utilise an effective virtual working environment, with employees of construction organisations given relevant facilities, such as laptops and cell phones, to allow them to work remotely (Ogunnusi et al., 2021). Nonetheless, Simpeh et al. (2021) noted some reluctance in the broad implementation of COVID-19 safety measures amongst construction organisations around the world, particularly in developing countries like Nigeria, with superstitions and lack of personal protective equipment supply being the most identified barriers. On this premise, the chapter aims to highlight the safety, health and wellbeing of construction workers in Nigeria, drawing on opportunities and challenges associated with the COVID-19 pandemic.

## 2.0   The impact of COVID-19 on health and wellbeing of construction employees

The health and wellbeing of employees relates to all facets of life at work, constituting safety and quality of the physical work environment, workers' psychology towards their work, social interactions, climate and the broader work organisation. Such wellbeing of employees translates into a major factor that can determine organisations' effectiveness. When organisations fail to recognise the need to promote workers' wellbeing, it ultimately leads to workplace glitches that may lead to stress accumulation, bullying, mental health disorders and addiction. Although the COVID-19 pandemic has had a significant impact on every sector of the global economy as evidenced in previous studies (Gamil and Alhagar, 2020), very limited focus has been placed on the safety and wellbeing of employees outside the healthcare sector, especially in developing countries like Nigeria.

The construction sector, especially in the global south, has witnessed almost a complete shutdown of its operations with resulting impacts on both the site operators and office employees. As the pandemic resulted in a downshift of the global economy, several construction organisations were pushed to lay off a large portion of their employees (Koh, 2020). This has tremendously affected the psychological wellbeing of workers, which in turn affected their social security. In the case of Nigeria, the majority of construction workers are employed in small and medium-sized organisations with limited levels of job security, which further exacerbated the nation's burden of disease via its direct psychological effects and long-term socio-economic impact among these workers (Kola et al., 2021). The lack of social protection is often seen as largely due to the industry's lack of a formalised structure, with a high rate of labour mobility due to temporary and casual employments (ILO, 2018). Thus, in the advent of a crisis such as the COVID-19 pandemic, there was a lack of social benefits to cater for employees, thereby adding to their anxiety and stress levels (Frimpong et al., 2022).

While there is a paucity of studies on construction workers' safety and wellbeing in the country as a result of the pandemic, lessons from other parts of the world reveal the extent to which employees in the construction sector have been mentally impacted by the pandemic resulting from the furlough and uncertainty around employment. The need to learn new technical skills and adapt to different schedules, remote working, etc., have added to the call for a closer look at the state of health and wellbeing among workers within the sector. In addition, the growing evidence regarding workers' wellbeing, such as suicide, depression, pollutant exposure and increased fatalities within the sector, is on the rise (Bowen et al., 2014; Pollock et al., 2020); this in turn is an indication of a lack of health and wellbeing awareness and services among the employees for coping with both work and personal crises. A high number of employees have been reported to have had health-related issues that also affected their wellbeing. Several factors, including fear of contracting the virus, furlough of workers, job demand, limited transportation modes, etc., account for the high number of employees with issues of health and wellbeing during this period (Koh, 2020; Stiles et al., 2021). To expand on this, an earlier study on young workers' physical and mental health in the sector reported high prevalence with regards to the nature of the work demand in the sector, which often resulted in substance abuse, thereby impacting their general quality of life (ILO, 2018; Frimpong et al., 2022).

## 2.1    *Managing the impact of COVID-19 pandemic on safety, health and wellbeing of workers*

Considering the operational changes brought about by the pandemic to the construction workplace and the organisations at large, there are positives: the pandemic has further contributed towards the promotion of positive safety culture and behaviour across the sector, as several organisations, especially in the global south, instituted a strict safety regime to help respond to work challenges brought about by the pandemic (Ogunnusi et al., 2021). To help build on such progress, organisations will need to ensure other good practices that help strengthen the safety, health and wellbeing of its employees are maintained.

### 2.1.1    *Promotion of wellbeing among construction workers*

Most studies on the subject have focused on rates of accidents and prevention within the nation's construction sector. There is, however, the need for researchers to consider employees' mental health and wellbeing, partly impacted by the pandemic, and develop strategies to build worker resilience and coping mechanisms within the construction industry in Nigeria. Symptoms such as anxiety, stress, irritation, depression, overwhelm and sleep difficulties are associated with employees' mental health and, where this goes unchecked, can lead to debilitating impacts to the workers, their families and employers. As enshrined in the third sustainable development goal (SDG 3) proposed by the United Nations (2015), employers of labour are charged with the responsibility to promote wellbeing among their employees. Poor working conditions, amongst other related factors in construction, can impact employees' state of wellbeing. Thus, to ensure the success of SDG 3, organisations are required to ensure occupational safety and health risk control measures are implemented. For instance, the provision of appropriate welfare facilities such as conveniences, changing and break areas should be considered as site planning, to prioritise the wellbeing and health of workers (ILO, 2015). Hence, there is a need for the construction sector in the country to consider the adoption of specific programmes that will complement existing safety and health measures at the workplace.

### 2.1.2    *Stakeholders' commitment*

The success of any occupational health and wellbeing programme aimed at tackling construction workplace disease and workers' wellbeing will rely heavily on the involvement of all stakeholders. These include the employers, employees, trade unions, company insurance funds and relevant ministries at state and federal levels.

While it was acknowledged earlier that most employers in Nigeria may struggle to address workers' wellbeing, management support is seen as critical towards this uptake and sustainability of a health and wellbeing programme; a robust partnership with external organisations at local, state and national levels must be maintained to guarantee the development of an open wellbeing culture at the centre of any developed policy (Bevan and Cooper, 2021; Moda et al., 2022). Therefore, every stakeholder has specific roles to perform to help in managing the impact of the COVID-19 pandemic on the health and safety of workers. The following are core stakeholders whose inputs will tremendously help in managing health and safety of workers in the post-pandemic period.

### 2.1.3 *Role of employers in promoting safety and wellbeing*

Employers of labour provide good working conditions to ensure the wellbeing of employees. They provide appropriate welfare facilities and fund all health and safety facilities required on construction sites (ILO, 2015). Furthermore, health and safety trainings are also included and funded by the client to maintain safety within the construction environment. In addition, labour organisations play critical roles in ensuring health, safety and wellbeing of workers. For example, the international labour organisation code of practice defines employers' general duties on employee health and safety. Section 2.2 charges employers to provide "a suitable programme on the safety and health of workers consistent with national laws and regulations and should comply with the prescribed safety and health measures at the workplace" alongside the provision of employees' general welfare onsite, as enshrined in Section 19 of the Code of Conduct (ILO, 1992). With the passing into law of the Labour Safety, Health Welfare Bill (Umeokafor et al., 2014) in Nigeria, it is hoped that active promotion of safe and healthy work environments within the construction sector will take into consideration the provision of welfare facilities that cater to the employees' wellbeing by every organisation, while erring organisations will be enforced to comply with such provisions by the regulatory agencies (Adeyemo and Smallwood, 2017). To understand the depth of the mental health issues associated with the absence of employees' wellbeing as exacerbated by the COVID-19 pandemic, research is further needed that focuses on physical and psychological wellbeing related to working conditions and other external factors (e.g., extreme heat exposure, low wage and lack of progression, etc.) among construction workers in the country. Therefore, the critical role of trade unions and regulatory agencies, such as the Department of Occupational Safety and Health, Federal Ministry of Labour and Productivity, in the post-pandemic era should be on monitoring and ensuring workers' welfare and other rights are not jettisoned or denied.

#### 2.1.3.1 CONTRACTORS AND SUPPLIER'S SAFETY AND WELLBEING COMMITMENT

The pandemic did impact the industry supply chain from operational perspectives by disrupting supply and demand, either due to the slowdown of activities by the manufacturers or difficulty in coordinating logistics, labour, supply chain, etc. (Ogunnusi et al., 2021). However, despite the disruption witnessed in the supply shortages and demand during the pandemic, there was an increase in certain chains; for instance, the supply of PPE within the industry. This in turn allowed the growth of new capacities (Baldwin and Tomiura, 2020) to which contractors are expected to maintain to promote the control of workplace hazards. Contractors and suppliers are vital stakeholders who, at the point of execution of the project, should implement all safety provisions and laws to help promote worker safety and wellbeing. Osei-Asibey et al. (2021) outlined the key roles of contractors towards ensuring safety, health and wellbeing of workers as provision of adequate welfare facilities and developing and implementing practicable health and safety plans and policies. Other important roles include organising health and safety trainings for workers and appointing health and safety officers on site. These roles, if properly undertaken, would promote workers' health and safety in the post-pandemic period.

### 2.2   *Application of information and communications technologies in safety and health management*

Technology is one promising solution capable of managing the impact of the COVID-19 pandemic on health, safety and wellbeing of construction workers. A variety of tools was deployed to manage construction safety during the pandemic. Around the globe, it has been reported that information and communication technology (ICT) tools played a significant role in providing solutions to the health and safety challenges posed by the pandemic in different sectors (Yang et al., 2021). There was a plethora of new and existing innovative technologies utilised to improve the safety and wellbeing of workers. During the pandemic, many construction organisations, especially in the developed countries, were reported to have increased their levels of adopting technologies for the execution of their projects (Bartlett et al., 2020). In view of this, it is envisaged that developing countries may be encouraged to also fast-track the level of adopting such technologies towards ensuring a safe working environment for their work force.

Considering the nature of the COVID-19 virus, artificial intelligence (AI) application was used in monitoring workers body temperature and social distance tracking to ensure the safety and wellbeing status of construction workers was guaranteed at the peak of the pandemic (Yang et al., 2021). Similarly, AI-driven image recognition machines were used to detect the compliance of workers with safety measures, specifically the proper use of personal protective equipment (Nath et al., 2020). In addition, technological solutions that include virtual meetings and cloud management prevented the spread of the virus whilst maintaining the conduct of customary work procedures. Other technological solutions, such as Building Information Modelling (BIM), were applied to model work processes to aid in preventing construction site accidents and improve safety on construction sites (Akinlolu et al., 2020). Visualisation technologies, such as Virtual Reality (VR) and Augmented Reality (AR), enabled workers to detect safety-related risks while working on their respective jobsites (Akinlolu et al., 2020).

Nonetheless, it is instructive to note that these technologies, as effective as they are, may not at present be consistently applied on construction projects in developing countries like Nigeria. The apparent barriers to their adoption for improved performance and safety in construction include high costs of software and hardware, high costs of implementation, lack of skilled resources, poor or nonexistent regulatory support and lack of ICT infrastructure (Ebekozien and Aigbavboa, 2021).

In Nigeria, there are challenges of a poor enabling environment, inadequate resources available for construction health and safety issues and general dogmatism towards the use of technology to address construction safety issues. By their inherent nature, construction organisations in Nigeria often lack the resilience to ensure the safety of their employees amidst safety challenges such as the COVID-19 pandemic (Abubakar et al., 2021). The industry is largely dominated by small and medium-sized organisations handling small and medium-sized projects with little to no budget for construction safety management (Moda et al., 2022), which makes meaningful investment to manage the safety of workers during pandemics difficult.

### 3.0   Construction 4.0 and health and safety enhancement opportunities

The idea of a 'smart construction site' promoted by the concept of Industry 4.0 is considered the most effective way of enhancing safety climate and employees' safety behaviour. Industry 4.0 was an initiative of the German government that aimed at digitising the manufacturing sector in Germany. This project signalled the emergence of the 4th industrial revolution, which today is seen as the continuation of previous industrial revolutions that featured mechanisation, electrification and digitalisation in the manufacturing sector (Osunsanmi et al., 2018). Taher (2021) described Construction 4.0 as an innovative technique that creates smart and decentralised construction sites by connecting the physical site with cyberspace via ubiquitous connections. The concept of construction industry revolution 4.0 is underpinned by four core principles: interconnection and interoperability; information transparency; decentralised decision making through BIM and cloud computing; and technical support with drones, robots and 3D printers. The smart construction site is characterised by the presence of physical-to-digital platforms that helps coordinate, design and execute construction projects in an effective and efficient manner (Dallasega et al., 2018). Despite the construction industry being slow in terms of adopting technological developments, it has witnessed the application of various technologies at different project lifecycle phases in recent times. Technological innovations, including the Internet of Things, Building Information Modelling (BIM), artificial intelligence, augmented and virtual reality and big data have all been responsible for reshaping the industry (Dallasega et al., 2018). One critical problem associated with communication by different machines is interoperability challenges (the ability of heterogeneous systems to seamlessly share and exchange information). With the aid of interconnectivity and information transparency supported by various technologies, decision-making will become decentralised, reducing human interference to the barest minimum and reducing workplace incidents.

To create an intelligent construction site that reaps the full benefits of automation, the use of these technologies will need to be integrated and made to work as a complete system. Construction 4.0 is one such solution that is poised to integrate information and communication technologies together, just as it set out to create a smart and digital construction environment that leverages information and communications technology to plan, execute and monitor activities and processes across the project life cycle (Rastogi, 2017). However, the high cost of investment, inadequate awareness and knowledge of the tools, resistance to change and several other factors make such actions not implementable. To fully explore this opportunity, it is crucial for employers and other stakeholders to proactively engage in capacity building that is capable of responding to the use of technology. This will help increase productivity and enhance workplace safety and wellbeing among employees.

### 3.1   Construction 4.0 technologies

Over the last decades, various technologies have been deployed to support the implementation of Construction 4.0. The construction industry has witnessed the application of these technologies at different phases of the project lifecycle using an integrated and holistic approach. The common technologies that support automation at this stage include Cyber-Physical Production Systems (CPPS), robots, sensors and drones that aid in monitoring construction sites. However, at the operational phase, BIM and Internet of Things (IoT) are combined with other sensor devices to constantly monitor the performance of the facility and its maintenance (Choi et al., 2020; El Jazzar et al., 2021). The adoption of Construction 4.0 technologies can provide better means of managing health and safety risk, alongside the optimisation of operations and improvement around process efficiency on projects. However, it is evident that such a move towards technology integration is likely to introduce new health and safety risks which require closer attention to ensure employees are trained and aware of these new risks. Also, among the regulatory agencies, such scenarios present further opportunities to redevelop their approach to their present inspection regime, as well as development of robust risk assessment strategies across the industry while working with associated bodies on the development of new industry standards (Malomane et al., 2022)

The industry, even though considered slow in technology adoption, has witnessed tremendous success over the last decades in technology acceptance and implementation. The Nigerian scene is yet to witness a similar level of transition towards the adoption of technology in construction projects. However, there is potential for such integration, especially where investment is encouraged.

### 3.1.1   Building Information Modelling (BIM)

BIM has instituted changes in information management in the construction industry. BIM technologies produce parametric models that represent the building products in virtual forms (Arayici and Aouad, 2010). 3D-BIM models serve as input for cyberspace that can be connected to physical products onsite. BIM is made up of three elements: the integration architecture, the product model and the process model. With BIMs, a cyber-physical world is created to serve as the foundation for creating a smart and connected construction site.

Overall, there is a growing interest amongst project practitioners towards the application of BIM around the globe, changing construction processes at various levels. It is observed that the rate of BIM adoption across construction environments around the world correlates to academic efforts through BIM-focused studies, usually in advanced environments. In construction environments such as the UK and US, BIM has been reported to have triggered operational efficiencies and high productivity levels across the industry. Despite the high volume of construction activities carried out in developing countries, numerous challenges limit the rate of BIM adoption in such construction environments. Factors such as lack of trained resources, lack of technological infrastructure and high cost of adoption are often seen to limit BIM adoption in the country. McGraw (2014) reported the penetration of BIM across the construction sector, where high rates of adoption in the United Kingdom, France and the United States were synonymous with commercial projects (Table 16.1).

### 3.1.2   Augmented reality

Augmented reality (AR), according to Wang et al. (2014), is the virtual augmentation of real-life environmental elements using computer-generated imaging technology. Typically, establishing an augmented reality requires a display gadget, data gloves, GPS and smart boards. In addition, software is utilised to create the augmented virtual reality scene. AR has general applications which Omar and Nehdi (2016) categorised to include simulation, information access, communication and safety evaluations. However, there is an absence of data regarding its application in the Nigerian construction sector, and current development in the application of AR to progress monitoring is in the use of portable mobile augmented systems.

### 3.1.3   Robotics and other Unmanned Aerial Vehicles (UAVs)

With the right atmosphere, developing countries like Nigeria can benefit from this technology as it holds the potential of fast-tracking and undertaking construction tasks using robotic hands. This may include bricklaying robots, automatic rendering robots, climbing robots, spray painting robots, building inspection robots, etc. The application of drones in construction site has been used for surveying purposes, project site inspection and monitoring (Fleming et al., 2016; Akinade, 2017) and facilities management (Fernandez et al., 2015).

### 3.1.4   Wearable technologies

These are smart automated devices that can be worn on the body as implant or accessories to support construction workers in hazard recognition. They are used to gather real-time data through direct tracking of on-site activities and workers'

*Table 16.1* Country profile where contractors engage with BIM on specific project types.

| Building Projects | UK | France | Germany | US | Canada | Brazil | Japan | S/Korea | Aus/NZ |
|---|---|---|---|---|---|---|---|---|---|
| Commercial (Offices, Retail, Hotels) | 69% | 68% | 59% | 66% | 54% | 53% | 63% | 48% | 70% |
| Institutional (Education, Healthcare, Religious) | 61% | 32% | 31% | 77% | 41% | 31% | 23% | 35% | 39% |
| Government/Publicly Owned (Courthouses, Embassies, Civic/Sports and Convention) | 54% | 10% | 22% | 68% | 44% | 12% | 0% | 51% | 37% |
| Multifamily Residential | 33% | 35% | 44% | 18% | 26% | 19% | 23% | 20% | 26% |
| Single family Residential | 17% | 19% | 22% | 1% | 10% | 16% | 0% | 1% | 4% |
| *Civil Projects* | | | | | | | | | |
| Infrastructure (Roads, Bridges, Tunnels, Dams, Water/Wastewater) | 33% | 19% | 16% | 14% | 31% | 28% | 13% | 24% | 25% |
| Industrial/Manufacturing | 26% | 23% | 19% | 35% | 36% | 31% | 47% | 24% | 34% |
| Industrial/Energy (Primary Power Generation, Oil/Gas facilities) | 20% | 13% | 3% | 18% | 28% | 12% | 0% | 21% | 16% |
| Mining/Natural Resources | 6% | 0% | 0% | 4% | 18% | 6% | 0% | 1% | 11% |

wellbeing. They enable the real-time tracking of workers' physiological status, which is integrated into safety systems for monitoring and improving safe performance (Awolusi et al., 2018). Likewise, real-time location can be integrated into safety vests to provide workers' locations for hazard recognition and prevention. Warning audio signals are sometimes integrated to provide audible alarms in proximity to danger.

### 3.2   Construction 4.0 and potential safety, health and wellbeing benefits to construction workers

Construction 4.0, if well implemented and applied in managing construction sites, will systematically address the fear of outbreak of any pandemic in the post-COVID-19 pandemic period. Works may not completely stop due to outbreaks of any disease on construction sites where robots take charge of most of site activities. The following are some of the area Construction 4.0 would support in managing safety, health and wellbeing of workers on site:

With Construction 4.0 technologies implemented on site, the overall safety of workers on construction sites is greatly enhanced. For example, by combining artificial intelligence (AI), Internet of Things (IoTs) and other sensor technologies, construction hazards can be identified and controlled to prevent accidents on sites. Nath et al. (2020) developed an AI-driven image recognition machine that can monitor workers' compliance with safety measures, specifically the proper use of personal protective equipment. In addition, Construction 4.0 solutions can be used to support virtual meetings, thus preventing the spread of the virus whilst maintaining the conduct of customary work procedures. An integrated system with Building Information Modelling (BIM) connected to other visualisation technologies such as Virtual Reality (VR) and Augmented Reality (AR) was reported to have the potential to reduce accidents and improve safety on construction sites (Akinlolu et al., 2020). Where fully integrated construction sites are created, all human elements can completely be eliminated, thus avoiding the spread of COVID-19 and other diseases.

Construction is a labour-intensive industry full of risks that must be managed to ensure the health and safety of personnel. Integrated systems based on artificial intelligence, sensor technologies and the Internet of Things can be used to identify and analyse risks on sites. These systems can estimate the likelihood of occurrence and impact of accidents on sites. For example, Akinlolu et al. (2020) developed Virtual Reality- (VR) and Augmented Reality- (AR) enabled systems to help workers detect safety-related risks on sites. Further integration of such technology will aid in managing safety on site and enhance workplace productivity.

The integration of Construction 4.0 will add new roles and responsibilities in addition to provision of opportunities that will allow workers, especially supervisors managing smart construction sites, to work remotely, as well as increase of worker morale and loyalty. Workers must not necessarily be on site to monitor work or check health and safety compliance. This opportunity gives workers some flexibility, thus allowing them to attain a better work/life balance, which naturally promotes their emotional health and wellbeing.

**4.0    Sustainability approach for the Nigerian construction industry**

The pandemic has left behind further room for improvement within the construction sector globally, including the need for standardised work-related health and safety trainings for employees, a platform that can support long-term physical and mental health of its employees and the need to improve work environments to help build resilience within the sector. While the Nigerian construction industry is steadily bouncing back to normal operations after the impact of the COVID-19 pandemic, various strategies are needed to shape the delivery of projects safely.

Organisations within the Nigerian construction sector need to ensure the existence of holistic frameworks that support workers' safety, physical health and wellbeing. The organisations should also ensure that counselling and occupational health services are in place to cater to their workers' needs. In addition, line managers/supervisors should be trained to support their teams and have the requisite skills to have sensitive conversations on coping strategies.

Industrial Revolution 4.0 presents the opportunity for the adoption of cutting-edge strategies that would ensure sustainable practices are maintained within the construction industry during future pandemics. Timely investment around construction technologies 4.0 can benefit the sector in managing construction safety during future pandemics. This will help avoid the complete shutdown of operations witnessed in several projects. For instance, machines can replace humans during lockdown periods. IoT can connect multiple robots working onsite and transmit any alerts on any safety hazards detected. Geospatial and imagery technologies can be used to accumulate real-time safety data from sites during pandemics and alert safety officers monitoring progress from home. Similarly, real-time tracking and monitoring of construction activities can also be supported by technologies such as RFID, GPS and GIS.

In addition, stakeholders in the construction industry must realise the need to invest in information and communications technologies to help with early warnings and preparation to minimise the disruption witnessed during the COVID-19 pandemic. In this regard, it is believed that integrating digital technologies in the supply chain could help avoid delays with instant communication and service delivery due to pandemics in the chain, as transactions such as payment for construction materials can be done with ease (Ogunnusi et al., 2021).

**5.0    Conclusion**

Industry players in Nigeria must invest proportionately in developing newer skills and roles for stakeholders whose jobs may be taken away by digital technologies, for which the need for strategic and systematic upskilling of the entire workforce with regular training on new tools and technologies (such as BIM) and operating procedures is considered imperative. More focused construction project planning and management can tremendously help address incessant disruptions due to pandemics in the future. The COVID-19 pandemic clearly justifies the need for a robust risk management plan in construction projects, with resilient contract administration plans to accommodate such unprecedented challenges. Proactive planning, such as flexible construction teams that are resilient to change and crisis, is considered necessary. In addition, safety and health measures should be put in place to protect construction workers on-site to avoid future outbreaks of disease and promote workforce wellbeing on construction sites.

Ensuring the safety and wellbeing of workers in Nigeria as operations begin to return to normalcy after the pandemic remains a major challenge. Any improvement considered will require adequate legislation that is backed up with active enforcement while encouraging the broad participation of all stakeholders.

# References

Abubakar, M., Zailani, B.M., Abdullahi, M., & Auwal, A.M. (2021). Potential of adopting a resilient safety culture toward improving the safety performance of construction organizations in Nigeria. *Journal of Engineering, Design and Technology*, 20(5), 1236–1256.

Adeyemo, O., & Smallwood, J. (2017). Impact of occupational health and safety legislation on performance improvement in the Nigerian construction industry. *Procedia Engineering*, 196, 785–791.

Agyekum, K., Kukah, A.S., & Amudjie, J. (2021). The impact of COVID-19 on the construction industry in Ghana: The case of some selected firms. *Journal of Engineering, Design and Technology*, 20(1), 222–244.

Akinade, O.O. (2017). *BIM-based software for construction waste analytics using artificial intelligence hybrid models.* Doctoral dissertation, University of the West of England.

Akinlolu, M., Haupt, T.C., Edwards, D.J., & Simpeh, F. (2020). A bibliometric review of the status and emerging research trends in construction safety management technologies. *International Journal of Construction Management*, 1–13.

Alsharef, A., Banerjee, S., Uddin, S.J., Albert, A., & Jaselskis, E. (2021). Early impacts of the COVID-19 pandemic on the United States construction industry. *International Journal of Environmental Research and Public Health*, 18(4), 1559.

Arayici, Y., & Aouad, G. (2010). Building information modelling (BIM) for construction lifecycle management. In *Construction and building: Design, materials, and techniques, 2010* (pp. 99–118). Hauppauge, New York, USA: Nova Science Publishers.

Awolusi, I., Marks, E., & Hallowell, M. (2018). Wearable technology for personalized construction safety monitoring and trending: Review of applicable devices. *Automation in Construction*, 85, 96–106.

Baldwin, R., & Tomiura, E. (2020). Thinking ahead about the trade impact of COVID-19. *Economics in the Time of COVID-19*, 59, 59–71.

Bartlett, K., Blanco, J.L., Johnson, J., Fitzgerald, B., Mullin, M., & Ribeirinho, M.J. (2020). *Rise of the platform era: The next chapter in construction technology.* Available at www.mckinsey.com/industries/private-equity-and-principal-investors/ourinsights/rise-of-the-platform-era-the-next-chapter-in-construction-technology (Accessed 14 March 2022).

Bevan, S., & Cooper, C.L. (2021). Workplace health interventions to improve productivity. In *The healthy workforce*. Bingley, United Kingdom: Emerald Publishing Limited.

Bowen, P., Edwards, P., Lingard, H., & Cattell, K. (2014). Occupational stress and job demand, control and support factors among construction project consultants. *International Journal of Project Management*, 32(7), 1273–1284.

Choi, M., Ahn, S., & Seo, J. (2020). VR-Based investigation of forklift operator situation awareness for preventing collision accidents. *Accident Analysis & Prevention*, 136, 105404.

Dallasega, P., Rauch, E., & Linder, C. (2018). Industry 4.0 as an enabler of proximity for construction supply chains: A systematic literature review. *Computers in Industry*, 99, 205–225.

Ebekozien, A., & Aigbavboa, C. (2021). COVID-19 recovery for the Nigerian construction sites: The role of the fourth industrial revolution technologies. *Sustainable Cities and Society*, 69, 102803.

El Jazzar, M., Schranz, C., Urban, H., & Nassereddine, H. (2021). Integrating construction 4.0 technologies: A four-layer implementation plan.

Fernandes, N. (2020). Economic effects of coronavirus outbreak (COVID-19) on the world economy. IESE Business School Working Paper No. WP-1240-E. Available at SSRN: https://ssrn.com/abstract=3557504 or http://dx.doi.org/10.2139/ssrn.3557504.

Fernandez Galarreta, J., Kerle, N., & Gerke, M. (2015). UAV-based urban structural damage assessment using object-based image analysis and semantic reasoning. *Natural Hazards and Earth System Sciences*, 15(6), 1087–1101.

Fleming, K.L., Hashash, Y.M., McLandrich, S., O'Riordan, N., & Riemer, M. (2016). Novel technologies for deep-excavation digital construction records. *Practice Periodical on Structural Design and Construction*, 21(4), 05016002.

Frimpong, S., Antwi, A.B., Sunindijo, R.Y., Wang, C.C., Ampratwum, G., Dansoh, A., Boateng, E.S., Hagan, J.A., & Mensah, P.A. (2022). Health status of young construction workers in the Global South: The case of Ghana. *Safety Science*, 148, 105673.

Gamil, Y., & Alhagar, A. (2020). The impact of pandemic crisis on the survival of construction industry: A case of COVID-19. *Mediterranean Journal of Social Sciences*, 11(4), 122–122.

ILO. (1992). Safety and health in construction. *An ILO Code of Practice*. Available at www.ilo.org/global/topics/safety-and-health-at-work/normative-instruments/code-of-practice/WCMS_107826/lang-en/index.htm (Accessed 2 March 2022).

ILO. (2015). Good practices and challenges in promoting decent work in construction and infrastructure projects. Issues paper for discussion at the Global Dialogue Forum on Good Practices and Challenges in Promoting Decent Work in Construction and Infrastructure Projects. Available at www.ilo.org/sector/Resources/publications/WCMS_416378/lang-en/index.htm (Accessed 2 March 2022).

ILO. (2018). *Improving the safety and health of young workers*. Available at Improving the Safety and Health of Young Workers (ilo.org) (Accessed 1 March 2022).

King, S.S., Rahman, R.A., Fauzi, M.A., & Haron, A.T. (2021). Critical analysis of pandemic impact on AEC organizations: The COVID-19 case. *Journal of Engineering, Design and Technology*, 20(1), 388–383.

Koh, D. (2020). Occupational risks for COVID-19 infection. *Occupational Medicine*, 70(1), 3–5.

Kola, L., Kohrt, B.A., Hanlon, C., Naslund, J.A., Sikander, S., Balaji, M., Benjet, C., Cheung, E.Y.L., Eaton, J., Gonsalves, P., & Hailemariam, M. (2021). COVID-19 mental health impact and responses in low-income and middle-income countries: Reimagining global mental health. *The Lancet Psychiatry*, 8(6), 535–550.

Malomane, R., Musonda, I., & Okoro, C.S. (2022). The opportunities and challenges associated with the implementation of fourth industrial revolution technologies to manage health and safety. *International Journal of Environmental Research and Public Health*, 19(2), 846.

McGraw, H. (2014). The business value of BIM for construction in major global markets: How contractors around the world are driving innovation with building information modeling. *SmartMarket Reports*. Available at www.construction.com/toolkit/reports/bim-business-value-construction-global-markets (Accessed 3 January 2015).

Moda, H.M., Ofodile, N., Zailani, B.M., Abubakar, M.A., & Ibrahim, Y.M. (2022). Management support as a critical success factor (CSF) for changing worker's safety attitude: A case of the Nigerian construction industry. *International Journal of Construction Management*, 1–7.

Nath, N.D., Behzadan, A.H., & Paal, S.G. (2020). Deep learning for site safety: Real-time detection of personal protective equipment. *Automation in Construction*, 112, 103085.

National Bureau of Statistics (NBS). (2021). Annual abstract on statistics, summary of survey findings, 87–94.

Ogunnusi, M., Omotayo, T., Hamma-Adama, M., Awuzie, B.O., & Egbelakin, T. (2021). Lessons learned from the impact of COVID-19 on the global construction industry. *Journal of Engineering, Design and Technology*, 20(1), 299–320.

Omar, T., & Nehdi, M.L. (2016). Data acquisition technologies for construction progress tracking. *Automation in Construction*, 70, 143–155.

Osei-Asibey, D., Ayarkwa, J., Acheampong, A., Adinyira, E., & Amoah, P. (2021). Framework for improving construction health and safety on Ghanaian construction sites. *Journal of Building Construction and Planning Research*, 9(2), 115–137.

Osuizugbo, I.C. (2021). Disruptions and responses within Nigeria construction industry amid COVID-19 threat. *Covenant Journal of Research in the Built Environment*, 8(2).

Osunsanmi, T.O., Aigbavboa, C., & Oke, A. (2018). Construction 4.0: The future of the construction industry in South Africa. *International Journal of Civil and Environmental Engineering*, 12(3), 206–212.

Pollock, A., Campbell, P., Cheyne, J., Cowie, J., Davis, B., McCallum, J., McGill, K., Elders, A., Hagen, S., McClurg, D., & Torrens, C. (2020). Interventions to support the resilience and mental health of frontline health and social care professionals during and after a disease outbreak, epidemic or pandemic: A mixed methods systematic review. *Cochrane Database of Systematic Reviews*, (11).

Rastogi, S. (2017). Construction 4.0: The 4th generation revolution. Indian Lean Construction Conference, ILCC.

Simpeh, F., Bamfo-Agyei, E., and Amoah, C. (2021). Barriers to the implementation of COVID-19 safety regulations: Insight from Ghanaian construction sites. *Journal of Engineering, Design and Technology*, 20(1), 47–65.

Stiles, S., Golightly, D., & Ryan, B. (2021). Impact of COVID-19 on health and safety in the construction sector. *Human Factors and Ergonomics in Manufacturing & Service Industries*, 31(4), 425–437.

Taher, G. (2021). Industrial revolution 4.0 in the construction industry: Challenges and opportunities. *Management Studies and Economic Systems*, 6(3/4), 109–127.

Umeokafor, N., Isaac, D., Jones, K., & Umeadi, B. (2014). Enforcement of occupational safety and health regulations in Nigeria: An exploration. *European Scientific Journal*, 3, 93–104.

United Nations. (2015). *The 17 goals | sustainable development*. Available at https://sdgs.un.org/goals (Accessed 30 May 2022).

Wang, X., Truijens, M., Hou, L., Wang, Y., & Zhou, Y. (2014). Integrating augmented reality with building information modeling: Onsite construction process controlling for liquefied natural gas industry. *Automation in Construction*, 40, 96–105.

Yang, Y., Chan, A.P., Shan, M., Gao, R., Bao, F., Lyu, S., Zhang, Q., & Guan, J. (2021). Opportunities and challenges for construction health and safety technologies under the COVID-19 pandemic in Chinese construction projects. *International Journal of Environmental Research and Public Health*, 18(24), 13038.

Yusuf, S.O., Adindu, C.C., Badmus, A., & Muhammed, H. (2021, March). Curbing the effect of Covid-19 pandemic in the Nigeria construction industry through digitalization of operations and processes. Proceedings of the 5th CU Construction Conference 2021, School of Energy, Construction and Environment, Coventry University, UK.

# 17 Construction site management during COVID-19 in Myanmar

*Aung Paing and Bonaventura Hadikusumo*

## Introduction

This chapter centres on construction site management in four different types of construction projects during COVID-19 in Myanmar. The inception of COVID-19 in Myanmar was at the end of March 2020. During the first wave of COVID-19 in Myanmar, the government was able to cope with the situation. However, due to mandated regulations to prevent the spread of the virus, constructions were required to be postponed from March 2020 until May 2020 (MOHS, 2020). Construction projects, especially big projects, were disturbed by the COVID-19 outbreak in various aspects such as late delivery of shipped materials, labour scarcity and overall construction project management, including safety (MOC, 2020). In the course of the second wave of COVID-19, which started at the end of August 2020, the construction industry reached a perilous point as hundreds of positive cases, including most construction workers, were reported daily (MOHS, 2020).

Consequently, rules and regulations for different sectors, including construction, were issued and administered by the Ministry of Health and Sports of Myanmar government. Examples of COVID-19 safety standards for construction in Myanmar are physical distancing of 6 feet, not allowing more than 50 workers at a particular workplace, condition to wear masks all the time, monitoring the temperature of workers and employees and so on (MOHS, 2020). These commandments allowed constructions to recommence partially in the COVID-19 era. Most of the time, contractors were responsible for supplying adequate COVID-19 prevention-and-protection facilities onsite and in-office. These covered hand-washing stations, hand sanitisers, regular disinfection of common areas and, if necessary, accommodation for workers, which could be in-site or off-site labour camps; sometimes both were provided, depending on the situation of the project (MOC, 2020).

Because of COVID-19 legal obligations, it affected labour's productivity, especially on group tasks (Tekin, 2022). Management of construction projects became distressing due to COVID-19 rules and regulations, which led to problems such as shortages of labour and materials and delays in material delivery and coordination (Alenezi, 2020). Construction site management and approaches to bringing some of these issues under control are learnt in this study. The following sections will discuss the details of four case studies to fulfil two objectives of this research,

DOI: 10.1201/9781003278368-19

which are to study the impact of COVID-19 and its regulations on construction sites and to study how an owner and a contractor managed problems related to COVID-19. Some of the unique management and approaches which were found in the case study were feasible and could be adopted by other construction projects in the COVID-19 and post-COVID-19 eras.

## Impact of COVID-19 on the construction sector

COVID-19 affected the construction industry in many ways. The research of Alsharef et al. (2021) found that in America, the degree of COVID-19 impacts on a construction sector differed between states. There were projects where construction was carried out as usual, while some other projects had been fully stopped. Their research highlighted that different states in America had imposed different levels of restrictions, depending on how they defined construction projects in each state as either essential or non-essential.

In preparation for the continuity of construction projects, safety management had to be transformed and adapted according to a particular region and its regulations. Due to this, it affected construction projects directly and indirectly, including construction site management involving workforce management, material management, coordination management and so on.

In the cost aspect, JLL Research (2020) reported that construction sites demanding more safety practices and equipment created significant rises in the project costs. These extra costs, according to Emmett (2022), included needing to build additional site offices and the need to provide facilities for hygiene of workers, such as hand sanitisers and hand-washing stations. The research of Abinraj (2020) emphasised the addition of the total project cost due to COVID-19. It stated that COVID-19 cost up four to five percent of the project cost in constructions in India. The time aspect was affected from day-to-day work to specific events of work, such as delays in material delivery (Kerr, 2020). For example, waiting and queuing time during the time of workers' arrival at an entrance gate of construction sites was extended as they had to practise physical distancing and undergo temperature monitoring and disinfection.

In the aspect of workforce management, implementation of safety protocols made working conditions more difficult and intricate. For example, it was compulsory that every worker and employee had to put their personal masks on during working hours and in work places. This multiplied the number of workers having heat stress in hot regions. Even before COVID-19, the number of construction workers who died due to heat stress was found to be over eight hundred in the US (Fulcher and Abrams, 2020). During COVID-19, when workers were strongly recommended not to work face-to-face, wearing personal masks increased the risk of heat stress for construction workers. O'Sullivan (2020) recommended replacing masks with face shields and allowing more frequent breaks. It was also suggested that providing proper air circulation and ventilation in workplaces can be beneficial in addressing the problem of heat stress and the spread of COVID-19. Staggering different groups of workers was sometimes necessary to reduce the number of workers in a particular workplace when it was crowded. As a result, this affected the productivity and performance of projects.

In the aspect of material management, because of the lockdown of regions, imported materials and equipment lagged in most construction projects, and the critical path of the project timeline depending on these materials was impacted. In India, according to Nandan (2020) and Abinraj (2020), fit-out materials and HVAC equipment were normally brought in from China, the US, Italy, Germany, Spain and South Korea before COVID-19. However, as these countries were rapidly spreading and severely affected by COVID-19, India shut its nation in, thus delaying the delivery of overseas construction materials. According to JLL Research (2020), the construction industry in the United States encountered problems because many manufacturing companies that supplied construction materials, equipment and others were closed temporarily. Apart from materials shipment, materials such as rebars required on-site fabrication. However, during COVID-19, when manpower was critical and needed to be efficiently utilised, it was not a prudent approach to use manpower in on-site fabrication activities. In order to minimise the necessity of manpower, Nandan (2020) suggested implementing alternate strategies such as automation and off-site fabrication and using technology more often. It also pointed out that source materials alternatives should have flexibility when suppliers encountered disruptions in the supply chain.

In the aspect of coordination, normal face-to-face meetings were substituted with virtual meetings using online platforms such as Zoom, Microsoft Teams and Google Meet. However, construction usually entails building permits and inspections, which cannot be done virtually. According to Alsharef et al. (2021), it induced delays to have projects inspected by local authorities and hence, delayed the completion of projects. Moreover, due to COVID-19, the original baseline of a project schedule required several revisions, which needed time-consuming coordination and cooperation of the many parties involved in a project. As a result, it affected the productivity of employees and performance of projects.

## Case study

A case study was carried out in order to fulfil purposes of this research. As two objectives of this research are to study the impacts of COVID-19 and its regulations on a construction site and how owners and contractors managed problems related to COVID-19, research questions were "what" and "how". Moreover, this research entailed in-depth understanding and explanation of how construction projects carried on safely during COVID-19. According to Yin (2018), case study research methodology is most relevant to be applied because research questions in this research require the explanation of "what", "how" and "why".

### *Methodology*

The research methodology framework used in this research is described in Figure 17.1. It consists of four main stages: conceptualisation, data collection, data analysis and conclusions and recommendations. Each main stage is discussed in detail.

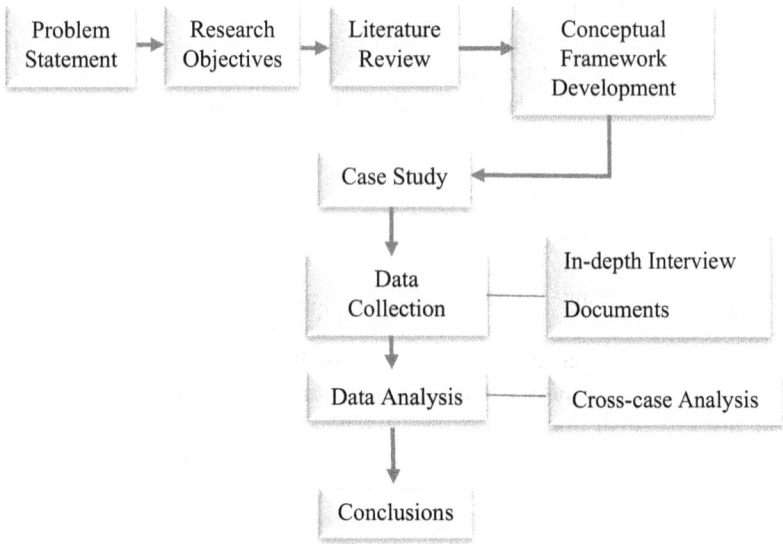

*Figure 17.1* Research methodology framework.

### Data collection

Data for this research was mainly collected by interview, which allowed research-ers to have in-depth investigation of problems. Open-ended questions with three sections were used for in-depth interviews. The first section is about general infor-mation about the project. The second and third sections are to fulfil objectives of the study. Four construction projects were selected that met the main criteria of this research. The first criterion was that the project must be located in a COVID-19-affected country or region. The second criterion was that construction opera-tion must be continued partially or fully during COVID-19. The selected four projects were of different types: housing project, building project, factory project and road project. The data collection procedure is described in Figure 17.2. After interviews, necessary data and documents were collected via email.

Case A is a housing project. The scope of the project consisted of 20 six-storeyed building units. The construction was in progress and the project continued partially during COVID-19. The overall project area is 4.17 acres. The name of the project is "Lan Thit Mixed Use Development Project". The type of building struc-ture is a traditional reinforced concrete structure. Case B, "Yoma Central Project", is a building project with an area of 10.5 acres. It has 24 storeys and the project continued fully during COVID-19, except during the lockdown period. Case C is a factory project with a land plot of 0.78 acres. It is "Shwe Wah Nadi Agriculture Production Co., Ltd" project. It has only one storey with a steel structure. Similar to Case B, this project continued fully except during the lockdown period. Case D is a highway project which is 80 miles long. It connects Yangon-Pyay-Magway region. This project continued partially during COVID-19.

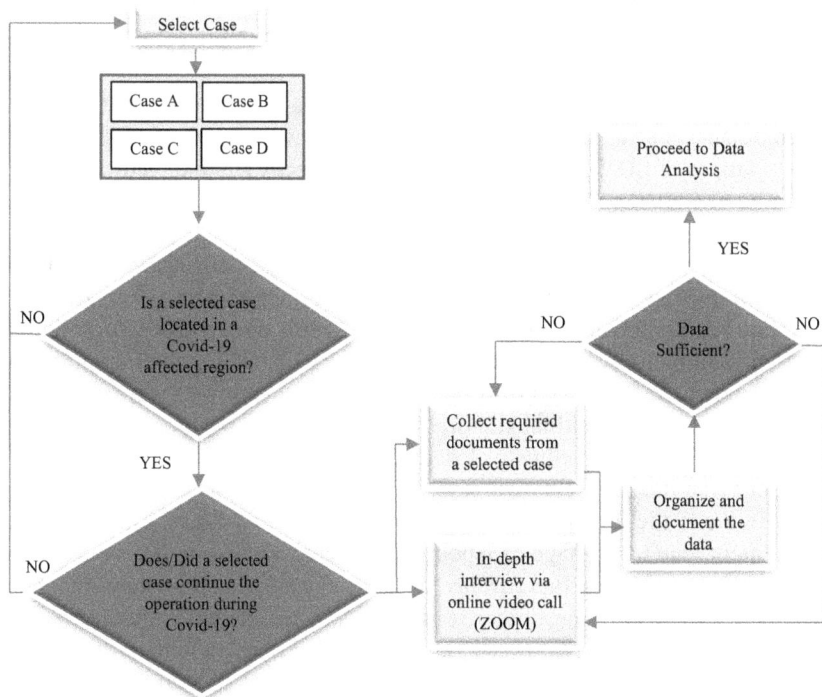

*Figure 17.2* Data collection procedure.

### *Data analysis*

There are two parts of the data analysis. The first is case-wise analysis, which was used to analyse the individual cases. In the case-wise analysis, researchers did in-depth analysis for each case under five main topics: safety management, lockdown management, workforce management, material management and coordination management. After case-wise analysis, researchers carried on with the next part of analysis, which is cross-case analysis. According to Yin (2018), cross-case analysis is suitable for multiple-case studies. This analysis was carried out to compare and differentiate between cases. Unique and common management, unique and common problems and changes in construction site from normal to the COVID situation were all discussed after cross-case analysis.

### **Results and discussion**

From the case-wise analysis and cross-case analysis, unique and common issues, unique and common management and approaches and changes in construction site from normal to the COVID-19 era were major findings.

### Unique and common issues during COVID-19

Unique and common issues that all cases A, B, C and D had to come across during the COVID-19 era were found in five areas: COVID-19 prevention and safety management, lockdown, workforce management, material management and coordination management. All these issues were mostly consequences of safety rules and regulations of COVID-19 in Myanmar, both directly and indirectly.

Firstly, in COVID-19 prevention and safety management, it was discovered in all cases that it was impractical to comply with six feet of physical distancing all the time. Similarly, wearing masks continuously during working hours was also nonviable in practice. In Case B (Building Project), workers of different trades had to use the same facilities, such as lifts and toilets, which created direct and indirect physical contact. During the lockdown, construction works were not able to be continued fully. Only some minor activities were carried out during that time. In addition, imported materials were postponed from being dispatched on time to sites due to closed borders. For Case D (Highway Project), the main issue during lockdown was that workers from another region could not commute to the region where the work was currently located. In workforce management, due to shortage of labours, only critical trades and activities were focused to be finished on time. Delayed start and early finish of work happened every day due to the long queue resulting from temperature monitoring and physical distancing at the entrance gate. In material management, at the time of material delivery, it was difficult to prevent congregation of workers and suppliers. For Case C (Factory Project), as the structure was steel, they had to depend on imported steel from China.

For coordination management, as virtual communication and meetings played the most crucial role in minimising physical contact and reducing the number of employees working in office, productivity and daily routines were badly affected due to the bad internet connection in Myanmar, and miscommunication often occurred. Moreover, it was difficult to manage and coordinate with work-from-home employees. In some cases, it was found that online meetings were not efficient at first because of unfamiliarity with technology and software. Except for Case B, the rest preferred face-to-face meetings.

### Common management and approaches during COVID-19

The following section summarises common management and approaches in order to prevent the spread of COVID-19 and to mitigate losses in terms of time and cost in four projects during the outbreak of COVID-19 in Myanmar.

#### Physical distancing

Although not all cases could practise the required physical distance all the time, they practised physical distancing as much as and whenever possible. Practises of physical distancing were found in all projects at entrance gates to construction sites and during lunchtime and toolbox meetings. In the office, not only was the sitting plan rearranged with enough distance, but they also practised a work-from-home system alternatively to reduce physical contact. The lesson learned in physical distancing is that on construction sites, it is almost impossible to practise physical distancing during working hours due to limited working space and the need for teamwork in some activities.

*Safety management and COVID-19 prevention*

Disinfection was conducted in all projects as it is an effective way to prevent COVID-19. Moreover, sanitisers were sufficiently provided on site and in the office. Wearing masks and other safety equipment was mandatory in every-day site operation whenever possible, and safety officers and supervisors were responsible for checking daily. Apart from that, to enhance the awareness of COVID-19 among workers and employees, knowledge sharing was often performed during every toolbox meeting, and there were vinyl and signboards posted on site which described how to work safely during COVID-19. The temperature of everyone who entered the site was also monitored. Therefore, the lesson learned in this section is that COVID-19 prevention practices such as disinfection, providing masks, hand sanitisers and temperature monitoring can be conducted at most construction sites, although these practices may affect productivity and delay work.

*Workforce management*

All of the projects studied accommodated their workers on-site or off-site or both. This required additional management. They had to assign their trusted workers or representative workers to control the rest of the workers. They had to provide bathing areas and arrange food supplies for workers. Although they provided shelter for their workers within a safe compound, they still monitored each worker's temperature during toolbox meetings in the morning. Those workers who had to come from outside were transported by ferries which had seats with physical distancing markings. Therefore, the lesson learned in workforce management during COVID-19 is that accommodating workers can help to reduce the risk of labour shortage and can even eliminate some safety requirements. Thus, accommodation of workers should be considered in construction projects during COVID-19.

*Coordination management*

Basic communication and coordination were done and instructed via the Viber chat application, which is widely used in Myanmar. Work-from-home employees were also monitored via Viber. For online meetings, Zoom and Microsoft Team were used most frequently. During the COVID-19 period, virtual communication was crucial in eliminating physical contact, and employees should be well-trained to become familiar with online platforms.

### Unique management and approaches during COVID-19

In addition to these common management and approaches of construction site operation tables, there were some unique management and approaches from each case, which are described categorically.

#### Case A (housing project)

In the housing project, the advantage was that different trades can be assigned to different building units, thus creating less congregation of workers. The dining area, where congregation of workers mostly occurred, was also expanded. Moreover, workers were given different lunch breaks to reduce physical contact. Toolbox meetings were carried out with three different groups of workers in different areas.

The contractor of this project used one of their previous projects as a quarantine centre for Myanmar Government and this project. Any workers who showed symptoms of COVID-19 were sent to their quarantine centre. Moreover, they had a full-time doctor on-site to check workers who showed potential COVID-19 symptoms. They also had a registration form to record daily manpower and to trace COVID-19 cases if they happened. Working hours were also reduced so that workers would not be stressed out during this pandemic time.

The material management in this project was eccentric. They made sure to have materials from different suppliers delivered to site at different times. Moreover, they requested suppliers to pack materials whenever possible. This made unloading of materials trouble-free, and more importantly, it reduced the number of workers required to unload and hence reduced the potential transmission of COVID-19.

#### Case B (building project)

By the time COVID-19 happened in Myanmar, construction was already at a high level, which provided workers with good ventilation. Moreover, it allowed them to take rests during breaktime at different floor levels. In this project, workers were highly restricted from mingling with other workers from different towers, teams and/or floors.

In addition to disinfecting the common area and offices, like other projects, they also sprayed alcohol on everyone who entered the site. They strongly enforced workers to wash hands and legs before and after work. For that, they provided a washing area in front of the site. For material procurement, they sourced from different suppliers and pre-ordered much earlier. Therefore, there was no material delay on this project.

#### Case C (factory project)

Workers were accommodated in the site in this project. Therefore, they did not focus too much on physical distancing. Another reason why they did not put too much effort into practising physical distancing was because the land area of the project is large and had open spaces. However, they had to provide necessary facilities, such as a temporary canteen and bathing area. They were also connected with Ayeyarwady COVID Control Center, where they sent any workers who were diagnosed with COVID-19.

As already mentioned, workers in this project were accommodated at the site. Workers had to sign an agreement form which stated rules and regulations to be followed during their stay at the site. Safety officers or site supervisors always monitored workers and warned those who violated these safety rules. For the physical health of workers, they had to do exercise every morning during toolbox meetings. There were two rest days in a week. Materials were delivered just outside the site to reduce physical contact with outsiders.

*Case D (highway project)*

This project also did not focus too much on physical distancing, as it was an outdoor project and the space was not confined. However, safety officers still monitored workers to maintain physical distancing. In this project, they strongly focused on enhancing knowledge and awareness of workers during toolbox meetings. COVID-19 personal protections, such as masks and gloves, were burnt on site.

### Changes in construction site from normal to the COVID-19 era

Table 17.1 highlights how the construction in Myanmar changed during the COVID-19 era.

*Table 17.1* Changes in construction from normal to COVID-19 era.

| Normal construction site | Construction site during COVID-19 era |
| --- | --- |
| Toolbox meetings were conducted every day with all workers | Different groups of workers have toolbox meetings on different days or in different areas |
| Site office provided space for all site office employees | Separate site office and/or distanced seating |
| Hygiene was not taken seriously | Hygiene was at its highest priority |
| Crowded lunchtime | Different lunch breaks and dining areas were expanded |
| Workers felt safe to work in construction | Workers were demotivated, stressed and worried to go to construction during COVID-19 era, affecting their work performance |
| Workers came to construction site from their home or dormitories | Workers were accommodated in-site or at labour camp |
| Fewer distractions and less non-value-added works | Less productive because workers had to practise COVID-19 safety measures (for example, late start and early finish of work due to long queue with physical distancing and temperature monitoring at the entrance gates) |

*(Continued)*

*Table 17.1* (Continued)

| Normal construction site | Construction site during COVID-19 era |
|---|---|
| Employees and workers can move from one work area to another efficiently | Movement of employees and workers was constrained due to physical distancing and the limited use of facilities, such as lifts |
| Materials were delivered to construction site traditionally | During COVID-19, whenever possible and applicable, materials were delivered with packages and/or delivered outside of the site |
| Easy coordination and communication among each other as employees worked at office | Employees worked from home alternatively. It affected performance and productivity and it also caused miscommunications |
| Face-to-face meetings | Virtual meetings and communications |

**Implications for practise and research**

Unique management and approaches found in the data analysis can be functional and continue to be practised during the COVID-19 and post-pandemic period. This research has highlighted the importance of characteristics and the nature of construction projects. Construction projects which give good air ventilation can reduce the risk of COVID-19 as in Case D's Highway Project. For Case A's Housing Project, which has many building units, different trades of workers were assigned to different building units. Therefore, construction works were continued with minimal impact and disturbance. Since construction projects are unique, understanding of their nature and characteristics is crucial. Apart from characteristics of projects, management and an approach where materials were delivered in Case A and Case C are remarkable, including packing materials and delivering outside of the site. It may affect productivity of workers, although from the safety perspective, it is a lot safer than the traditional method of material delivery. Another practice is the use of virtual communication and meetings. In this digital age, construction projects should continue to practise and get familiar with advanced technologies as much as and whenever possible. Virtual meetings save a lot of time and help to reduce physical contact with each other. Hence, it should also continue to be practised during the post-COVID-19 era. Depending on the needs and situation of a construction project, accommodating workers should be considered whether to practise or not in the post-pandemic period because from a safety aspect, it may prevent COVID-19-like diseases in the future, which is unlikely to happen, but it requires additional management and costs which may concern project stakeholders of a project. Nevertheless, it may enhance productivity of workers and if it is what a project needs, accommodation of workers should be considered.

For further study and improvement, as this research was conducted on only four types of project, which are housing, building, factory and highway projects, other construction projects such as bridge, dam, offshore and tunnel projects should be studied because each has different characteristics.

## Conclusions

COVID-19 rules and regulations enforced by Myanmar Ministry of Health were practised on all four projects as much as possible. The two objectives of this research as mentioned in the earlier section were to study the impact of COVID-19 and its regulations on construction sites and how owners and contractors managed problems related to COVID-19.

For the first objective of studying the impacts of COVID-19 and its regulations on construction sites, it can be seen from the data analysis and findings that some safety practices, such as physical distancing and wearing masks, were found to be difficult to practise all the time. Moreover, during the lockdown period, construction was not able to perform efficiently, which caused delays in the arrival of imported materials. Workers were not able to travel from one region to another during the lockdown period. Because of COVID-19 safety requirements and measures such as temperature monitoring and physical distancing, it also affected the working hours of workers. Overall, it affected the productivity of workers and impacted critical activities, thus impacting the project completion dates.

For the second objective of studying how owners and contractors managed problems related to COVID-19, they all had to reduce physical contact, reduce the number of workers and employees in a particular area, share knowledge and enhance awareness of COVID-19, focus more on workplace hygiene and add required facilities to site and office for the convenience of workers and employees. In communication and coordination, virtual platforms such as Zoom and Microsoft Teams were widely used, although most employers were still trying to get familiar with this software at that time. One of the unique approaches in handling COVID-19 found in the research was the material delivery methods of Case A and Case C. In Case A, they asked suppliers to pack materials whenever possible so that unloading was much easier. In Case C, the delivery method was to deliver materials just outside of the site. By practising this, physical contact with outsiders can be reduced. To mitigate the delay of material delivery, material should be sourced from different suppliers and should have alternative options for flexible material procurement, as found in Case B. Accommodating workers in-site and/or labour camps was also a trending and efficient approach in controlling the spread of COVID-19 among project communities and reducing the risk of labour shortage. However, it required additional care and extra facilities for workers.

These unique and common management and contractor approaches were found to be effective both to practise and to prevent the spread of the virus in construction projects during the COVID-19 era. Some of them – for instance, the use of virtual meetings – would still be appropriate to practise in some projects in the post-pandemic period.

# References

Abinraj, R.S. (2020). *India: Impact of Covid-19 on construction and engineering sector.* [Online]. ResearchGate. Available at www.researchgate.net/publication/340966338_INDIA_IMPACT_OF_COVID-19_ON_CONSTRUCTION_AND_ENGINEERING_SECTOR.

Alenezi, T.A.N. (2020). COVID-19 causes of delays on construction projects in Kuwait. *IJERGS*, 8(1), 6–9.

Alsharef, A., Banerjee, S., Uddin, S., Albert, A., & Jaselskis, E. (2021). Early impacts of the COVID-19 pandemic on the United States construction industry. *International Journal of Environmental Research and Public Health*, 18(4), 1559.

Emmett, T. (2020). *COVID-19 and the impact on Australian construction projects* [Online]. Available at www.turnerandtownsend.com/en/perspectives/COVID-19-and-the-impact-on-australian-construction-projects/.

Fulcher, J., & Abrams, M. (2020). *Protecting workers from heat stress and COVID-19* [Online]. Public Citizen. Available at www.citizen.org/article/protecting-workers-from-heat-stress-and-COVID-19-recommendations-for-employers/.

JLL Research. (2020). *COVID-19 construction industry impacts* [Online]. Available at www.us.jll.com/en/coronavirus-resources/construction-industry-impacts-and-considerations (Accessed 31 May 2022).

Kerr, K. (2020, July 21). Alberta's construction industry: Physical distancing on the girder? *The Globe and Mail* [Online]. Available at www.theglobeandmail.com/business/industry-news/property-report/article-albertas-construction-industry-physical-distancing-on-the-girder/ (Accessed 31 May 2022).

Ministry of Construction. (2020). *Minister's office/news* [Online]. Available at https://construction.gov.mm/news-show/f87c94b0-d396-11ec-a8be-e9291a621227.

Ministry of Health and Sports. (2020). *COVID-19 (coronavirus disease 2019) acute respiratory disease* [Online]. Available at https://mohs.gov.mm/Main/content/publication/2019-ncov.

Nandan, A. (2020). *COVID-19: Building again Brick by Brick* [Online]. Available at www.savills.co.th. https://en.savills.co.th/research_articles/166413/181475-0 (Accessed 31 May 2022).

O'Sullivan, T. (2020). *Avoiding heat illness risks due to facial coverings* [Online]. LHSFNA. Available at www.lhsfna.org/avoiding-heat-illness-risks-due-to-facial-coverings/#:~:text=Using%20face%20coverings%20makes%20it (Accessed 31 May 2022).

Tekin, H. (2022). The impact of COVID-19 on construction labor productivity: The case of Turkey. Engineering, Construction and Architectural Management, (ahead-of-print).

Yin, R.K. (2018). *Case study research and applications: Design and methods* (6th ed.). Thousand Oaks, CA: Sage Publications, Inc.

# Implications of the COVID-19 pandemic for construction project performance

# 18 Intricacies and lifeline for the construction industry amidst the coronavirus pandemic

*Samuel A. Adekunle, Clinton O. Aigbavboa,
Obuks A. Ejohwomu, Babatunde Fatai Ogunbayo
and Matthew Ikuabe*

## Introduction

In 2019, the coronavirus (also known as COVID-19; 2019-nCoV) was detected in Wuhan, China. It is considered novel in nature and manifests by attacking the lower respiratory tract, resembling pneumonia (Huang et al., 2020b). Because of its novelty, several studies have been conducted to understand this disease (Ataguba Ochega and Ataguba, 2020; Huang et al., 2020a; Lai et al., 2020). This disease was declared a pandemic by the World Health Organization (WHO) on 11 March as it claimed many lives, and the infection rate was growing exponentially around the world. It was declared a public health emergency of international concern on 30 January. The occurrence of this disease impacted many aspects of human living. It caused significant destabilisation globally (Schindler et al., 2020) to every facet of life. One is that it has been touted to have economically extreme impacts (Bartik et al., 2020). Every sector of the economy was affected, and losses were suffered in different magnitude. For instance, according to Bartik et al. (2020), 43% of small businesses were reported to have closed due to COVID-19.

The outbreak of COVID-19 was declared to be novel; the complications remain totally unclear as new complications were unravelled from time to time, thus making its treatment a bit difficult (Lai et al., 2020). Hence, it claimed many casualties across ages and regions of the world. Globally 18,354,342 cases and 696,147 deaths were reported by the WHO in July (WHO, 2020a). It is evident that ages 25–64 are mostly hit by this pandemic globally (Figure 18.1).

To curb the spread of COVID-19, a general policy adopted by many countries was the curfew (Benítez et al., 2020), shutting down the economy through a total lockdown, social distance and restriction of movement and activities (closure of airports and schools, among others). Other measures adopted include the use of protective equipment, including nose masks, and regimented essential service access, among others. These measures were enacted to help flatten the curve. However, the impact of these restrictions due to COVID-19 has been observed to increase stress, promote gender-based violence (WHO, 2020b), and affect the stock markets (Aslam et al., 2020).

The construction industry is an important one, vital to the growth of the economy, and is not immune to these effects. Traditionally, it is a busy industry

DOI: 10.1201/9781003278368-21

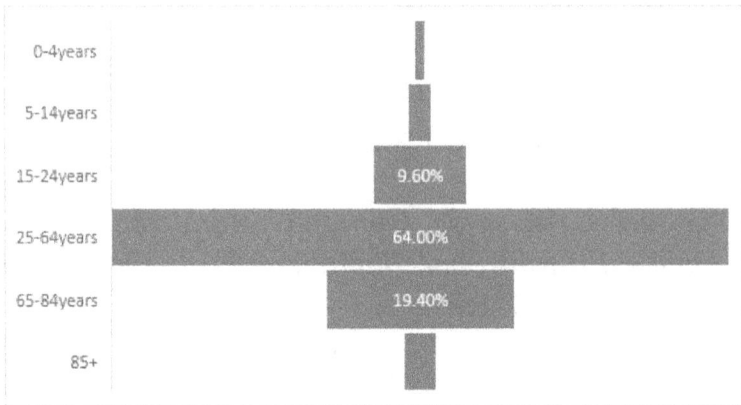

*Figure 18.1* Age distribution of COVID cases (January to July 2020) (WHO, 2020a).

employing a vast number of hands working concurrently; hence human contact is inevitable. Moreover, it is an essential industry as it provides shelter to people and health facilities, among others. For instance, several structures were constructed during the pandemic to accommodate victims, among which are the high-standard isolation units in Shenzhen, China (Zhou et al., 2020). However, this must be done without compromising the health of workers.

Beyond the value delivered by the construction industry, it is also impacted by the many COVID-19 policies and regulations enacted. For instance, some challenges facing construction include labour shortage, 15% productivity loss, Health, Safety and Environment issues, especially the procurement of face masks for workers (CIOB, 2020), and nonexistent COVID-19 protocols for site workers. The ripple effect of these prevalent challenges portends a huge threat to safety and productivity for the construction industry. For instance, the closure of construction sites by the main contractor, cancellation of projects, and projects being placed on hold (Constructionline, 2020) have been reported as some of the effects of the pandemic in the construction industry. Meanwhile, many governments worldwide announced support that included bailout funds, extended working hours, rebate systems, corporate financing facilities, and others to assist the construction industry during the COVID-19 pandemic.

## COVID-19 in industries

Consequently, the study opted to map the studies on the impact of COVID-19 on other industries and adopt a lesson learnt approach. Hence, a total of 15 publications were selected, focusing on industries like mining, investments, and waste management (Table 18.1). A critical look at the selected publications reveals that existing publications focus on the economic and labour implications through studying the stock markets, supply, demand, etc., of COVID-19.

*Table 18.1* Literature on COVID-19 impacts on industries.

| Title | Reference | Findings |
|---|---|---|
| The impact of Coronavirus (COVID-19) outbreak on faith-based investments: An original analysis | (Sherif, 2020) | Using the Dow Jones market index in the UK, the study observed the impact of the pandemic on sharia-compliant investments. The findings observed a negative but insignificant effect as compared to other non-compliant investments. |
| The economic impact of the Coronavirus 2019 (Covid-2019): Implications for the mining industry | (Laing, 2020) | The study articulates the pandemic's short-, medium-, and long-term effects on the mining industry. |
| Preventing COVID-19 from the perspective of industrial information integration: Evaluation and continuous improvement of information networks for sustainable epidemic prevention | (Yin et al., 2020) | The industrial sector information integration was explored as a way to fight against pandemics. |
| Challenges, opportunities, and innovations for effective solid waste management during and post-COVID-19 pandemic | (Sharma et al., 2020) | The increase of solid waste management and the attending challenges were studied. Also, the study suggested waste management priorities in the COVID-19 era. |
| Challenges and strategies for effective plastic waste management during and post-COVID-19 pandemic | (Vanapalli et al., 2020) | The study raised environmental concerns due to dependence on plastic. The paper suggested sustainable plastic waste management through individual behavioural, social, and institutional changes. |
| Investigating the emerging COVID-19 research trends in the field of business and management: A bibliometric analysis approach | (Verma and Gustafsson, 2020) | The study observed the emerging research trends through visualising bibliographic data. |
| The Coronavirus crisis in B2B settings: Crisis uniqueness and managerial implications based on social exchange theory | (Mora Cortez and Johnston, 2020) | The study discussed B2B settings in the light of the coronavirus and suggested a model for survival. |
| Understanding the impact of COVID-19 intervention policies on the hospitality labour market | (Huang et al., 2020a) | Through the observation of the effect of COVID-19 measures on small businesses, the study discussed impacts and implications and suggested recommendations. |

(*Continued*)

*Table 18.1* (Continued)

| Title | Reference | Findings |
|---|---|---|
| Impacts of COVID-19 on global tourism industry: A cross-regional comparison | (Uğur and Akbiyik, 2020) | The study adopted text mining to observe the pandemic's impact on the tourism industry by comparing the selected locations globally. The effect of technology was also discussed, and the study suggested plans to reanimate the industry. |
| Supply and demand shocks in the COVID-19 pandemic: An industry and occupation perspective | (Maria Del Rio-Chanona et al., 2020) | The study from an industry and occupation level observed the effect of demand and supply shocks due to the pandemic. It was observed that low-wage occupations, not high-wage occupations, are more vulnerable to the adverse impacts of demand and supply and also identified the same at the industry level. |

This study articulates the impacts (short-, medium-, and long-term) of COVID-19 on the construction industry. The study looks at the coronavirus issues as it affects the construction industry from a holistic perspective. To achieve this, the study has two objectives: (1) To conduct a scientometric analysis of the COVID-19 research in the construction industry, and (2) To carry out an in-depth discussion of the COVID-19 pandemic in developing countries. The result of this study is significant because it allows for proper planning. This is because the COVID-19 impact is not expected to be eroded immediately, but subsequently in years to come.

**Research method**

This study is an enquiry into an area that is relatively new; an objective approach was adopted, whereby the authors are neutral observers in the collected social reality data (Inaba and Kakai, 2019). The study adopted a two-stage approach. Firstly, a bibliometric review was conducted, and secondly, a critical discussion of the impact of COVID-19 pandemic on the construction industry in developing countries through the lens of two selected developing countries was performed. The first stage was adopted to identify the research focuses regarding COVID-19 in the construction industry. The impact of COVID-19 in developing countries was assessed by adopting two countries. The study observed the implications of COVID-19 on the economies of developing countries. To achieve this, two African countries were selected (South Africa and Nigeria) to observe the impact on the construction industry.

*Bibliometric analysis*

This study adopted a Systematic Literature Review approach to gathering data using scientometrics. The systematic review of the literature was conducted using the Scopus database. The Scopus database has enjoyed wide adoption by researchers for similar studies (Newman et al., 2020; Adekunle et al., 2021a). The Scopus database is considered rich and presents current research outputs across fields. To achieve the research objectives, the study conducted a search of the database through the use of keywords. The following keywords were adopted: "2019-nCOV" OR "COVID-19" OR "Coronavirus disease 2019" OR "Novel Coronavirus Pneumonia" OR "NCP" OR "2018 novel coronavirus" OR "SARS-CoV-2" OR "2019 Novel Coronavirus Diseases" OR "novel coronavirus" OR "pneumonia" AND "Construction industry". This returned 93 documents for the search on research publications on COVID-19 in the construction industry. The documents cover various research publications on the construction industry during the pandemic. As earlier stated, the adopted documents were returned based on the keywords found in their title, abstract, or keywords.

The returned results are expected due to the new nature of the studies in this area. The data was analysed using VOSviewer (van Eck and Waltman, 2019). This was done to achieve visualisation of the data collected; various researchers have extensively adopted this for this purpose (Adekunle et al., 2021b; Aghimien et al., 2021). VOSviewer, through visualisation, identifies clusters, items in a cluster, their similarities, and the relationships (Jan van Eck and Waltman, 2006; Eck and Waltman, 2007). For this study, it was adopted to identify the COVID-19 research focus in the construction industry.

*Impact of COVID-19 on the construction industry in developing countries*

The second aspect of the study involves the identification of the impact of COVID-19 on the construction industry in developing countries. To achieve this, the study adopted two developing countries for the in-depth discussion of the impact of COVID-19 on their construction industry. These countries are Nigeria and South Africa, respectively.

*Construction industry research focus during COVID-19*

To achieve an articulated identification of the research focus in the construction industry during the COVID-19 pandemic, a keyword search using the study-related keywords was conducted in the Scopus database. The search was carried out in August 2021. As earlier stated, the Scopus database is considered to contain recent publications and is always current. The retrieved data was analysed using VOSviewer to identify the COVID-19 research clusters in the construction industry (Figure 18.2).

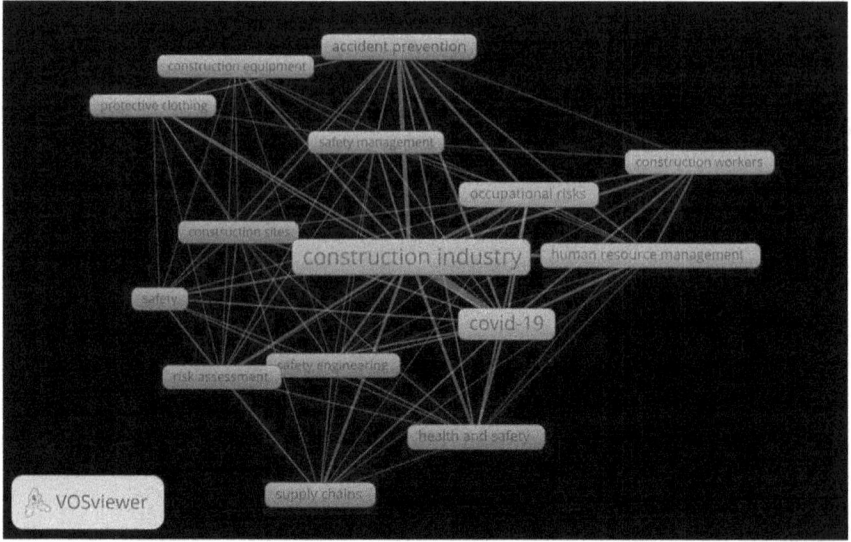

*Figure 18.2* COVID-19 research focus in the construction industry.

The study identified three research focuses. This is represented by the clusters defined by colours in Figure 18.2. These are briefly explained here:

Cluster 1-The cluster is represented by the colour red. The keywords in this cluster can be classified as supply chain and health and safety.
Cluster 2-This cluster is represented with the colour green. This cluster is named occupational health and safety and human resource management.
Cluster 3-This is shown with the colour blue, and it is named construction employ-ment and safety management.

The identified clusters (research focus) reveal that the pandemic accentuated some of the long-standing challenges in the construction industry, especially concern-ing construction industry productivity, labour, and safety. The pandemic, therefore, challenges the construction industry to adopt innovative ways to prevent accidents and ensure worker safety. Furthermore, the COVID-19 pandemic also challenges the construction industry to adopt technology and quit the over-reliance on inten-sive human labour. This ensures productivity, efficiency, and also ensures that work continues despite the restrictive measures instituted to avoid human transmission of the virus.

From Figure 18.3 and Table 18.2, it is evident that most COVID-19 research in the construction industry has been conducted in the United States of America, the United Kingdom, China, Australia, and Malaysia, consequently, making them more advanced and organised in the research. It is worthwhile to note that in Africa, COVID-19 research in the construction industry is observed to emanate from three

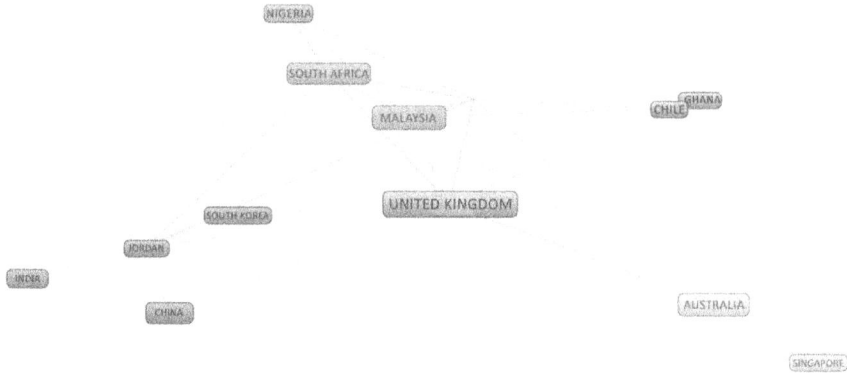

*Figure 18.3* COVID-19 research countries.

*Table 18.2* Publications by country.

| S.N | Territory | Documents | Citations |
|---|---|---|---|
| 1 | Australia | 13 | 38 |
| 2 | Chile | 3 | 36 |
| 3 | China | 11 | 8 |
| 4 | Finland | 3 | 2 |
| 5 | Ghana | 3 | 18 |
| 6 | Hong Kong | 6 | 5 |
| 7 | India | 7 | 6 |
| 8 | Jordan | 3 | 20 |
| 9 | Malaysia | 14 | 56 |
| 10 | Nigeria | 4 | 37 |
| 11 | Singapore | 3 | 7 |
| 12 | South Africa | 10 | 59 |
| 13 | South Korea | 3 | 6 |
| 14 | Turkey | 3 | 0 |
| 15 | United Kingdom | 18 | 65 |
| 16 | United States | 14 | 79 |

countries: South Africa, Nigeria, and Ghana. Although these countries are identified on the visualisation map, the number of documents per country (Ghana-3, Nigeria-2, and South Africa-8) show that the research on COVID-19 in these construction industries is still in its infancy. By implication, these countries require more research on how COVID-19 affects the construction industry, especially in developing countries.

## Impact of COVID-19 on developing countries

The effect of COVID-19 on the construction industry of developing countries was examined. To achieve this, South Africa and Nigeria were selected. South Africa and Nigeria are referred to as the largest economies in sub-Saharan Africa (Siemens, 2017); they are also referred to as the two leading African countries (Ogwueleka and Ikediashi, 2017). Moreover, South Africa and Nigeria has been identified as developing countries by previous studies (Adekunle et al., 2021a).

### Nigeria

The impact of COVID-19 was felt in Nigeria. The Gross Domestic Product (GDP) reportedly decreased by – 6.10% (year-on-year) in real terms in the second quarter of 2020 (National Bureau of Statistics, 2020). This was attributed to financial issues (Nwannekanma, 2021). On a sector analysis, the construction industry was also not immune to the effects. The construction industry during the second period was reported to have experienced a decrease in output nominally by −3.2% (year-on-year). Furthermore, it also shrunk compared to the preceding quarter. Thus, it has a lower contribution to the GDP.

A critical look at the construction industry shows that its growth was fluctuating before 2020 (pre-COVID-19) (Figure 18.2), but plummeted in Q2 of 2020, which is unconnected with the effects of the COVID-19 pandemic and the attendant measures implemented to curb it. The real estate was also hit as it shrunk; likewise, both the "supply" and "demand" sides of the construction sector were hit.

It can therefore be inferred that the construction industry has been on a steady decline and has been worsened by the pandemic. It is safe to say that the Nigerian construction industry requires systematic, strategic, and sustainable measures and policies in order to rescue it from the long-term effects of this impact. This might

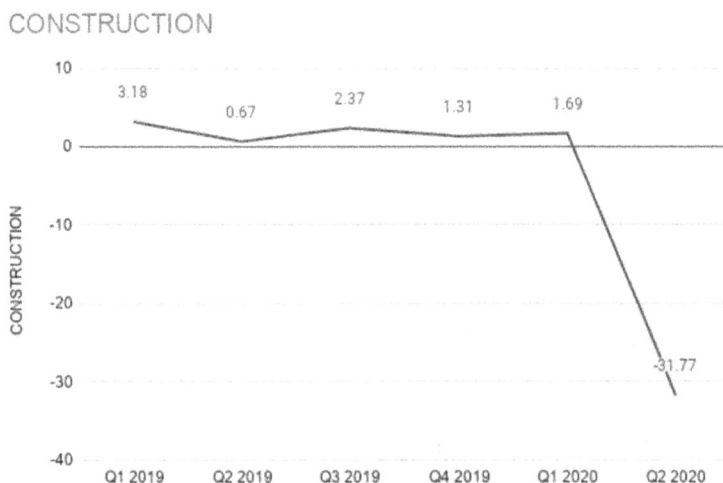

*Figure 18.4* Construction industry in Q2 (National Bureau of Statistics, 2020).

include government intervention in terms of bailout funds and a review of the value added tax, among others. The World Bank (2020) opined that the economic recovery would require not just the government but the public and private sectors. This is important to curb further losses and recover the losses experienced by the industry and the economy. Lockdown measures were reported to lead to a 13.0% loss in the GDP (Andam et al., 2020).

### South Africa

Many businesses (84.5%) in South Africa reported a decrease in turnover, and this included the construction industry (StatsSA, 2020). The South African construction industry did not fare any differently from other countries' experiences during the COVID-19 pandemic. According to StatsSA (2020), the South African economy shrunk by 16%, and the construction industry was not spared as it experienced a 76.6% drop in output (Figure 18.3). However, this is not unexpected because the construction industry in South Africa was far from its optimum pre-COVID-19 (StatsSA, 2020). From Figure 18.3, the construction industry appears to be the hardest hit by the COVID pandemic in South Africa. During the pandemic, 0% of construction organisations operated at full capacity, about 26% operated partially, while about 74% were temporarily closed or paused trading (StatsSA, 2020). As in the case of Nigeria, an urgent but systematic solution is required to achieve a sustainable recovery pathway. Considering the vital role of the construction industry, it is necessary for the economic recovery of many nations around the globe. The construction industry is essential to provide mass employment; thus, investment in this sector is required.

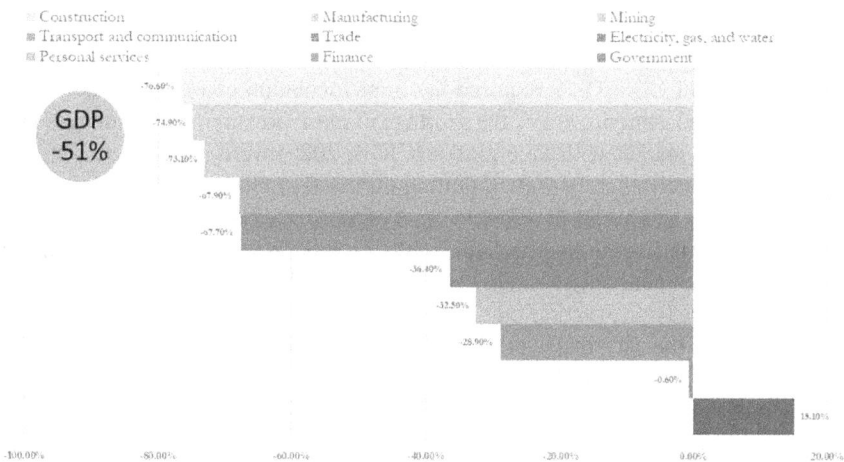

*Figure 18.5* Section-based growth (StatsSA, 2020).

## Discussion

From the collected data articulating the impact of COVID-19 on different industries, the focus has been on the economic and labour implications. However, for the construction industry, this study will discuss the impact under the following headings: economic, safety, legal, and labour availability.

## Economic

The shock created by the COVID-19 pandemic affected many economies due to the different strategies deployed to curb its spread. Due to the lockdown measures, many workers inevitably worked from home (Office for National Statistics, 2020). However, unlike other industries, the construction industry cannot rely on working from home, as activities in the construction industry are mostly on-site. Following this and movement restriction, there will be a drop in productivity. This is due to the low availability of labour and a decline in investment (OECD, 2020), which might not be unconnected to the drop in GDP. GDP in advanced countries were hit; hence during this period, the construction industry was hit as the spending power of clients was also impacted. Consequently, there is a drop in consumer investments, and one of the implications is several uncompleted projects; some might not recover from this shock. Also, the construction industry might not experience new projects, especially from private clients post-COVID-19 for some years.

However, many strict rules regarding statutory remittances require relaxation and incentives provided for stakeholders. This is to support the construction, consulting organisations, and other stakeholders. This includes the relaxation of VAT payment and incentives on taxes, among other measures (for instance, bailout funds) to accommodate the new realities and assist stakeholders. Most importantly, there must be a systematic and all-inclusive recovery pathway designed for the construction industry.

## Safety

The incidence of COVID-19 required the implementation of wearing face masks to curb its spread. Among others, the shortage of mask procurement challenges and flooding of the market with fake masks (CIOB, 2020) were reported as some of the attendant challenges. However, putting on the face mask is greeted by different perspectives and myths in different parts of the world (Wang et al., 2020). This presented an implementation problem. Another regulation that has been difficult to implement in the construction industry is the inability to maintain the mandatory 2-metre distance (Constructionline, 2020).

Considering the fact that work on-site is energy-intensive, especially for the labourers, and requires a lot of perspiration, this might work against workers' productivity and might also result in difficulty breathing compared with when no masks are being worn by workers. Also, some workers will decline their use on the basis of their beliefs. In terms of cost for the construction companies, this is an additional cost which trickles into the overall building cost.

In light of the pandemic and its attendant measures, there is a need to restructure the site safety protocols to ensure the protection of workers and eliminate transmission. Stricter implementation of safety rules is being proposed based on the nature of the construction sites in order to prevent transmission. Periodic tests must be conducted on-site so as not to be caught off-guard.

## Labour availability

From Figure 18.1, it is evident that COVID-19 is affecting the labour age group in the construction industry more. Thus, the construction industry is positioned to be hit by a severe labour shortage. For example, most suppliers could not make supplies due to staff shortages (Constructionline, 2020). The worst to be hit will be skilled jobs that require some level of skill; this is because the required job fits recruitment for replacement. However, the labour shortage will affect every aspect of the construction industry, including the supply chain.

On the other hand, attempting to activate the work-from-home rule will not work perfectly in the construction industry as construction labourers, masons, heavy equipment operators, among others, cannot work from home. The introduction of a staggered work approach to achieve a smaller number of workers on-site per time will adversely affect construction project completion time. Post-COVID-19, due to the high rate of job loss, there will be unemployment and pay cuts for the same job. Worker satisfaction and motivation are going to be a challenge.

COVID-19 therefore requires the adoption of technology to achieve information management and site activities. During the lockdown period, technological tools were adopted to achieve many processes, including organising and conducting meetings. By extension, to achieve a resistant construction industry to similar pandemics in future, the construction industry must adopt technology and digitise its processes. Also, it is the right time to consider automating the construction industry process, especially for on-site activities.

## Legal

The post-COVID-19 era will experience many legal battles due to project delay and budget overrun, although this is dependent on the contract conditions. However, most existing contract conditions never envisaged the novel COVID-19 in their clauses. For instance, most will want to rely on the *force majeure* clauses; however, this might become a matter of interpretation relative to the COVID-19 pandemic. This is because most references to this clause referred to natural disasters and unrest, among others.

According to Squire Patton Boggs (2020), in their analysis of some existing conditions like JCT design and build (DB) 2016 and NEC, observed that there are different perspectives to defining *force majeure* clauses, and some existing contract conditions did not make provisions nor did they give a proper definition for it. Hence, post-pandemic might see many contracts progressing not strictly based on the letters but with amicable and logical resolutions to save the project. Also, many existing contract conditions will require a total revision to accommodate the new realities.

## Conclusion

The effect of COVID-19 has been felt across countries regardless of economic status, and there is an urgency to open up the economy without compromising health. However, this must be done cautiously without eroding the pre-pandemic sustainability gains. Furthermore, although the construction industry has always been crucial to the rejuvenating economies, it will be hard for it to be engaged immediately post-COVID-19 because many economies are struggling and consumer spending is low. Hence, the effects of this pandemic will not easily erode in the next 2–3 years; however, a systematic roadmap is required in the construction industry to provide employment and infrastructure. The pandemic is also a catalyst for the adoption of automation in the construction industry, especially in the area of information management. This will drastically reduce workers' need for physical contact, thus reducing transmission. This study is vital to the industry stakeholders and policymakers as it will enable them to plan adequately through sustainable aggressive fiscal policies and strategies for reopening the economy. These policies must be specific and accommodating in nature, as a blanket strategy will not be effective given the peculiar nature of the construction industry.

## References

Adekunle, S.A., Ejohwomu, O., & Aigbavboa, C.O. (2021a). Building information modelling diffusion research in developing countries: A user meta-model approach. *Buildings*, 11(7), 264. doi: 10.3390/buildings11070264.

Adekunle, S.A., Aigbavboa, C.O., Ejohwomu, O., Adekunle, E.A., & Thwala, W.D. (2021b). Digital transformation in the construction industry: A bibliometric review. *Journal of Engineering, Design and Technology*, (2013). doi: 10.1108/JEDT-08-2021-0442.

Aghimien, D., Aigbavboa, C.O., Oke, A.E., Edwards, D., & Roberts, C.J. (2021). Dynamic capabilities for digitalisation in the AECO sector-a scientometric review. *Engineering, Construction and Architectural Management*. doi: 10.1108/ECAM-12-2020-1012.

Andam, K., Edeh, H., Oboh, V., Pauw, K., & Thurlow, J. (2020). *Estimating the economic costs of COVID-19 in Nigeria* (No. 63; Strategy Support Program).

Aslam, F., Mohmand, Y. T., Ferreira, P., Memon, B. A., Khan, M., & Khan, M. (2020). Network analysis of global stock markets at the beginning of the coronavirus disease (Covid-19) outbreak. *Borsa Istanbul Review*, 141926. doi: 10.1016/j.scitotenv.2020.141926.

Ataguba Ochega, A., & Ataguba, J.E. (2020). Social determinants of health: The role of effective communication in the COVID-19 pandemic in developing countries. *Global Health Action*, 13(1), 1788263. doi: 10.1080/16549716.2020.1788263.

Bartik, A.W., Bertrand, M., Cullen, Z.B., Glaeser, E.L., Luca, M., & Stanton, C.T. (2020). *How are small businesses adjusting to COVID-19? Early evidence from a survey*. Available at www.nber.org/papers/w26989 (Accessed 11 September 2020).

Benítez, M.A., Velasco, C., Sequeira, A.R., Henríquez, J., Menezes, F.M., & Paolucci, F. (2020). Responses to COVID-19 in five Latin American countries. *Health Policy and Technology*, (xxxx), 449. doi: 10.1016/j.hlpt.2020.08.014.

CIOB. (2020). *60% of businesses struggle to obtain face masks: Construction manager.* Available at www.constructionmanagermagazine.com/60-of-businesses-struggle-to-obtain-face-masks/ (Accessed 21 September 2020).

Constructionline. (2020). *The impact of COVID-19 across the construction industry [Infographic]: Constructionline.* Available at www.constructionline.co.uk/insights/news/covid-19-infographic/ (Accessed 25 September 2020).

Eck, N.J. Van, & Waltman, L. (2007). Bibliometric mapping of the computational intelligence field nees. *International Journal of Uncertainty, Fuzziness and Knowledge-Based Systems*, 15(5), 625–645.

Huang, A., Makridis, C., Baker, M., Medeiros, M., & Guo, Z. (2020a). Understanding the impact of COVID-19 intervention policies on the hospitality labor market. *International Journal of Hospitality Management*, 91(July). doi: 10.1016/j.ijhm.2020.102660.

Huang, C., Wang, Y., Li, X., Ren, L., Zhao, J., Hu, Y., Zhang, L., Fan, G., Xu, J., Gu, X., Cheng, Z., Yu, T., Xia, J., Wei, Y., Wu, W., Xie, X., Yin, W., Li, H., Liu, M., . . . Cao, B. (2020b). Clinical features of patients infected with 2019 novel coronavirus in Wuhan, China. *www.thelancet.com*, 395, 497. doi: 10.1016/S0140-6736(20)30183-5.

Inaba, M., & Kakai, H. (2019). Grounded text mining approach: A synergy between grounded theory and text mining approaches. In A. Bryant & K. Charmaz (eds.), *The SAGE handbook of current developments in grounded theory*. Thousand Oaks, CA: SAGE Publications Ltd. doi: 10.4135/9781526485656.

Jan van Eck, N., and Waltman, L. (2006, April). VOS: A new method for visualizing similarities between objects. *Erim Report Series Research in Management*, 11. Available at www.erim.eur.nl.

Lai, C.-C., Shih, T.-P., Ko, W.-C., Tang, H.-J., & Hsueh, P.-R. (2020). Severe acute respiratory syndrome coronavirus 2 (SARS-CoV-2) and coronavirus disease-2019 (COVID-19): The epidemic and the challenges. *International Journal of Antimicrobial Agents*, 55, 105924. doi: 10.1016/j.ijantimicag.2020.105924.

Laing, T. (2020). The economic impact of the coronavirus 2019 (Covid-2019): Implications for the mining industry. *The Extractive Industries and Society*, 7(2), 580–582. doi: 10.1016/j.exis.2020.04.003.

Maria Del Rio-Chanona, R., Mealy, P., Pichler, A., Lafond, F., & Doyne Farmer, J. (2020). Supply and demand shocks in the COVID-19 pandemic: An industry and occupation perspective. *Oxford Review of Economic Policy*. Available at www.insee.fr/en/statistiques/4473305?sommaire=4473307 (Accessed 11 September 2020).

Mora Cortez, R., & Johnston, W.J. (2020). The coronavirus crisis in B2B settings: Crisis uniqueness and managerial implications based on social exchange theory. *Industrial Marketing Management*, 88(April), 125–135. doi: 10.1016/j.indmarman.2020.05.004.

National Bureau of Statistics. (2020). *Nigerian gross domestic product report Q2 2020, national bureau of statistics quarterly report, 2016.* Available at www.nigerianstat.gov.ng/nanapages/download/329.

Newman, C., Edwards, D., Martek, I., Lai, J., Thwala, W.D., & Rillie, I. (2020). Industry 4.0 deployment in the construction industry: A bibliometric literature review and UK-based case study. *Smart and Sustainable Built Environment*, (June). doi: 10.1108/SASBE-02-2020-0016.

Nwannekanma, B. (2021). Construction sector slumps amid shrinking funds. The Guardian Nigeria News – Nigeria and World News – Property – The Guardian Nigeria News – Nigeria and World News, Guardian Property. Available at https://guardian.ng/property/construction-sector-slumps-amid-shrinking-funds/ (Accessed 10 August 2021).

OECD. (2020). Evaluating the initial impact of COVID-19 containment measures on economic activity Introduction and key messages. Tackling Coronavirus Contributing to a Global Effort.

Office for National Statistics. (2020). Coronavirus and homeworking in the UK labour market: 2019. In ONS (Issue April). Available at https://www.ons.gov.uk/employmentandlabourmarket/peopleinwork/employmentandemployeetypes/articles/coronavirusandhomeworkingintheuklabourmarket/2019

Ogwueleka, A.C., & Ikediashi, D.I. (2017). The future of BIM technologies in Africa: Prospects and challenges. In *Integrated building information modelling* (pp. 307–314). UAE: Bentham Science Publisher. doi: 10.2174/9781681084572117010016.

Schindler, S., Jepson, N., & Cui, W. (2020). Covid-19, China and the future of global development. *Research in Globalization*, 2, 100020. doi: 10.1016/j.resglo.2020.100020.

Sharma, H.B., Vanapalli, K.R., Cheela, V.S., Ranjan, V.P., Jaglan, A.K., Dubey, B., Goel, S., & Bhattacharya, J. (2020). Challenges, opportunities, and innovations for effective solid waste management during and post COVID-19 pandemic. *Resources, Conservation and Recycling*, 162(July). doi: 10.1016/j.resconrec.2020.105052.

Sherif, M. (2020). The impact of Coronavirus (COVID-19) outbreak on faith-based investments: An original analysis. *Journal of Behavioral and Experimental Finance*, 126175. doi: 10.1016/j.knosys.2020.105893.

Siemens. (2017). *African digitalization maturity report*. Available at www.siemens.co.za/pool/about_us/Digitalization_Maturity_Report_2017.pdf (Accessed 5 June 2019).

Squire Patton Boggs. (2020). Termination notice requirements/obligations.

StatsSA. (2020). *GDP falls by 2,0% | Statistics South Africa*. Available at www.statssa.gov.za/?p=13401 (Accessed 25 September 2020).

StatsSA. (2020). Business impact survey of the COVID-19 pandemic in South Africa. *Pretoria*. Available at www.statssa.gov.za,info@statssa.gov.za,Tel+27123108911 (Accessed 10 August 2021).

Uğur, N.G., and Akbiyik, A. (2020). Impacts of COVID-19 on global tourism industry: A cross-regional comparison. *Tourism Management Perspectives*, 36(April), 100744. doi: 10.1016/j.tmp.2020.100744.

Vanapalli, K.R., Sharma, H.B., Ranjan, V.P., Samal, B., Bhattacharya, J., Dubey, B.K., & Goel, S. (2020). Challenges and strategies for effective plastic waste management during and post COVID-19 pandemic. *Science of the Total Environment*, 750. doi: 10.1016/j.scitotenv.2020.141514.

van Eck, N.J., & Waltman, L. (2019). Manual for VOS viewer version 1.6.10. *Univeristeit Leiden*. The Netherlands. Available at www.vosviewer.com/documentation/Manual_VOSviewer_1.6.1.pdf.

Verma, S., & Gustafsson, A. (2020). Investigating the emerging COVID-19 research trends in the field of business and management: A bibliometric analysis approach. *Journal of Business Research*, 118(June), 253–261. doi: 10.1016/j.jbusres.2020.06.057.

Wang, J., Pan, L., Tang, S., Ji, J. S., & Shi, X. (2020). Mask use during COVID-19: A risk adjusted strategy. *Environmental Pollution*. Elsevier Ltd, 115099. doi: 10.1016/j.envpol.2020.115099.

WHO. (2020a). Coronavirus disease (COVID-19).

WHO. (2020b). *COVID-19 and violence against women what the health sector/system can do*. Available at www.womensaid.org.uk/the-impact-of-covid-19-on-women-and-children-experiencing-domestic-abuse-and-the- (Accessed 11 September 2020).

The World Bank. (2020). *Nigeria development update: Rebuilding after COVID-19*. Available at www.worldbank.org/en/country/nigeria/publication/nigeria-development-update-rebuilding-after-covid19 (Accessed 10 August 2021).

Yin, S., Zhang, N., & Dong, H. (2020). Preventing COVID-19 from the perspective of industrial information integration: Evaluation and continuous improvement of information networks for sustainable epidemic prevention. *Journal of Industrial Information Integration*, 19(June). doi: 10.1016/j.jii.2020.100157.

Zhou, Y., Zhang, Z., Wang, B., Ren, G., Qi, H., & Wang, X. (2020). Construction time, cost and testing data of a prefabricated isolation medical unit for COVID-19. *Data in Brief*, 32. doi: 10.1016/j.dib.2020.106068.

# 19 Assessment of COVID-19 control and prevention measures

## Lessons learned at construction sites

*Mírian Caroline Farias Santos*
*and Dayana Bastos Costa*

## Introduction

COVID-19 has spread rapidly worldwide. The first confirmed case of COVID-19 in Brazil took place on February 25, 2020, and since then, the number of cases has grown considerably. Until October 28, 2020, 5,468,270 cases and 158,456 deaths were recorded at 74.83 deaths per 100,000 inhabitants (Geocovid, 2022). Although the recommendations are to minimise human interactions through social distancing, some activities, such as construction, play a fundamental role in society and are impossible to be carried out online (Araya, 2021). Furthermore, as the construction industry is recognised as one of the most dangerous activities for its workers (Albert et al., 2020), it requires rapid response and risk mitigation measures (Bruin et al., 2020).

Some impacts of COVID-19 on the construction industry are absenteeism, interruption of supply (OSHA, 2020), reduction in the number of workers allowed inside the sites, and changes in how they work, along with impacts on how managers organise the workforce (Araya, 2021). However, the nature of these impacts depends on the location of the works, as the rules and policies adopted by many countries may differ from region to region (Bruin et al., 2020). For example, the Supreme Court of Brazil decided on states' and municipalities' autonomy to decide on measures to control the spread of COVID-19 in 2020 (Supreme Federal Court of Brazil, 2020). Thus, several decrees were issued in cities, including Salvador City (Bahia-Brazil), where some determined general and specific protocols for construction activities.

Simpeh and Amoah (2021) pointed out the need for further study to determine why some organisations have lapses in implementing the basic COVID-19 measures. Furthermore, given the diversity of recommendations, the scarcity of studies, and the uniqueness of the COVID-19 pandemic, it is crucial to understand the problems associated with the coronavirus to refine the recommendations implemented.

This chapter presents an assessment of COVID-19 control and prevention measures, discussing difficulties and lessons learned in a sample of construction projects in the metropolitan region of Salvador (State of Bahia- Brazil) from April to October 2020.

DOI: 10.1201/9781003278368-22

## Measures to prevent and control COVID-19 applied in the construction industry context

Different countries, states, and municipalities have been adopting various risk mitigation measures to control the spread of COVID-19. According to their objective, Bruin et al. (2020) grouped the main measures applied to worldwide society into categories such as:

- **Mobility Restrictions** – aims to limit the movement of people to contain or slow down the spread of the virus. For example, closing or restricting public transport and outdoor activities.
- **Socio-economic Restrictions** – aims to restrict social and economic activities in which people gather for educational, recreational, sporting, or work-related purposes. For example, closing or limiting schools and mandatory telecommuting.
- **Physical Distancing** – also called social distancing, aims to maintain adequate distance between people without losing social connections.
- **Hygiene Measures** – aims to limit the risk of spreading the infected virus directly or indirectly to third parties. For example, wash hands and use Personal Protective Equipment (PPE).

Although this classification of measures is not specific to construction sites, it can mostly be recommended to the construction industry. Simpeh and Amoah (2021) identified some of these measures as commonly implemented by construction companies. The measurements were related to (a) Social distancing, (b) Hygiene (sanitisation), (c) Screening, (d) PPE, (e) Creating awareness, (f) Site access, (g) Handling of deliveries, and (h) Compliance, which were based on the recommendation of the World Health Organization (WHO) and the Government of South Africa.

Assaad and El-Adaway (2021) reviewed the updated guidelines and industry best practices developed by various USA organisations, government entities, and cities. These include the Associated General Contractors of America (AGC), the Occupational Safety and Health Administration (OSHA), the Centers for Disease Control and Prevention (CDC), the Department of Labor (DOL), and the City of Boston. Their work states the practices recommended by the AGC and OSHA, categorised into (a) Personal responsibilities, (b) Social distancing, (c) Jobsite/office practices, (d) Management of sick employees, (e) Engineering controls, (f) Administrative controls, (g) Safe work practices, and (h) Personal protective equipment (PPE).

In Brazil, the first federal government document, named CIRCULAR LETTER SEI n° 1088/2020/ME (Brazil Federal Ministry of Economics, March 27, 2020) established general guidelines for workers and employers due to the pandemic of COVID-19. Other documents were CIRCULAR LETTER SEI No. 1247/2020/ME (Brazil Federal Ministry of Economics, April 14, 2020), and JOINT ORDINANCE n° 20 (Brazil Federal Ministry of Economics, June 18, 2020), which contains specific guidelines for the construction sector. Some of these national recommendations for the construction sector include the establishment of a symptom control protocol for workers; notifications by employees if any family member has COVID-19; daily attendance record of all workers and visitors with contact information; installation of more washing stations/hand sanitisers and alcohol dispensers, among others.

In addition to these government national and local measures, there were also recommendations from the Construction Industry Chamber – SINDUSCON-BA and Industry Social Service – SESI-BA. Therefore, many countries' rules and policies will likely have different results (Bruin et al., 2020).

## Methodology

This study adopted a qualitative research approach and used primary and secondary data collection. According to Hox and Boeije (2005), primary data is collected for a specific research problem, in contrast to secondary data, where other researchers collect the data and make it available for the research community's reuse. This research comprises three main steps: (a) literature review, (b) data collection, and (c) data analysis and interpretation (Figure 19.1), as described here. The Ethics Committee of the Research Office from the Federal University of Rio Grande do Sul – ProPESQ-UFRGS approved this study (Ethics Committee approval number: 45035121.1.0000.5347).

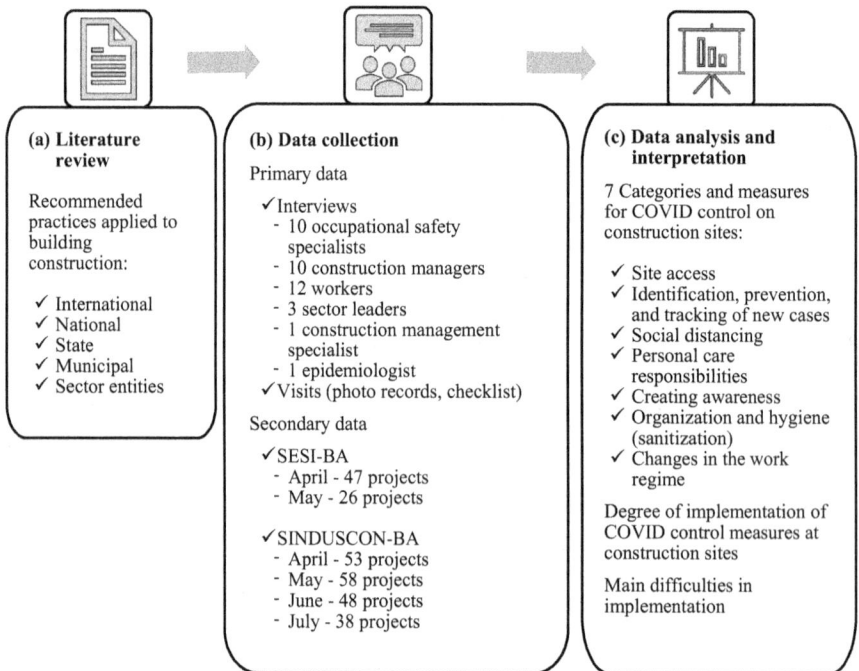

**(a) Literature review**

Recommended practices applied to building construction:

✓ International
✓ National
✓ State
✓ Municipal
✓ Sector entities

**(b) Data collection**

Primary data

✓ Interviews
- 10 occupational safety specialists
- 10 construction managers
- 12 workers
- 3 sector leaders
- 1 construction management specialist
- 1 epidemiologist
✓ Visits (photo records, checklist)

Secondary data

✓ SESI-BA
- April - 47 projects
- May - 26 projects

✓ SINDUSCON-BA
- April - 53 projects
- May - 58 projects
- June - 48 projects
- July - 38 projects

**(c) Data analysis and interpretation**

7 Categories and measures for COVID control on construction sites:

✓ Site access
✓ Identification, prevention, and tracking of new cases
✓ Social distancing
✓ Personal care responsibilities
✓ Creating awareness
✓ Organization and hygiene (sanitization)
✓ Changes in the work regime

Degree of implementation of COVID control measures at construction sites

Main difficulties in implementation

*Figure 19.1* Research steps.

### Literature review

The first stage of the research was to investigate measures recommended by the international, national, state, and municipal levels and those recommended by local sector entities. For this, the San Francisco Order of the Health Officer No. C19–07c (April 29, 2020), LA Building & Safety Announcement No. 5 Revised (April 15, 2020), and Official Letter SEI Circular No. 1247/2020/ME from the Brazil Ministry of Economy (April 14, 2020) were used as references. In addition, municipal Decrees from March 31 to August 8 were investigated (cities of Salvador, Porto Alegre, Passo Fundo, Caxias do Sul, and Fortaleza), as well as the construction industry documents: Brazilian Construction Industry Chamber – CBIC (March 2020), Regional Construction Industry Chamber such as Bahia (April 2020), Rio Grande do Sul (March 2020) and Ceará (May 2020). The criterion for choosing the materials was the relevance, meaning, and appropriate documents in which the recommendations could be applied to the researchers' local context.

### Data collection

This stage aimed to collect primary and secondary data by characterising the degree of implementation of the measures in a sample of construction projects from the metropolitan region of Salvador-Brazil. In addition, this data allowed us to identify the main difficulties and lessons learned in implementing COVID-19 measures.

#### Primary data collection

In September 2020, the SINDUSCON-BA provided a list of 23 construction companies with projects in progress in the Salvador region. Ten construction companies agreed to participate in the study from this list, and one construction project per construction company was selected. Table 19.1 shows the characteristics of 10 construction projects studied.

Interviews with 10 safety specialists and 10 construction managers from each construction project occurred to inquire about measures adopted at the sites. All interviews happened in an open-question format, in which the interviewees freely answered the questions by video call or by telephone contact. Furthermore, there were three interviews with construction industry leaders' representatives and a specialist in construction management. They shared their perspectives on how the sites and companies faced COVID-19, including adopted measures and their implementation difficulties. Finally, the last interviewee was an epidemiologist who provided the view of a health specialist regarding measures adopted during construction.

#### Secondary data collection

Secondary data were collected from surveys carried out by SINDUSCON-BA and from SESI-BA. In the SINDUSCON-BA survey, construction project representatives answered electronic questions related to site typologies, suspected COVID-19

*Table 19.1* Characterisation of the sample of the construction projects studied.

| Project | Building system | Multi-story buildings | Building area (m²) | Number of workers | Construction phase during the study |
|---|---|---|---|---|---|
| 1 | Cast in-place concrete wall | Residential | 16.916 | 130 | Structure, Masonry, Roof, and Finishing |
| 2 | Cast in-place concrete wall | Residential | 36.767 | 84 | Foundation and Structure |
| 3 | Structural masonry | Mixed | 2.140 | 15 | Finishing |
| 4 | Reinforced concrete, Ceramic block masonry, and Drywall | Residential | 64.992 | 280 | Structure and Masonry |
| 5 | Reinforced concrete, Ceramic block masonry, and Drywall | Residential | 22.604 | 110 | Finishing |
| 6 | Reinforced concrete, Ceramic block masonry, and Drywall | Residential | 47.939 | 200 | Structure |
| 7 | Reinforced concrete, Ceramic block masonry, and Drywall | Residential | – | 46 | Structure |
| 8 | Facade renovation | Hospital | 2.000 | 30 | Finishing |
| 9 | Reinforced concrete and Ceramic block masonry | Residential | 12.284 | 60 | Structure |
| 10 | Reinforced concrete, Ceramic block masonry, and Drywall | Residential | 9.966 | 75 | Structure; Plumbing; Finishing |

cases, deaths, absenteeism at the sites, suggestions, and best practices adopted. This data involves 53 to 38 construction projects and data from four months (April to July 2020). Most of this data was presented in bar graph format, and some answers had to be inferred through interpretation.

Concerning the SESI-BA data, inspections were made of 47 sites in April, and 26 sites were reinspected in May. In both inspection rounds, interviewees answered questions about implementing current Decrees and Ordinances recommendations.

### Data analysis and interpretation

The data analysis involved assessing measures identified in the reviewed recommendation from the literature review phase. Initially, the study identified 54 measures, from which 32 were selected based on two criteria. The first criterion was the frequency of the practice occurrence in the different sources of the recommended practices reviewed (at least more than 50% of sources), except for the measure regarding the use of elevators in the sites since there were not enough primary and secondary data available for analysis. The second criterion was selecting other actions that were less relevant in the different sources of the recommended practices reviewed but valuable to enrich the results since this study collected primary and secondary data for this assessment.

Since some measures identified had everyday purposes, this study proposed seven categories to classify those measures according to their application, thus improving data interpretation: Site access, Identification, prevention, and tracking of new cases, Social distancing, Personal care responsibilities, Creating awareness, Organisation and hygiene (sanitisation), and Changes in the work regime. The categories were based on the following works: Bruin et al. (2020), Simpeh and Amoah (2021), and Assaad and El-Adaway (2021).

The assessment involved whether the implementation of each measure was "Total," meaning that all sources of evidence confirm the implementation of the measure, or "Partial," meaning that at least one source of evidence does not confirm the implementation of the measure. Next, the degree of implementation was calculated for each category of measures, and the main difficulties were discussed, considering the primary and secondary data. The degree of implementation calculation was the ratio of measures implemented (partial or total) to the total number of measures in each category.

## Results and discussion

Table 19.2 presents the results concerning the degree of implementation of COVID-19 control and prevention measures. Based on the results, the organisation and hygiene category had the highest implementation (60% of the measures implemented), while personal care responsibilities, creating awareness, and changing the work regime achieved partial implementation (100% of partial implementation). Next, the results and discussion of each category will be presented.

*Site access*

The Site access category had 67% partial implementation and 33% full implementation of the measures for the construction projects studied. In April, according to the data from SESI-BA, the construction projects had difficulties acquiring thermometers at the beginning of the pandemic, mainly due to the shortage of equipment in the market. Thus, some interviewees reported using a screening questionnaire to help identify symptomatic workers. There was a growing adoption of temperature measurement over May, when the SINDUSCON-BA survey was carried out, until October, during the primary data site visits, when 90% of the interviewees mentioned using a thermometer at the sites.

Alsharef et al. (2021) and Zheng et al. (2021) also identified a lack of thermometers to measure temperature during the initial period of the pandemic. Although data from SESI-BA indicated that the sites were restricting visitor access (47% in April and 62% in May), only one construction site implemented protocols for the daily registration of visitors. Some of these visitors are suppliers and deliverers,

*Table 19.2* Degree of implementation of COVID-19 control and prevention measures based on primary and secondary data.

| Category | Measures | Degree of implementation per measures | Degree of implementation per category | |
|---|---|---|---|---|
| | | | Partial | Implemented |
| **Site access** | Temperature measurement | Partial | 67% | 33% |
| | Daily attendance record of all workers and visitors with contact information | Partial | | |
| | Restrict or minimise the access of people who do not work on the site, especially material suppliers | Total | | |
| **Identification, prevention, and tracking of new cases** | Immediately remove the employees with symptoms or confirmed cases | Total | 60% | 40% |
| | In positive cases for COVID-19: active search for workers who had contact with the contaminated for evaluation | Partial | | |
| | Designate a supervisor for COVID-19 | Total | | |
| | Establish a symptom control protocol for employees | Partial | | |
| | Develop and ensure a correction plan to address any non-compliance | Partial | | |
| **Social distancing** | Maintain minimum distance for social distancing | Partial | 67% | 33% |
| | Identify the agglomeration and high-risk contamination points | Total | | |
| | Avoid face-to-face meetings | Partial | | |
| | Prioritise the immediate removal of risk groups | Partial | | |
| | Stagger the working times (entry to and exit from the site, changing rooms, and dining hall) | Partial | | |
| | Adopt measures to reduce the intensity and duration of personal contact between workers | Total | | |
| **Personal care responsibilities** | Use of masks or PPE provided | Partial | 100% | 0% |
| | Change uniforms daily, sharing them is prohibited, and determining that they do not use them on the way to and from work | Partial | | |

| Category | Measures | Degree of implementation per measures | Degree of implementation per category | |
|---|---|---|---|---|
| | | | Partial | Implemented |
| **Creating awareness** | Training, recording, and monitoring the use of PPE | Partial | 100% | 0% |
| | Informational posters at the site | Partial | | |
| | Make daily safety briefings | Partial | | |
| **Organisation and hygiene (sanitisation)** | Install more wash stations/ hand sanitisers and alcohol dispensers | Total | 40% | 60% |
| | Adequacy of facilities such as dining hall and changing rooms | Total | | |
| | Sanitise shared materials before use | Total | | |
| | Frequently clean and disinfect all high-touch areas | Partial | | |
| | Reinforcement in the cleaning of environments | Total | | |
| | Check if the hygiene, distancing, and cleaning guidelines are being met | Total | | |
| | Provision of 70% alcohol gel and/or soap in work areas | Total | | |
| | Keep all areas ventilated, including the dining hall and rest places for workers | Partial | | |
| | Prohibit drinking fountain with an inclined jet | Partial | | |
| | Do not share phones, desks, tools, and PPE | Partial | | |
| **Changes in the work regime** | Reduced working hours | Partial | 100% | 0% |
| | Division of teams into work shifts if necessary | Partial | | |
| | Identify the functions that can perform your activities from home | Partial | | |

which, according to Alsharef et al. (2021)'s work, represents a greater risk of spreading the virus since they visit different places.

*Identification, prevention, and tracking of new cases*

Measures related to identifying, preventing, and tracking new cases categories had 60% partial implementation and 40% full implementation. Although during the interviews, all safety specialists and workers reported that when symptoms or cases were confirmed, the workers were removed from work, some safety specialists said they expected workers to have more symptoms before referring them to the medical sector. This is due mainly to the diversity of the disease's symptoms and the uncertainties of other less severe illnesses. Thus, there is a risk of having workers with active viruses generally working at the sites as a contamination vector.

Based on SESI-BA data, in 84% of the projects studied in April and 85% of projects in May, the workers had a way to communicate COVID-19 symptoms. They could inform their immediate leader, the health and safety sector, and the administrative or HR sector. According to primary data, the first communication usually was with the safety COVID-19 supervisor. Many companies had difficulties resolving non-compliance. To solve that, safety specialists established actions, such as informal conversation (100%), warning (40%), suspension (20%), or new training (20%). Although 90% of the safety specialists reported the possibility of tracking the workers in a specific zone of work, and 20% said that they could map common areas, searching for workers who had contact with contaminated was a difficulty.

*Social distancing*

The social distancing category had 67% partial implementation and 33% full implementation of the measures. According to the safety specialists, the high-contact areas and high risk of contamination locations were the dining hall (60%), changing room (30%), entrance and exit of the sites (30%), and during construction activities with necessary high personal contact, such as transporting heavy materials (40%) and concreting (20%). In addition, workers also pointed out the time register (25%) as a location of agglomeration.

Furthermore, 50% of the safety specialists responded that they had difficulty maintaining social distancing. Some practices adopted by the sites to keep the social distance include using signs and posters, changes in layout, redistribution of tables and chairs in the dining hall, and boundaries on benches, among others.

Regarding changes in the work routine to maintain distance, 40% of construction managers changed the planning process to keep a safe distance between workers, and 20% redistributed teams in different work zones. Another measure to enhance social distancing was the reduction of face-to-face meetings and increased caution during these meetings.

According to SESI-BA data, the scaling of the dining hall and changing rooms increased from 28% (April) to 54% of the works (May). From September to October, 100% of respondents confirmed this practice on the sites from September to October.

From April to July 2020, data from SESI-BA and SINDUSCON-BA showed a high priority (almost 90% of respondents) to remove people in the risk group from the sites. However, from September to October 2020, the percentage was around 60%, based on the primary data. This behaviour may be associated with the drop in the number of cases and the greater flexibility of the municipal government regarding commercial activities and some construction activities.

*Personal care responsibilities*

The personal care responsibilities category had 100% partial implementation of the measures regarding masks and PPEs use and daily change of uniforms. Although all workers responded that they used the mask provided, a few sites had workers not using the PPE properly during the visits. In addition, 70% of safety specialists confirmed difficulties in making workers wear or change their masks. The low frequency of correct protective elements corroborates Moreno-Sueskun et al. (2020) findings. According to Alsharef et al. (2021), several workers frequently removed their masks due to discomfort and fogging in the safety glasses. Regarding the daily uniform change, one company provided extra uniforms and bags to pack the uniforms; some workers responded that they do not change their uniforms daily (42%).

*Creating awareness*

Creating awareness measures had 100% partial implementation. From April to June 2020, according to the SINDUSCON-BA data, 100% of respondents reported that companies provided specific training to prevent COVID-19. From September to October, 70% of respondents, during primary data collection, reported that they offered particular training on the use of PPE. During the site visits, there were informational posters in 90% of the sites visited. Although most companies provide PPE, increasing information about the disease and its prevention is essential; 80% of safety specialists reported that one of the recurrent difficulties was the awareness of workers.

*Organisation and hygiene (sanitisation)*

For the rrganisation and hygiene category, 40% of the measures were partially implemented, and 60% were fully implemented. The measures successfully implemented, according to SESI-BA data, were: (a) Install more wash stations/hand sanitisers and alcohol dispensers; (b) Adequacy of facilities such as dining hall and changing rooms; (c) Sanitise shared materials before use; (d) Reinforcement in the cleaning of environments; (e) Check if the hygiene, distancing, and cleaning guidelines are being met; and (f) Provision of 70% alcohol gel and/or soap in work areas. Other good practices observed in this work were providing face shields, delivering individual hygiene kits to workers, cleaning team training for correct hygiene, and cards to signal sanitised or non-sanitised tables.

We noted that some changing rooms, where workers took off their masks to clean themselves and change clothes, had little or no ventilation. The administrative sector also lacked better ventilation since, in some sites, the windows were kept closed and the air conditioning was turned on. Some construction sites also did not prohibit drinking fountains with an inclined jet. The lack of isolation of these devices allowed workers to put their mouths in the drinking fountains.

Moreover, 90% of safety specialists reported that high contact points were clean, such as handrails, door handles, elevator buttons, chair arms, and telephones. However, there was no consensus on the frequency of cleaning.

*Changes in the work regime*

Changes in the work regime measures had 100% partial implementation. As these measures depended on administrative decisions and production organisation, they were implemented differently in each project. In October, 30% of the construction managers reported redistributing teams in different shifts at their sites. The division into work shifts was also reported by 25% of workers in this study and some sectoral entities. SESI-BA data showed that approximately 75% of the construction projects used the home office modality in April and May. The remote work activities were generally restricted to the risk group and the administrative departments.

Reducing the workload, employees, and staggering shifts can reduce the risk of contamination. However, productivity can be reduced, especially if there are absences for medical requests. According to Araya (2021), while it is intended to reduce the risks related to the dissemination of COVID-19, it is natural to expect a reduction in productivity.

## Implications for practice

Table 19.3 summarises lessons learned regarding COVID-19 control and prevention measures at construction sites based on the empirical study and literature review. Adopting these measures can positively impact construction workplaces in the long term, such as cleaning, organisation, and creating a safer environment.

*Table 19.3* Lessons learned about COVID-19 control and prevention measures.

| Categories | Lessons learned |
|---|---|
| **Site access** | – Avoid unnecessary contact between construction site workers and suppliers' workers during deliveries.<br>– Use of questionnaires to identify symptomatic and asymptomatic workers. |
| **Identification, prevention, and tracking of new cases** | – Create communication channels for workers to clarify doubts and report possible symptoms.<br>– Keep an updated record of the teams and the workplace, including any relocation of workers.<br>– Safe route boundaries can help to map paths in common areas, when possible, using different routes for different teams or workplaces. |
| **Social distancing** | – For activities in which it is difficult to keep a social distance, establish a rigorous protocol, such as separating people by team or work zone and monitoring possible symptoms after executing these critical services.<br>– Implementing the practice of staggering in entrances, exits, time registers, changing rooms, and dining halls to reduce possible agglomerations. |
| **Personal care responsibilities** | – Companies can provide extra uniforms and bags to pack the uniforms. |

| Categories | Lessons learned |
|---|---|
| **Creating awareness** | – Increase information about COVID-19 and its prevention, besides carrying out practical training on using PPE and other protectors.<br>– Closer monitoring, corrective actions, and actions of encouragement, such as the appointment of exemplary employees. |
| **Organisation and hygiene (sanitisation)** | – Install hand-washing stations with disinfectants at the entrance and various locations on the construction sites; disinfection of tools and surfaces, avoiding sharing tools and equipment; and daily cleaning record.<br>– Provide individual hygiene kits to workers, additional locations to register in, cleaning team training for correct hygiene, and cards to signal sanitised or non-sanitised tables.<br>– Keep areas well-ventilated, especially the changing rooms and administrative sectors, which generally lack open spaces for natural ventilation. |
| **Changes in the work regime** | – Reducing the workload and employees can reduce the risk of contamination, making teams leaner and often optimised.<br>– Consider changes in the work regime strategies together with the planning. |

## Conclusions

This chapter presented an overview of the degree of implementation of COVID-19 control and prevention measures at sites in the metropolitan region of Salvador (Bahia-Brazil). Most of the lessons learned regarding personal care responsibilities, creating awareness, organisation and hygiene, and identification, prevention, and tracking of new cases may be adopted independently of the end of this pandemic.

Similar problems in literature, such as temperature measurement for site access, identifying symptoms in workers, controlling visitors' and suppliers' access to sites, and workers' awareness of using the PPR correctly, were also identified. Besides this, other measures successfully adopted include installing more wash stations/hand sanitisers and alcohol dispensers.

The main limitations of this study are the small number of participants in primary data collection and the short time of visits, as it sought to reduce the risk of contamination for researchers. Thus, verifying the entire COVID-19 prevention routine at the sites during working hours was impossible.

For future works, it is suggested to propose and implement solutions with the support of digital technologies, such as BIM, to help re-establish construction activities and minimise the impacts imposed by the COVID-19 pandemic. Finally, new studies should investigate the long-term effects of COVID control and prevention measures on the sites' health, safety, and productivity.

## Acknowledgement

This study was supported by the Ministry of Science, Technology, Innovation, and Communication of Brazil through CNPq (Conselho Nacional de Desenvolvimento Científico e Tecnológico) (Grant Number 02963/2020–2).

## References

Albert, A., et al. (2020). Does the potential safety risk affect whether particular construction hazards are recognised or not? *Journal of Safety Research*, 75, 241–250.

Alsharef, A., et al. (2021). Early impacts of the COVID-19 pandemic on the United States construction industry. *International Journal of Environmental Research and Public Health*, 18, 1559.

Araya, F. (2021). Modeling the spread of COVID-19 on construction workers: An agent-based approach. *Safety Science*, 133, 105022.

Assaad, R., & El-adaway, I. (2021). Guidelines for responding to COVID-19 pandemic: Best practices, impacts, and future research directions. *Journal of Management in Engineering*, 37(3), 06021001.

Brazil Federal Ministry of Economics. (2020, March 27). *Official letter SEI n° 1088/2020/ME*. Brasília, DF: Ministério da economia. Available at www.sindusconpa.org.br/arquivos/File/1088-2020-ME.pdf (Accessed 3 July 2021).

Brazil Federal Ministry of Economics. (2020, April 14). *Official letter SEI n° 1247/2020/ME*. Brasília, DF: Ministério da economia. Available at www.gov.br/trabalho/pt-br/inspecao/covid-19-1/covid_19_construcao_civil_orientacoes_gerais.pdf (Accessed 3 July 2021).

Brazil Federal Ministry of Economics. (2020, June 18). *Joint ordinance N° 20*. Brasília, DF: Ministério da economia. Available at www.in.gov.br/en/web/dou/-/portaria-conjunta-n-20-de-18-de-junho-de-2020-262408085 (Accessed 3 July 2021).

Bruin, Y., et al. (2020). Initial impacts of global risk mitigation measures taken during the combatting of the COVID-19 pandemic. *Safety Science*, 128, 1047773.

Geocovid. Available at https://covid.mapbiomas.org/cases/ (Accessed October 8 2022).

Hox, J.J., & Boeije, H.R. (2005). Data collection, primary vs. secondary. In K. Kempf-Leonard (ed.), *Encyclopedia of social measurement* (pp. 593–599). Atlanta, GA: Elsevier Science.

Los Angeles. (2020, April 15). *Los Angeles building & safety announcement no. 5*. Available at www.ladbs.org/docs/default-source/publications/misc-publications/construction-site-guidance.pdf?sfvrsn=8f6ef753_18 (Accessed 1 April 2020).

Moreno-Sueskun, I., et al. (2020). Reincorporación al trabajo en el contexto de la pandemia de COVID-19 en sectores de industria y construcción en Navarra (España). *Archivos de prevención de riesgos laborales*, 23(4), 443–457.

Occupational Safety and Health (OSHA). *Guidance on preparing workplaces for COVID-19*. Available at www.osha.gov/Publications/OSHA3990.pdf. (Accessed 3 December 2020).

San Francisco. San Francisco order of the health officer no. C19–07c. Available at https://sf.gov/sites/default/files/2020-04/2020.04.29%20FINAL%20%28signed%29%20Health%20Officer%20Order%20C19-07c-%20Shelter%20in%20Place.pdf (Accessed 15 December 2020).

Simpeh, F., & Amoah, C. (2021). Assessment of measures instituted to curb the spread of COVID-19 on construction site. *International Journal of Construction Management*, 1–19. doi: 10.1080/15623599.2021.1874678.

Supreme Federal Court of Brazil. (2020). *STF recognises concurrent competence of states, DF, municipalities and the Union in combating COVID-19*. Available at www.stf.jus.br/portal/cms/verNoticiaDetalhe.asp?id Conteudo=441447 (Accessed 3 March 2021).

Zheng, L., Chen, K., & Ma, L. (2021). Knowledge, attitudes, and practices toward COVID-19 among construction industry practitioners in China. *Front. Public Health*, 8, 599769. doi: 10.3389/fpubh.2020.599769.

# 20 COVID-19 and shock events in the AEC sector

## Perspectives on mitigating measures

*Innocent Musonda, Adetayo Onososen,*
*Thembani Moyo and Motheo Meta Tjebane*

### 1.0 Introduction

The emergence of the COVID-19 pandemic has caused a global change and forced social, cultural, and economic systems to modify their organisational frameworks and operational procedures. The effects of the pandemic were apparent, and numerous industries had to modify their workflow and operating practices. Within the construction industry, managers had to adapt to the new environment by being aware of the influence of COVID-19 on various aspects of construction projects, issues and considerations, and preparedness levels of related entities (Rokooei et al., 2022). Additionally, the pandemic brought problems with contract administration, particularly regarding project notices for delays, scheduling, and schedule recovery; project suspension, termination, and reinstatement; and workplace safety compliance, among others (Osman and Ataei, 2022). At the height of the pandemic, complete lockdowns and quarantine prevented individuals from moving or working. Among the issues the sector is currently facing are the labour and critical people shortages on construction projects that resulted from the relaxation of those laws, the proliferation of COVID-19, and the dynamic changes to the construction work environment such as social distancing (Assaad and El-adaway, 2021). Due to the uncertainties the pandemic caused, many construction companies were finding it difficult to deal with the economic effects of this epidemic, such as market disruption, decreased investment, and decreased government spending on building (Raoufi and Fayek, 2020). Although some preliminary studies address the backdrop of COVID-19 within the construction industry and how the height of COVID-19 has affected it in developing countries (Olatunde et al., 2021; Agyekum et al., 2022), relatively few current implications on project performance and future directions are available. Thus, this research explored mitigating the effect of COVID-19 in Africa's construction industry by looking at the effect and mitigating measures for future shock events.

### 2.0 Perspectives/concepts

In tracing the implications of COVID-19 in the construction sector, it is evident that the new regulations imposed by governments to control the spread of the virus were implemented without a reservoir of knowledge on strategies to mitigate

DOI: 10.1201/9781003278368-23

negative implications on various economic sectors (Marco-Franco et al., 2021). The impact of the COVID-19 pandemic cannot be over-emphasised, as it brought severe social and economic challenges that have had a significant impact on the construction sector. Globally, operations in the construction sector were negatively affected by the COVID-19 pandemic, as construction workers normally operate within proximity, putting them at a higher risk of exposure to COVID-19 (Sierra, 2022). Kukoyi et al. (2022) have also articulated how the sector is generally labour-intensive and requires well-defined health and safety protocols. Introducing new health and safety regulations led construction industries to redesign their health and safety regulations to align with the new regulations (Roziqin et al., 2021).

Due to the minacious fashion of rapid spread and extreme transmission rate, COVID-19 impacted the availability of the workforce as an affected person had to isolate (Gbadamosi et al., 2020). In South Africa, the stipulated time was two weeks. Evidence suggests that construction sites sometimes had to continue operations with a labour shortage (Wang et al., 2020). This triggered the need to develop new systems to mitigate the risk and challenges associated with the pandemic. One of the earlier strategies was record-keeping and developing a follow-up plan for sick workers (Kukoyi et al., 2022). Through such initiatives, it became evident that some workers did not comply with the COVID-19 safety regulations or used COVID-19 personal protective equipment (PPE) incorrectly and ignored the health and safety protocols (Amoah and Simpeh, 2021). Accordingly, studies have demonstrated the implications of the need for the construction sector to adhere to the lockdown health and safety protocols (Sierra, 2022) (Kukoyi et al., 2022; Dobrucali et al., 2022). Notable implications have been operational delays as construction workers undergo training on new protocols (Alsharef et al., 2021) and additional costs on the projects due to increased procurement expenses to adhere to the new regulations on health and safety (Lidia Pinti and Bonelli, 2022).

## 3.0   Methodology/framework/case study

### Study design

The qualitative method was used to analyse data without numerical measurements to get respondents' descriptors, observations, attitudes, thoughts, and motivations (Ramírez-Montoya et al., 2021). A focus group of postgraduate students (doctoral candidates) with experiences of construction trends during the pandemic and from six countries were considered valuable in sharing their insights for the study. This is because focus groups are a popular technique for gathering data since they utilise team dynamics to examine interprofessional perspectives. In a focus group, participants are chosen as a deliberate, though not necessarily representative, selection of a certain community and the interviews are "focused" on a specific issue (Takashima et al., 2020). Physical distance presents particular difficulties for this technique because it depends on bringing groups together. Individual interviews might be possible as limitations are eased, but focus groups will probably be affected for a longer time. Online focus groups have been investigated in qualitative research and may be a practical tool (Sy et al., 2020; Makhathini et al., 2023). An online focus group was employed to collect in-depth answers to questions from a diverse set of participants spread out geographically and to take advantage of group interaction (Blake et al., 2021; Dahab et al., 2020).

### Sampling

The respondents were construction professionals from various Sub-Saharan African countries. The respondents are chosen through convenience sampling. Convenience sampling is a non-probability sampling strategy that makes it easier to choose construction industry professionals convenient to the researcher (Badamasi et al., 2021). Figure 20.1 shows the spatial distribution of participants.

### Session administration

The focus group session lasted for about 150 minutes. Before the session, participants were briefed about the study and their consent to partake. The briefing was done in English. The session consisted of a moderator, a timekeeper, and two members helping collect information. The session took place on Microsoft Teams and was recorded.

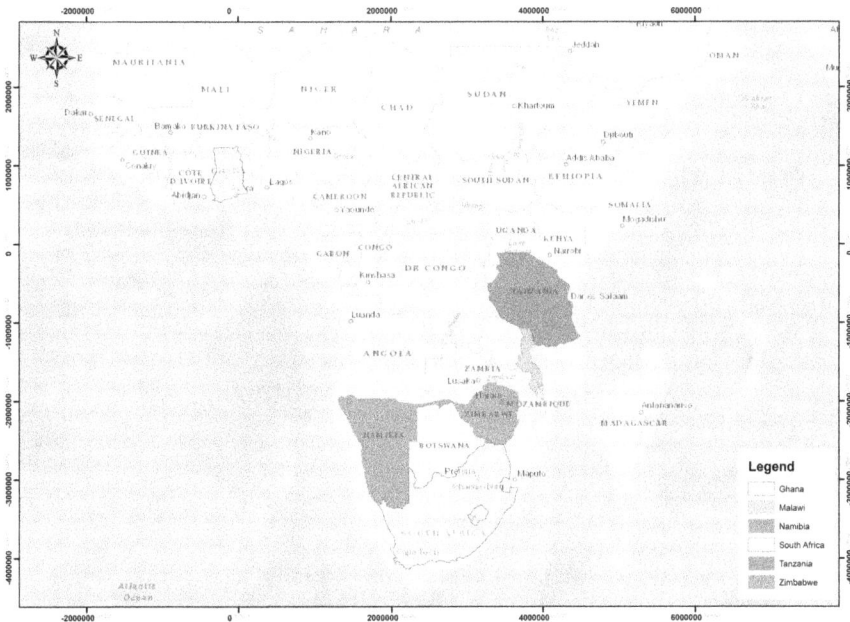

*Figure 20.1* Spatial distribution of focus group participants.

**Transcription and thematic analysis**

Two researchers transcribed the audio file using online Microsoft Word for accuracy. The data was analysed using Atlas.ti. The study adopted a thematic analysis approach. This is coding major themes and checking for consistency. To analyse the interview responses thematically, the procedures adopted include familiarisation with the data, developing initial codes, generating themes, reviewing the themes, and defining and naming the themes. This approach was coded using Atlas.ti. Coding the themes involved checking the assessment of the interviewees' feedback to the group and tagging the responses in line with the code to facilitate easy retrieval. The responses from the respondents of this study were coded in nodes (themes) by identifying patterns in them. From the data analysis, five themes were generated under the effects of the COVID-19 pandemic on construction, while seven were generated on measures to mitigate future shock events. These themes are discussed and supported by verbatim extracts from the data to highlight important issues.

## 4.0   Findings

*Profile of respondents*

Table 20.1 summarises the demographic details of the participants in the focus group discussion.

*Table 20.1* Demographic details of the focus group participants.

| Participants | Profession | Gender | Organisation | Position | Years of experience | Countries |
|---|---|---|---|---|---|---|
| **Participant 1** | Quantity Surveyor | Female | Academia | Lecturer | 5 | Malawi |
| **Participant 2** | Project Manager | Male | Construction | Director | 8 | South Africa |
| **Participant 3** | Civil Engineer | Female | Government | Chief Executive Officer | 13 | South Africa |
| **Participant 4** | Quantity Surveyor | Female | Construction | Quantity Surveyor | 5 | Tanzania |
| **Participant 5** | Quantity Surveyor | Male | Consulting | Quantity Surveyor | 6 | Ghana |
| **Participant 6** | Estate manager | Female | Consulting | Estate manager | 9 | Namibia |
| **Participant 7** | Architects | Female | Construction | Quantity Surveyor | 4 | South Africa |
| **Participant 8** | Project Manager | Male | Construction | Director | 20 | Zambia |
| **Participant 9** | Quantity Surveyor | Male | Construction | Director | 9 | South Africa |
| **Participant 10** | Civil Engineer | Male | Academia | Student | 3 | Zimbabwe |

## 5.0　Discussion

### 5.1　*Effect of the COVID-19 pandemic on construction*

The coronavirus, or COVID-19, severely impacted the nature of work in the built environment and productivity, and the effects are still reflected today. The built environment was not spared, as all sectors were severely impacted. The participants were asked to briefly describe the pandemic's effect on day-to-day operations as they experienced it (Sierra, 2022). All participants affirmed that the pandemic heavily impacted construction activities.

### 5.1.1　*Construction operations*

The response from participants from the six countries represented revealed that while some countries implemented total lockdown, there were no lockdowns in some, such as Tanzania. Thus, some construction activities in some countries were carried out, but they also felt the impact of the pandemic. However, a similar trend noticed based on discussion from the participants is that African countries experienced a lot of suspended or cancelled projects as budgets had to be reviewed. This is confirmed by Ogunnusi et al. (2022). A few examples of the responses are provided:

> In Malawi, some projects were still running in the private sector, but the rules were quite strict whereby masks were required and were quite expensive since the N95 masks were specified. Contractors, therefore, complained about the cost associated with providing COVID-compliant sanitation requirements. Checks were also routinely carried out by the government on construction workers to confirm masks were changed.
>
> (P7)

A similar trend also noticed from the feedback from the participants revealed that the cost of compliance with the new health and safety regulations on site was expensive, especially for small and medium construction companies. While some of the participants indicated that health and safety compliance was not stringent prior to COVID-19, regular inspections by the government during the pandemic used military officers in some cases, as opposed to government inspectors, to enforce their usage of the COVID-19 safety requirements.

> Due to a high rate of workers getting drunk on site, we started using breath analysers on projects. However, with COVID-19, breadth analysers had to be used per individual.
>
> (P9)

> Health and safety pricing was introduced to be covid compliant, but its cost also affected the overall project cost and resulted in several disputes.
>
> (P2)

Delayed schedules, extended project times, delayed supply of materials, and uncertainty led to an unprecedented increase in the claims from project stakeholders.

> Contractors claiming for stoppage time and the effect of screening time on the productivity of workers also affected the progress of work.
>
> (P7)

This is ascertained by Friston et al. (2020). The quality of the project was affected on several fronts. The participant indicated that in some countries, such as Ghana, testing of concrete strength is carried out in universities. However, due to the pandemic and lockdown, the tests could not be carried out, and thus the quality of materials could not be ascertained. Secondly, the participants mentioned they knew several colleagues and highly skilled workers who died because of the pandemic. This gap in expertise and shortage of skills is further compounded by the fact that the institutions of learning and training were closed, and the industry had lost considerable skills which could have been developed within this period. The consequential effect of this besides delayed projects is that the already dwindling skills level in the built environment is now more compounded. Also, specialists or subcontractors for foreign nations could not travel into the country and thus heavily delayed the project.

The lack of proactive capacity within the government to respond to shock events also resulted in different negative outcomes of the lockdown policy. A participant mentioned that:

> From a public works perspective, in South Africa, there were no clear guidelines to inform the industry . . . there should have been proactive thinking during the lockdown in terms of guidelines for operations to follow lockdown . . . . budgets were also revisited, and resources for projects yet to be commenced were redirected to finance intervention programs. The reallocation of resources had a greater impact as projects were removed from national plans. There was an increase in domestic violence from mental health thereby requiring temporal health facilities.
>
> (P3)

Turnaround time on decision-making and services provided by the government was also slow. COVID-19 revealed a lot of loopholes in government, and we saw we are not prepared and have no knowledge on responding to shock events. There was no coherence in decision-making between the levels of government, hence projects were heavily delayed, extended, and cancelled. Projects that had not been started were reclassified as non-emergency, and only the emergency ones remained. A participant expressed his situation as follows:

> The schedules had to be revised. . . . The COVID policy was done for all projects that were never previously considered . . . procurement of concrete

and steel was difficult like other materials, and prices were high when gotten. Reworks were high due to low quality of work.

(P9)

The participant discussed delays in information management, such as payment certificates, as one of the effects of the pandemic. This is confirmed by Ogunnusi et al. (2022). A participant indicated that:

Payments were delayed and therefore also delayed the projects. . . . In Tanzania, there was no lockdown, but construction processes were still affected, e.g., compensation could not be processed due to delays in the arrival of supplied materials from other countries. (P4)
Delayed approval of documents by municipalities deferred the progress of work and increased time and cost. In Zambia, there were similar experiences on COVID-19 impacts (p7)

The psychological effect of the pandemic is also underreported. In some countries, the military was brought in to enforce the lockdowns, and some participants mentioned the experiences left sour effects on their disposition to work.

In Ghana, the military was used to enforce COVID-19 regulations and compliance on the streets, and therefore artisans feared going to site for fear of being punished or battered. (P5)
Restrictions were slowly introduced, and the stricter the rules were, the more the workers felt threatened by the inability to work. (P7)

Aside from the uncertainty associated with the pandemic and its resulting psychological effect, workers were also mentally affected by the inability to work and the need to afford basic needs (Sierra, 2022; Maharaj et al., 2023).
Summarised effects highlighted by the participants include failed projects, increased project cost, the decline in quality of projects, loss of productivity, uncertainties, contractual disputes/conflict, slow/unclear decision-making, delayed project completion time, high increase in claims, increase in the cost of safety compliance, shortage of labour, declining expertise, delayed/non-payments, amongst others.

### 5.1.2   Academia/research

As mentioned by the participants, the pandemic's highlighted effects on the built environment were disrupted academic training, delayed academic calendar, inability to teach practical modules, disruption to the supply of needed upskilling, and inability to undertake site visits.
Impact on Academia: Human resources were constrained as training was halted because of the pandemic. Students also had to stay home as academic activities

were suspended, implying classes could not be held, and in more severe examples, practical courses could not be taught. However, much later, during the pandemic, platforms such as Zoom, Facebook, MS Teams, etc., were introduced to offer academic learning to students (Gambo and Musonda, 2022).

> In Nigeria, the move to online learning to curb the impact of the covid was not as effective due to the cost of internet subscription and epileptic power supply in most places across the country. Students missed or could not prepare for examinations.
>
> (P9)

> Additional cost for changing the nature of work from physical to online.
>
> (P10)

The inability to produce graduates and trainees, however, also indicates that the human resources needed to support the industry were impacted throughout the pandemic. Also, in some cases, the quality of work done could not be ascertained as testing centres were closed.

> In Ghana, testing of construction materials was halted as in some cities, it is only the universities which offer such services.
>
> (P8)

### 5.1.3  Supply chain

As identified, the effects on the supply chain include reallocation of budgets, supply chain disruptions, material shortages, and increased cost of materials and transportation costs. Some of the participants noted that:

> Stores were closed, and materials could not be sourced.
>
> (P2)

The construction industry supply chain is traditionally known for its hierarchical structure that tends to flow from the client to the main contractor, who then pays the project's subcontractors, who in turn pay their subcontractors. This can easily translate into cash flow problems for these entities (Al-Mhdawi et al., 2022). This meant alternative and new supply chain strategies had to be developed to ensure all parties got the end of the bargain. The pandemic saw new standards, procedures, and relationships being developed to ensure goods and services were delivered. Moreover, SMMEs were hardest hit as prices increased and the number of service providers was limited. Hence, supplier diversification should be investigated when certain supplies or services are crucial to a project and cannot be easily delivered by local providers (Zamani et al., 2022).

*5.1.4  Livelihood*

In terms of livelihood, the effects were loss of jobs, low wages and salaries, rene-gotiation of employment conditions, etc.

> Day-to-day operations were affected and impacted the livelihood of workers as those with high temperatures were only sent home since there were no standard hospitals around, especially in the remote areas.
>
> (P1)

In addition, COVID-19 has affected employment variables like pay, work hours, workload, stress levels, relationships with co-workers and employers, and avail-ability of paid time off, all of which can have a direct bearing on workers' physical and mental health, as well as that of their families and communities (Pamidimuk-kala and Kermanshachi, 2021). The COVID-19 pandemic also saw job restructur-ing. Jobs were igitalizin to igitali exposure by encouraging workers to work side by side rather than face to face and by arranging shifts to igitali worker contact. This meant salaries and employment conditions changed to ensure the safety of people (Onubi et al., 2022).

*5.1.5  Socio-cultural effects*

Misinformation bred fear, leading to distrust/suspicion and constrained workspaces on-site. Misinformation also played a central role in confusion as some of the workers either disbelieved the pandemic was real or felt it was a global conspiracy. A participant also expressed the following:

> In Zambia, it was a huge impact as some companies and contractors had to close down. (P7)
> In the rural areas, it was widely believed that COVID-19 only affected those from the urban areas and so people wearing masks were mistaken for those who had COVID not knowing they were trying to protect them-selves. (P1)
> In hot areas with a lot of heat, wearing the PPE and the masks became very difficult to work with. (P1)
> Temperature checks became difficult for those in hot environments. (P9)

Socio-cultural elements in a society are crucial to understanding the success or fail-ure of implementing preventive public health policies. To ensure that public health initiatives are feasible and acceptable, particular consideration must be given to cultural and community norms (Zakar et al., 2021). This meant educating people about the effects of the pandemic. Moreover, social media and the internet played a role in the misconceptions and educating people on the pandemic (Khan et al., 2021).

*Table 20.2* Effect of COVID-19 pandemic in the Built Environment.

| Categories | Effects |
| --- | --- |
| Construction Operations | Failed projects |
| | Increased project cost |
| | Decline in quality of projects |
| | Loss of productivity |
| | Uncertainties |
| | Contractual disputes/conflict |
| | Slow/unclear decision-making |
| | Delayed project completion time |
| | High increase in claims |
| | Increase in cost of safety compliance |
| | Shortage of labour |
| | Declining expertise |
| | Delayed/non-payments |
| Academia/Research | Disrupted academic training |
| | Delayed academic calendar |
| | Inability to teach practical modules |
| | Disruption to supply of needed upskilling |
| | Inability to undertake site visits |
| Supply Chain | Reallocation of budgets |
| | Supply chain disrupted |
| | Material shortages |
| | Increased cost of materials |
| | Increased transportation costs |
| Livelihood | Loss of jobs |
| | Low wages and salaries |
| Socio-cultural Effects | Misinformation bred fear |
| | Fear led to distrust/suspicion |
| | Constrained workspaces on-site |

### 5.2    Measures to mitigate future shock events impact on construction project performance

#### 5.2.1    Digital transformation

Optimisation of systems/processes using technology (BIM, Digital Twins, CDE, Human-robot teams) is an important measure to mitigate future shock events. The participants indicated adopting digital solutions as a solution to mitigating shock events and mentioned the need for public-private collaboration to make digital transition accessible and affordable (Makhathini et al., 2023).

> Technology was a challenge and offer solutions, but it is still challenged and needs development. (P1)
> … cost-effective platforms to be deployed across the board to influence easy usage (P1)
> In South Africa, the government's existing systems were not suited for the digital technologies migration that COVID-19 as the type of equipment in computers were old and not suited for emerging digital tools. (P5)

Robotics would be useful for areas with few expertise/human-resource/ highly risky areas. (P6)

We cannot run away from igitalizing if we are to achieve a resilient infra- structure delivery. (P1)

### 5.2.2 *Proactive government policy*

Develop action plans to mitigate shock events by formulating appropriate policies and budgetary provisions to anticipate and plan for future shock events (Kuldo- sheva, 2021). Previous studies such as Gambo and Musonda (2022) have attributed the level of challenge experienced during COVID-19 to a lack of proactive gov- ernment policies on managing shock events. Therefore, policymakers must enact important policies on proactively dealing with shock events. This will include how organisations and individuals respond to these shock events, resilient systems to be put in place, and the efficiency of these systems.

### 5.2.3 *Forms of contract/standards/contract guidelines*

A review of contract guidelines to address shock events is imperative as a mitiga- tion measure (Bushman et al., 2021). Participants opined that some of the contracts were unclear and couldn't address the pandemic challenges, while there is also a deficit in workers' knowledge of the contracts' standards stipulations.

In Zambia, COVID exposed some of the critical gaps in the form of contracts being used, and some clients accepted COVID claims while some didn't accept, despite using the same form of contract, thus needing a look at how the forms of contract are formulated hence requiring formulating a detailed response to COVID.

On some projects, entire risks were transferred to the contractors.

(P7)

Lots of contracts were modified to accommodate costs incurred. In the begin- ning, a letter was issued nationally to all contractors to say COVID claims should not be entertained, but along the way, this could not be substantiated . . . some of the claims end up in adjudication as they were inflated.

(P8)

### 5.2.4 *Capacity development*

Increased investment in upskilling professionals for digital adoption is vital to drive awareness, generate interest, and prepare professionals to engage in infrastructure delivery using enhanced systems/methods (Gill et al., 2019).

Reskilling intervention is a bigger scope in the drive towards digital trans- formation. (p4)

[B]usiness as usual shouldn't continue, but move towards innovation. (P3)

### 5.2.5   Improved information management/awareness

Enhanced information sharing/awareness can eliminate misinformation leading to distrust/suspicion (Abdullahi, 2019). This would lead to better data management for enhancing compliance. The participants highlighted enhanced information management as critical in how we respond to shock events and mentioned the low adoption of digitalised information management systems in the built environment and the challenges this poses.

### 5.2.6   Health and safety

Due to the pandemic, there has been an increase in technology adoption for health and safety preventive strategies to curb the spread on and off construction sites. Notable tools were used where sensors linked with employee profiles were introduced at construction sites for fever monitoring and social distance tracking (Yang et al., 2021; Alsharef et al., 2021; Bou et al., 2021). Such novel developments can be leveraged, extended, and enhanced for the construction health and safety monitoring.

### 5.2.7   Training/upskilling

The use of emerging innovations in the built environment to improve skills, capacity development, and expertise is critical to the future nature of work in the sector and in responding to shock events (Onososen and Musonda, 2022).

Other measures indicated by the participants are using digital approaches to learning and training for skills development. Virtual reality has recently been identified to undertake research and practical training such as virtual visits. Also, financial support from the government, feedback, and dialogue during future shock events can absorb risk. Regulations can anticipate and plan for future shock events, revision of force majeure clause documents, revision of contractual documents, close communication, and elaborate planning to identify future risks.

> Need to upskill project managers in line with global best practices on contract administration as against a subjective approach to doing things. (P1)
>
> Fill gaps in training programs and not a general module disposed to scratching the surface. (P3)

*Table 20.3* Measures to mitigate future shock events on project performance.

| Measures | Key action points |
| --- | --- |
| Digital Transformation | Optimisation of systems/processes using technology (BIM, Digital Twins, CDE, Human-robot teams) |
| Policy | Development of action plan for mitigation of shock events; increased budget for shock events |
| | Guidelines on turnaround time during shock events |

| Measures | Key action points |
|---|---|
| Standards/Contract Guidelines | Review of contract guidelines to address shock events |
| Capacity Development | Increased investment in 4iR technologies; upskilling professionals; raising awareness of digital transformation; increased investment in STEM programs |
| Improved Information Management/Awareness | Enhanced information sharing/awareness can eliminate misinformation leading to distrust/suspicion |
| Health and Safety | Digital approach to health and safety monitoring; appropriate communication of the need for compliance |
| Training/Upskilling | Digital learning in training programs |
| Government Support | Financial support |
|  | Feedback and dialogue during future shock events to absorb risk |
|  | Regulations to anticipate and plan for future shock events |
|  | Revised force majeure clause documents |
| Employee-Workers Relationship | Close communication |
|  | Plan for uncertainties/risk |
|  | Address welfare concerns |
| Risk Identification | Identify future risks |
|  | Develop mitigation plan |

## Conclusion and implications for practice and research

This study identifies the effect of the pandemic on the built environment and lessons for mitigating measures for future shock events. It revealed that digital transformation, policy, standards/contract guidelines, capacity development, improved information management/awareness, health & safety, training/upskilling, employee-workers relationship, and risk identification are vital to preparing the built environment to be a resilient and responsive sector. It is recommended that the government properly and adequately maintain any completed work and review suspended projects. The pandemic has demonstrated a new approach to infrastructure delivery is imperative as existing systems have been proven unreliable. However, the cost of novel technological applications to enhance infrastructure delivery must not be detrimental to people's socio-economic concerns. This must also be done in an integrated approach that ensures necessary contractual obligations, standards, and guidelines anticipate and consider future shock events, lessons learnt, and current realities.

## Acknowledgement

This research is funded and part of collaborative research at the Centre of Applied Research and Innovation in the Built Environment (CARINBE).

## References

Abdullahi, S. (2019, July). Adoption of building information modelling in small and medium-sized adoption of building information modelling in small and medium-sized enterprises in developing countries: A system dynamics approach.

Agyekum, K., Kukah, A.S., & Amudjie, J. (2022). The impact of COVID-19 on the construction industry in Ghana: The case of some selected firms. *Journal of Engineering, Design and Technology*, 20(1), 222–244.

Al-Mhdawi, M.K.S., Brito, M.P., Abdul Nabi, M., El-adaway, I.H., & Onggo, B.S. (2022). Capturing the impact of COVID-19 on construction projects in developing countries: A case study of Iraq. *Journal of Management in Engineering*, 38(1).

Alsharef, A., Banerjee, S., Uddin, S.M.J., Albert, A., & Jaselskis, E. (2021). Early impacts of the COVID-19 pandemic on the United States construction industry. *International Journal of Environmental Research and Public Health*, 18(4), 1559. https://doi.org/10.3390/ijerph18041559.

Amoah, C., & Simpeh, F. (2021). Implementation challenges of COVID-19 safety measures at construction sites in South Africa. *Journal of Facilities Management*, 19(1), 111–128. https://doi.org/10.1108/JFM-08-2020-0061.

Assaad, R., & El-adaway, I.H. (2021). Guidelines for responding to COVID-19 pandemic: Best practices, impacts, and future research directions. *Journal of Management in Engineering*, 37(3), 06021001.

Badamasi, A.A., Aryal, K.R., Makarfi, U.U., & Dodo, M. (2021). Drivers and barriers of virtual reality adoption in UK AEC industry. *Engineering, Construction and Architectural Management*, ahead-of-print (ahead-of-print).

Blake, H., Knight, H., Jia, R., Corner, J., Morling, J.R., Denning, C., Ball, J.K., Bolton, K., Figueredo, G., Morris, D.E., Tighe, P., Villalon, A.M., Ayling, K., & Vedhara, K. (2021). Students' views towards sars-Cov-2 mass asymptomatic testing, social distancing and self-isolation in a university setting during the COVID-19 pandemic: A qualitative study. *International Journal of Environmental Research and Public Health*, 18(8), 4182.

Bou Hatoum, M., Faisal, A., Nassereddine, H., & Sarvari, H. (2021). Analysis of COVID-19 concerns raised by the construction workforce and development of mitigation practices. *Frontiers in Built Environment*, 66.

Bushman, D., Sekaran, J., Jeffery, N., Rath, C., Ackelsberg, J., Weiss, D., Wu, W., Van Oss, K., Johnston, K., Huang, J., Khatun, U., Sheikh, T., Sutcliff, J., & Tsoi, B. (2021). Coronavirus disease 2019 (COVID-19) outbreaks at 2 construction sites: New York city, October–November 2020. *Clinical Infectious Diseases*, 73(Supplement_1), S81–S83. https://doi.org/10.1093/cid/ciab312.

Dahab, M., van Zandvoort, K., Flasche, S., Warsame, A., Ratnayake, R., Favas, C., Spiegel, P.B., Waldman, R.J., & Checchi, F. (2020). COVID-19 control in low-income settings and displaced populations: What can realistically be done? *Conflict and Health*, 14(1), 1–54. https://doi.org/10.1186/s13031-020-00296-8.

Dobrucali, E., Sadikoglu, E., Demirkesen, S., Zhang, C., & Tezel, A. (2022). Exploring the impact of COVID-19 on the United States construction industry: Challenges and opportunities. *IEEE Transactions on Engineering Management*, 1–13. https://doi.org/10.1109/TEM.2022.3155055.

Friston, K.J., Parr, T., Zeidman, P., Razi, A., Flandin, G., Daunizeau, J., Hulme, O.J., Billig, A.J., Litvak, V., Price, C.J., Moran, R.J., & Lambert, C. (2020). Second waves, social distancing, and the spread of COVID-19 across America. *Welcome Open Research*, 5, 103. https://doi.org/10.12688/wellcomeopenres.15986.1.

Gambo, N., & Musonda, I. (2022). Influences of social media learning environments on the learning process among AEC university students during COVID-19 pandemic: Moderating role of psychological capital. *Cogent Education*, 9(1). https://doi.org/10.1080/2331186X.2021.2023306.

Gbadamosi, A., Oyedele, L., Olawale, O., & Abioye, S. (2020). Offsite construction for emergencies: A focus on isolation space creation (ISC) measures for the COVID-19 pandemic. *Progress in Disaster Science*, 8, 100130. https://doi.org/10.1016/j.pdisas.2020.100130.

Gill, N., Musonda, I., & Stafford, A. (2019). *Duality by design: The global race to build Africa's infrastructure*. Cambridge: Cambridge University Press.

Khan, M.N., Ashraf, M.A., Seinen, D., Khan, K.U., & Laar, R.A. (2021). Social media for knowledge acquisition and dissemination: The impact of the COVID-19 pandemic on collaborative learning driven social media adoption. *Frontiers in Psychology*, 12.

Kukoyi, P.O., Simpeh, F., Adebowale, O.J., & Agumba, J.N. (2022). Managing the risk and challenges of COVID-19 on construction sites in Lagos, Nigeria. *Journal of Engineering, Design and Technology*, 20(1), 99–144. https://doi.org/10.1108/JEDT-01-2021-0058.

Kuldosheva, G. (2021). Challenges and opportunities of digital transformation in the public sector in transition economies: Examination of the case of Uzbekistan. In Adbi (Issue 1248).

Lidia Pinti, R.C., & Bonelli, S. (2022). A review of building information modelling (BIM) for facility management (FM): Implementation in public organisations. *Applied Sciences*, 12(3), 1540. https://doi.org/10.3390/app12031540.

Maharaj, R., Musonda, I., Onososen, A. (2023). Construction Organisation's Planning and Implementation: The Case Between Conceptualization and Implementation Teams. In Haupt, T.C., Akinlolu, M., Simpeh, F., Amoah, C., Armoed, Z. (Eds.), *Construction in 5D: Deconstruction, Digitalization, Disruption, Disaster, Development. Lecture Notes in Civil Engineering*, vol 245. Springer, Cham. https://doi.org/10.1007/978-3-030-97748-1_22.

Makhathini, N., Musonda, I., & Onososen, A. (2023). Utilisation of remote monitoring systems in construction project management. In Z. Haupt, T.C. Akinlolu, M. Simpeh, F. Amoah, & C. Armoed (Eds.), *Construction in 5D: Deconstruction, digitalization, disruption, disaster, development*. Springer. doi: 10.1007/978-3-030-97748-1_8.

Marco-Franco, J.E., Pita-Barros, P., Vivas-Orts, D., González-de-Julián, S., & Vivas-Consuelo, D. (2021). COVID-19, fake news, and vaccines: Should regulation be implemented? *International Journal of Environmental Research and Public Health*, 18(2), 744. https://doi.org/10.3390/ijerph18020744.

Ogunnusi, M., Omotayo, T., Hamma-Adama, M., Awuzie, B.O., & Egbelakin, T. (2022). Lessons learned from the impact of COVID-19 on the global construction industry. *Journal of Engineering, Design and Technology*, 20(1), 299–320. https://doi.org/10.1108/JEDT-05-2021-0286.

Olatunde, N.A., Awodele, I.A., & Adebayo, B.O. (2021). Impact of COVID-19 pandemic on indigenous contractors in a developing economy. *Journal of Engineering, Design and Technology*, 20(1), 267–280.

Onososen, A., & Musonda, I. (2022). Barriers to BIM-based life cycle sustainability assessment for buildings: An interpretive structural modelling approach. *Buildings*, 12(3), 324. https://doi.org/10.3390/buildings12030324.

Onubi, H.O., Hassan, A.S., Yusof, N., & Bahdad, A.A.S. (2022). Moderating effect of project size on the relationship between COVID-19 safety protocols and economic performance of construction projects. *Engineering, Construction and Architectural Management*, ahead-of-print (ahead-of-print).

Osman, I., & Ataei, H. (2022). Studying construction claims due to COVID-19 for road and highway projects. *Journal of Legal Affairs and Dispute Resolution in Engineering and Construction*, 14(1).

Pamidimukkala, A., & Kermanshachi, S. (2021). Impact of Covid-19 on field and office workforce in construction industry. *Project Leadership and Society*, 2, 100018.

Ramírez-Montoya, M.S., Loaiza-Aguirre, M.I., Zúñiga-Ojeda, A., & Portuguez-Castro, M. (2021). Characterization of the teaching profile within the framework of education 4.0. *Future Internet*, 13(4), 91.

Raoufi, M., & Fayek, A.R. (2020). Identifying actions to control and mitigate the effects of the COVID-19 pandemic on construction organizations: Preliminary findings. *Public Works Management & Policy*, 26(1), 1087724X2096916.

Rokooei, S., Alvanchi, A., & Rahimi, M. (2022). Perception of COVID-19 impacts on the construction industry over time. *Cogent Engineering*, 9(1).

Roziqin, A., Mas'udi, S.Y.F., & Sihidi, I.T. (2021). An analysis of Indonesian government policies against COVID-19. *Public Administration and Policy*, 24(1), 92–107. https://doi.org/10.1108/PAP-08-2020-0039.

Sierra, F. (2022). COVID-19: Main challenges during construction stage. *Engineering, Construction, and Architectural Management*, 29(4), 1817–1834. https://doi.org/10.1108/ECAM-09-2020-0719.

Sy, M., O'Leary, N., Nagraj, S., El-Awaisi, A., O'Carroll, V., & Xyrichis, A. (2020). Doing interprofessional research in the COVID-19 era: A discussion paper. *Journal of Interprofessional Care*, 34(5), 600–606.

Takashima, R., Onishi, R., Saeki, K., & Hirano, M. (2020). Perception of COVID-19 restrictions on daily life among Japanese older adults: A qualitative focus group study. *Healthcare*, 8(4), 450.

Wang, Z., Liu, Z., & Liu, J. (2020). Risk identification and responses of tunnel construction management during the COVID-19 pandemic. *Advances in Civil Engineering*. https://doi.org/10.1155/2020/6620539.

Yang, Y., Chan, A.P., Shan, M., Gao, R., Bao, F., Lyu, S., . . . Guan, J. (2021). Opportunities and challenges for construction health and safety technologies under the COVID-19 pandemic in Chinese construction projects. *International Journal of Environmental Research and Public Health*, 18(24), 13038.

Zakar, R., Yousaf, F., Zakar, M.Z., & Fischer, F. (2021). Socio-cultural challenges in the implementation of COVID-19 public health measures: Results from a qualitative study in Punjab, Pakistan. *Frontiers in Public Health*, 9.

Zamani, S.H., Rahman, R.A., Fauzi, M.A., & Mohamed Yusof, L. (2022). Government pandemic response strategies for AEC enterprises: Lessons from COVID-19. *Journal of Engineering, Design and Technology*, Vol. ahead-of-print No. ahead-of-print. http://dx.doi.org/10.1108/JEDT-10-2021-0540.

# 21 Implication of COVID-19 SOP compliance to project-based construction workers in Malaysia

*Siti Rashidah Mohd Nasir*
*and Che Khairil Izam Che Ibrahim*

## Introduction

When the World Health Organization (WHO) declared the COVID-19 outbreak a pandemic in March 2020 (WHO, 2021), Malaysia was no exception, as it first hit Malaysia in January 2020. The increasing number of positive cases each day has made Malaysia among the highest numbers of positive COVID-19 cases in Southeast Asia. When the positive cases exceeded 553 incidents on 16 March 2020, the Malaysian government issued the first Movement Control Order (MCO) nationwide, intending to curb the spreading of the virus. Subsequently, various Standard Operating Procedures (SOP) were introduced, including MCO, MCO2, MCO3, EMCO, RMCO, CMCO, and TMCO. During the period of MCO, the Malaysian government ordered to close and lockdown all premises, including government and private sector, disrupting all types of businesses with no exception to the construction industry. Many countries have classified the construction industry as a highly affected sector because most of the ongoing projects were suspended or postponed due to the spread of the virus among construction workers. The national lockdown has resulted in operating at a lower productivity level, disruptions in supply chains (e.g., labour, materials, and equipment), and financial difficulty in continued funding of the projects (Assaad and El-adaway, 2021; Raoufi and Fayek, 2020). In addition, it has caused project delays and cost overruns (Alsharef et al., 2021).

According to Zamani et al. (2021), during MCO, construction projects were experiencing project interruption and suspension due to a lack of supplies, transportation, and labours. However, essential economic sectors were only allowed to operate under the third phase of the MCO but with strict SOP compliance. The National Security Council (NSC) and the Ministry of Health (MoH) established a new SOP with strict safety measures and monitoring procedures (Ministry of Health Malaysia, 2020). As for the construction industry, only critical activities and projects are allowed to operate, and a team of enforcement conducts duty checks for SOP compliance from time to time (Gara et al., 2022). A study conducted by the Construction Industry Development Board (CIDB) from April 2020 to December 2021 on 8,004 construction sites across Malaysia revealed that only 79 or about 1% of construction sites were

DOI: 10.1201/9781003278368-24

yet to begin operations (The Sun, 2020). Among the reasons for construction sites being unable to be fully operated is due to unavailability of workers, materials, capital, and concerns of infection risk. CIDB also stated that construction projects awarded had fallen 42% to RM55.3 billion for the period of January to October 2020, compared with RM94.6 billion in the same period the year before (The Sun, 2020).

Most existing studies have established the effect of COVID-19 and SOP challenges faced by construction practitioners. However, there is a need for further studies to explore the root cause of the problem, which can offer valuable insights into the causes, particularly within developing countries such as Malaysia. Thus, this chapter aims to extend this line of work by answering the question: who was affected the most in continuing site work during the pandemic? How does the SOP affect the performance of the project? The objectives of this chapter include (1) presenting a concise project incident in Malaysia during the pandemic related to SOP compliance; (2) establishing the subthemes and key themes of the incidents; and (3) discussing the effect of project performance in complying to SOP that could help the construction industry be more prepared for the transition toward the new normal and to ensure a smoother and better recovery from the pandemic related to health and safety of construction site workforce.

This section discusses the impact of the COVID-19 pandemic on construction projects within the context of project performance (cost and schedule) and compliance with the SOP by the site workforce.

### Cost performance

Gamil and Alhagar's (2020) studies revealed that the impacts of COVID-19 include the suspension of projects, time overrun, cost overrun, and financial impact. In addition, Wang et al. (2020) identified the impacts of COVID-19 on tunnel construction projects related to schedule delays and cost overruns. A study by Alsharef (2021) mentioned that contractors and subcontractors had faced substantial cash flow problems, failing to meet payment obligations. The series of MCO has contributed to a significant delay in most projects in Malaysia. Malaysia recorded a significant drop of 44.9% in the value of construction work done in the second quarter of 2020 (DOSM, 2020), resulting in a reduction of labour productivity per employee by 16% in that period (DOSM, 2020). Malaysia's construction industry contributes significantly to Malaysia's economic growth, with an annual total return of RM140 billion in construction projects (CIDB, 2020a, 2020b), making it a catalyst for Malaysia's GDP.

### Schedule performance

The COVID-19 pandemic has disrupted major construction activities, leading to project delays and cost overruns (Zamani et al., 2021). These delays consequently cause projects to deviate from their original scheduled completion stated in the contracts due to lockdowns and social distancing rules at construction sites (Alenezi, 2020). Construction projects faced slow progress owing to COVID-19 difficulties, and the project was further delayed if a significant number of construction workers tested positive for COVID-19 (Alsharef et al., 2021). In addition, construction projects idled down due to lockdowns, shortage of workforce, as well as deferred material delivery (Abdussalam et al., 2020). According to Gamil and Alhagar (2020), time overruns in building projects are linked to the government's movement control and prevention efforts. Alsharef et al. (2021) study the early impact of COVID-19 on the US construction industry, leading to project delays. Esa et al. (2020) stated that MCO enforcement has resulted in a delay in project delivery to the client, which has been linked to many issues, including a postponement in the raw materials and products supplies due to suspending the operation of the manufacturing sector. In addition, the issues of transportation and logistics restrictions due to the MCO period's border closures of states and regions. Delivering engineering deliverables was also related to the absence of key personnel due to COVID-19 difficulties (Jallow et al., 2020).

*Safety, health, and well-being of construction workers-related issues*

According to the International Labour Organization (ILO), the COVID-19 epidemic has affected around 2.7 billion workforces worldwide, accounting for 71% of global employment losses. In 2020, global unemployment increased by 33 million jobs (ILO, 2021). With the new SOP in place, working during the pandemic becomes more difficult for construction workers; for example, maintaining physical separation in construction workplaces, including sites, offices, and dorm rooms. In addition, the enforcement of SOP affects site workers, with mental health issues such as anxiety, exhaustion, and stress linked to the staff's misunderstanding of SOP compliance, resulting in a decrease in labour productivity (Tan and Abdul-Samad, 2022). These movement restrictions imposed as a pandemic-prevention tactic significantly impacted the planning and scheduling of construction projects (Bodenstein et al., 2020; CIDB, 2020a, 2020b).

## Research methods

The research adopts an inductive (i.e., bottom-up) perspective to identify critical incidents related to workers' issues faced by construction practitioners. Furthermore, it examines the corrective action taken in compliance with Standard Operating Procedures (SOP) for the construction workers' safety, health, and well-being during the COVID-19 pandemic. Accordingly, the research follows specific steps to identify those critical incidents and corrective actions, studies participants, collects data through interviews, and performs a thematic analysis.

*Study participants*

The primary data source for this study was 25 construction practitioners who routinely performed their work directly and indirectly on construction projects in 2021. They are from three different construction practitioners: contractors, consultants, and owners. Targeted subject matter experts were emailed the interview questions and requested to participate in the research. After each interview, transcripts were prepared for analysis. Interview eligibility also included the following criteria: (1) voluntarily willing to be interviewed, (2) handling the construction site in 2020, and (3) currently working as project manager (PM), project engineer (PE), site manager (SM), general manager (GM) and project director (PD). The 25 respondents (18 male and 7 female) interviewed consisted of 4 PEs, 17 PMs, 2 SMs, 1 GM, and 1 PD. Of the 25 respondents, 8% had less than five years of construction industry experience, 44% had 6–10 years of construction industry experience, 36% had 11–15 years of construction industry experience, 8% had 16–20 years of construction industry experience, and 8% had more than 21 years of construction industry experience. All participants were engaged in various building and infrastructure projects throughout Peninsular Malaysia, Sabah, and Sarawak.

*Data collection*

Data collection began using the semi-structured interview model of the incidents faced by the project personnel during the pandemic and corrective actions taken to overcome the poor project performance. The interviewer asked questions specific to the incident (e.g., Can you identify the incidents that led up to the project performance? What are the incidents that relate to the workers? Who was involved in the incident? Did you attempt to take corrective action after the incident? If so, what did you do? What was the outcome of the corrective action? Did anything change as a result of the corrective action?). All semi-structured interviews were held online using Google Meet or Zoom according to the interviewee's preference. Each interview lasted approximately 45 minutes to 1 hour. All interviews were digitally recorded, transcribed, and uploaded to ATLAS.ti 9 qualitative analysis software.

*Data analysis*

The interview notes were analysed using the thematic analysis procedure described by Braun and Clarke (2006). First, the interview notes for each group of cases were carefully reviewed to identify coded statements representing the most basic elements of the data that respect the note's context and could still be assessed in a meaningful way. Second, coded statements dealing with similar issues were grouped into preliminary categories and given temporary names. Coded statements found in project incidents and corrective actions during the COVID-19 pandemic could be included in separate categories based on the context surrounding the statement. These preliminary categories were then refined into conceptually distinct subthemes and given descriptive names. In creating these subthemes, the constructionist perspective was adopted as an inductive rather than deductive approach. Its purpose is to explain the context and conditions that enable the respondents' accounts of their projects. Lastly, the subthemes from the incidents and corrective actions were combined into broader key themes that represent the most incidents that occurred in projects related to safety, health, and well-being of the site workers during the COVID-19 pandemic.

## Results

A total of 16 coded statements for incidents related to workers at the site were derived from the interview notes; the frequency of coded statements and their prevalence for project incidents related to workers' issues are summarised in Table 21.1. The most common coded statement across the project incidents was "difficult performing site activities due to strict SOP" [1]. The coded statements were grouped by similarity, suggesting seven subthemes for the project incidents: (a) shortage of workers, (b) workers' utilities and test kit, (c) poor management during MCO, (d) working hour restriction at the site, (e) vaccination and quarantine, (f) safety awareness, and (g) SOP compliance. Table 21.2 shows the summary of these subthemes and examples from the interviewee associated with the coded statements.

*Table 21.1* Prevalence for project incidents related to workers' issues during the COVID-19 pandemic.

| Coded statements | Prevalence |
| --- | --- |
| [1] difficult in performing site activities due to strict SOP | 23 (92%) |
| [2] an additional cost of SOP compliance at the construction site | 21 (84%) |
| [3] lack of management skill | 20 (80%) |
| [4] lack of communication among project team members | 19 (76%) |
| [5] increase in-site workers' expenses (food and accommodation) | 18 (72%) |
| [6] delay to resume work due to documentation and approvals | 18 (72%) |
| [7] limited numbers of workers allowed at the site | 17 (68%) |
| [8] quarantine for staff and workers infected by COVID-19 | 16 (64%) |
| [9] vaccinated workers are only allowed to work at the site | 15 (60%) |
| [10] negligence and ignorance of SOP by site workers | 12 (48%) |
| [11] lack of SOP supervision at the site | 11 (44%) |
| [12] lack of safety measures, i.e., face mask, hand sanitiser, and body scan temperature | 10 (40%) |
| [13] burnout among workers | 8 (32%) |
| [14] confined space for site workers | 8 (32%) |
| [15] increase in workers' wages | 6 (24%) |
| [16] increase in workers' workloads | 5 (20%) |

*Note:* The percentage of total responses ($n = 25$) is given in parentheses

*Table 21.2* Summary of subthemes for site incidents related to workers' issues during the COVID-19 pandemic.

| Sub Theme | Codes statement | Examples of context by Interviewees |
|---|---|---|
| Shortage of Workers | [16] increase in workers' workloads | Some of the workers were required to work a double shift and a different work scope at the site (R1) |
| | [15] increase in workers' wages | Due to the shortage and additional workload, skilled workers took this as an opportunity to demand an increase in wages (R3 and R6) |
| Workers' Utilities and Test Kit | [5] increase in-site workers' expenses (food and accommodation) | The contractor has to look after the welfare of the foreign site workers because they were unable to return to their countries during MCO by providing them with food daily since most of the restaurants and food stalls were prohibited from operating in adhering to the NSC requirement (R3, R4, R12, and R14) |
| | [2] the additional cost of SOP compliance at the construction site | The contractor must provide comfortable and safe accommodation at the site using a Centralised Labour Quarter (CLQ) with basic facilities such as rooms, toilets, and other facilities that cost about RM30 thousand to RM40 thousand (R4) |
| Poor Management during MCO | [4] lack of communication among project team members | Much misleading information was received between the project team and other parties, which led to some work being postponed due to unclear instructions (R1, R5, R9, R14, R21, R22, R24, R25, and R14) |
| | [6] delay to resume work due to documentation and approvals | The contractor is required to conduct a site inspection and update related documents in seeking permission from the Ministry of International Trade and Industry (MITI) to resume site operation (R3 and R4) |
| | [3] lack of management skill | The contractor with lack of knowledge and poor management skill has resulted in work delays at the site (5) |
| | [11] lack of SOP supervision at the site | It was difficult for the site supervisor to ensure the allowable number of workers at the site (not more than 60%) and that workers were practising social distancing at all times (R9) |
| Working Hour Restriction at Site | [7] limited numbers of workers allowed at the site | The strict SOP limits 60% of the number of workers at the site at all times (R1, R2, R3, R4, R8, R9, R12, R15, and R22) |
| | [13] burnout among site workers | Due to the high workload, most of the workers were suffering from job burnout (R15) |
| Vaccination and Quarantine | [9] vaccinated workers are only allowed to work at the site | 60% of workers allowed to work at the site must be fully vaccinated (2 doses) and passed health screening (swab test and body temperature) before entering the site {R1 and R4) |
| | [8] quarantine for staff and workers infected by COVID-19 | Some of the workers were quarantined due to the infection of the virus, and all affected areas were sanitised, causing a delay to project progress (R10) |

| Sub Theme | Codes statement | Examples of context by Interviewees |
|---|---|---|
| Safety Awareness | [12] lack of safety measures, i.e., face mask and face shield | The workers were also often found to remove their face masks and face shields because of discomfort due to profuse sweat as a reaction to hot weather (R1) |
| | [10] negligence and ignorance of SOP by site workers | Attitude problems also contributed to the negligence and ignorance of the SOP. For example, the workers frequently argued with the contractor to perform swab tests, wear a face mask, and other SOP requirements (R21) |
| SOP Compliance | [14] confined space for site workers | Some work areas are in confined space, and the worker has to work with several workers to get the work done (R17) |
| | [1] difficult in performing site activities due to strict SOP | The contractor is to ensure workers comply with the SOP at all times, i.e., wear a face mask, perform swab tests, register to MySejahtera apps daily, and social distancing (R7, R10, R15, and R25) |

## Key themes and discussion

A set of three key themes were established that represent the main incidents faced by construction practitioners in coping with SOP compliance of COVID-19: (1) Cost Performance, (2) Schedule Performance, and (3) Health-Related Issues. Table 21.3 shows a summary of the key themes and their associated subthemes.

### *Theme 1: cost performance*

The first key theme that represents the most prevalent incidents at the site is related to cost performance. Most respondents agreed that the shortage of workers is the key issue that led to project cost performance. Kim et al. (2020) agreed that labour shortage is a serious issue because it increases labour wages, causing cost and schedule overruns in construction projects. The main cause of the shortage of workers is the lockdown measures, whether temporary or permanent, such as laying off some of the workers (Tan and Zainon, 2022) to sustain the project due to late payment from the project owner. Another cause of the reduction in the workforce is travel restrictions to curb the disease within its geographical location (The Sun, 2020). Malaysian governments had decided to close international borders and discourage intercity travels, which led to foreign workers' displacement. Several respondents agreed that most of the main contractors sourced workers through labour subcontractors. During the pandemic, these subcontractors could not supply the number of workers as agreed at the initial stage of the project. In addition, Ling et al. (2022) stated that the supply of migrant construction workers was insufficient to meet the demand on-site, and the cost of workers had increased. The cost of workers' utilities and test kits also affected the project cost. This extra cost, which was not part of the contract sum, has caused the contractor poor cash flow. As a result, conflicts,

*Table 21.3* Key themes for site incidents related to workers' issues during the COVID-19 pandemic.

| Theme | Sub Theme |
| --- | --- |
| Theme 1: Cost Performance | (a)  Shortage of Workers |
|  | (b)  Workers' Utilities and Test Kit |
| Theme 2: Schedule Performance | (c)  Poor Management During MCO |
|  | (d)  Working Hour Restriction at Site |
|  | (e)  Vaccination and Quarantine |
| Theme 3: Health-Related Issues | (f)  Safety Awareness |
|  | (g)  SOP Compliance |

claims, and disputes that account for substantial cost and schedule overruns were expected among the construction practitioners as construction organisations rely heavily on financial leverage for their performance to ensure their cash flows and financial stability (Alsharef et al., 2021).

### Theme 2: schedule performance

Even before the pandemic, the construction industry has been constantly faced with delay issues. Enforcing stricter on-site SOP due to COVID-19 worsened the issue (Ogunnusi et al., 2021).

The Malaysian government has instructed work hour restrictions and a limited number of workers allowed at the site to minimise the virus's spread. As a result, the project's progress was delayed, and the contractor could not deliver the project as scheduled. Almost half of the projects were expected to take 40% more time to complete than initially planned (Ling et al., 2022). The restricted working hours and the number of workers allowed at the site have somewhat reduced the productivity rate in a project's progress. This finding is consistent with Alsharef et al. (2021) and Esa et al. (2020) studies on the COVID-19 protocols, which has resulted in a significant drop in production. In addition to the strict SOP, work permits from the local authorities and MITI also contributed to the delay. Tan and Zainon's (2022) study confirmed that difficulty in obtaining permits and planning permissions during the pandemic is another reason for delays. Some authorities were not prepared for remote working and thus could not process the permit applications (Tan and Zainon, 2022). Communication issues among construction practitioners and site workers were also highlighted in this study. Jallow et al. (2020) confirmed that online communication and visualisation aids are not as effective as seeing the actual situation on-site. As a result, it was challenging to resolve project issues, which thus impeded the work progress. Jallow et al. (2020) also mentioned that a lack of communication among project teams leads to disagreements, resulting in project delays. The respondents also highlight that most contractors had applied for an Extension of Time (EoT) related to the force majeure clause and depended on the project owner to accept it as an excusable delay or impose them with liquidated damages for breaching the contract. Liquidated damages clauses are one of the most common legal and contractual causes of disputes in the construction industry (Assaad and El-adaway, 2021).

*Theme 3: safety and health-related issues*

The safe management measures practised at the site have an adverse effect on project progress due to the lower productivity. The contractor had to comply with the new regulation of SOP and get approval from the authorities to resume work. The SOP includes reducing physical interaction, practising social distance, implementing contact tracing by performing digital check-in and check-out using MySejahtera apps, implementing body scan temperature, maintaining regular sanitisation of the workplace, providing proper accommodation, and establishing a detailed monitoring plan to ensure the SOP compliance. Similar safety measures have also been practised in other countries (Assaad and El-adaway, 2021). Most interviewees agreed that the SOP had impacted the work progress, and this finding is consistent with that of Simpeh and Amoah (2021), who found that these measures are not easy to fulfil and are challenging to comply with. Ghandour (2020), in his studies, mentioned that in construction projects, remote working was unable to be practised and thus confronted several challenges that prevent on-time delivery. In Malaysia, the CIDB enforcement team regularly checks SOP compliance at the site and works to be forced to stop if it is in nonconformance (CIDB, 2022). Similar findings by Tan and Zainon (2022) stated that construction work must stop with penalties and fines for non-compliance. Construction work value for the Malaysian construction industry in Q2 2020 was recorded at the lowest of −44.9% due to the pandemic (DOSM, 2020). The interview findings revealed that the reduction was caused by MCO lockdown, shortage of workers, and SOP compliance, consistent with those identified by Ling et al. (2022).

## Research implications

The findings suggested that contractors faced the most incidents compared to the consultant and the project owner. As a result, contractors played a significant role in making the SOP compliance successful during the pandemic; for example, obtaining permits and approval from the local authorities to resume work starts with the contractor. Furthermore, the documentation for approval consumes considerable time due to the preparation in developing detailed safety measures according to the SOP, followed by the monitoring activities as a requirement for the permit's approval. In addition, these key themes set the root causes of poor project performance that can assist contractors in seeking solutions to problems they were facing, which include worker shortages, supply chain disruptions, project delays, and higher costs associated with project prolongation. As for the project owner, knowing the root causes of project delays would enable them to make a better decision regarding force majeure clauses. Using these clauses allows contractors to obtain an extension of time and a fair decision in exercising liquidated damages clauses, potentially driving contractor organisations to file for bankruptcy (Assaad and El-adaway, 2021). In continuation to this study, future research will study response action and its guidelines for the construction industry on the different short-term and long-term considerations to cope with the new way of doing the project activities. Furthermore, a topic will be conducted on the consequences of adopting post-pandemic-generation changes and incorporating new technologies.

## Conclusions

This study, which involves 25 construction practitioners with various backgrounds and projects, reveals that the COVID-19 pandemic worsened project performance due to the lockdown and actions taken in compliance with the SOP. The government enforced the SOP on the project practitioner to curb the spreading of the virus, thus creating many issues in the project, especially related to site workers. This research developed three key themes from studying a sample of the incidents at various project sites during the pandemic: (1) Cost Performance, (2) Schedule Performance, and (3) Safety and Health Related Issues. These key themes and their related subthemes represent in detail the issues related to site workers for SOP compliance, contributing to the literature relating to the effect on the project performance in the construction industry during the COVID-19 pandemic era. Future research opportunities exist to empirically validate these themes with practical response actions across a broader range of project contexts.

## Acknowledgement

This research was supported by Universiti Teknologi MARA under MyRA research grant [600-RMC/GPM ST 5/3 (047/2021)]

## References

Abdussalam, S., Dyaa, H., & Nehal, S. (2020). The effects of pandemic on construction industry in the UK. *Mediterranean Journal of Social Science*, 11, 48–60.

Alenezi, N.A.T. (2020). The impact of COVID-19 on construction projects in Kuwait. *International Journal of Engineering Research and General Science*, 8(4), 6–9.

Alsharef, A., Banerjee, S., Uddin, S.M., Albert, A., & Jaselskis, E. (2021). Early impacts of the COVID-19 pandemic on the United States construction industry. *International Journal of Environmental Research and Public Health*, 18, 1559.

Assaad, R., & El-Adaway, I.H. (2021). Guidelines for responding to COVID-19 pandemic: Best practices, impacts, and future research directions. *Journal of Management in Engineering*, 37(3).

Bodenstein, M., Corsetti, G., & Guerrieri, L. (2020). Social distancing and supply disruptions in a pandemic. *Finance and Economics Discussion Series*. doi: 10.17016/FEDS.2020.031.

Braun, V., & Clarke, V. (2006). Using thematic analysis in psychology. *Qualitative Research in Psychology*, 3(2), 77–101. doi: 10.1191/1478088706qp063oa.

CIDB. (2022). *NRP-permission to operate*. Available at www.cidb.gov.my/en/mco-permission-operate.

Construction Industry Development Board. (2020a). Embracing construction revolution. *CIDB Heights*, 3, 8–12.

Construction Industry Development Board. (2020b). Leadership in the time of pandemic. *CIDB Heights*, 2, 9–17.

Department of Statistics Malaysia. (2020). *Quarterly construction statistics: Second quarter 2020*. Available at www.dosm.gov.my/v1/index.php?r=column/cthemeByCat&cat=77&bul_id=TWxzVlA3L2lkYksxOWpjS3d6c3hHQT09&menu_id=OEY5SWtFSVVFVUpmUXEyaHppMVhEdz09 (Accessed 15 June 2022).

Esa, M.B., Ibrahim, F.S.B., & Kamal, E.B.M. (2020). Covid-19 pandemic lockdown: The consequences towards project success in Malaysian construction industry. *Advances in Science, Technology and Engineering Systems Journal*, 5(5), 973–983.

Gamil, Y., & Alhagar, A. (2020). The impact of pandemic crisis on the survival of construction industry: A case of COVID-19. *Mediterranean Journal of Social Sciences*, 11(4), 122–128. doi: 10.36941/mjss-2020–0047.

Gara, J.A., Zakaria, R., Aminudin, E., Yahya, K., Sam, A.R.M., Loganathan, R., Munikanan, V., Yahya, M.A., Wahi, N., & Shamsuddin, S.M. (2022). Effects of the COVID-19 pandemic on construction work progress: An on-site analysis from the Sarawak Construction Project, Malaysia. *Sustainability*, 14, 6007.

Ghandour, A. (2020). The impact of COVID-19 on project delivery: A perspective from the construction sector in the United Arab Emirates. *Humanities and Social Sciences Reviews*, 8(5). doi: 10.18510/hssr.2020.8516.

International Labor Organization. (2021). *Impact of COVID-19 on the construction sector*. Available at www.ilo.org/sector/Resources/publications/WCMS_767303/lang-en/index.htm (Accessed 15 June 2022).

Jallow, H., Renukappa, S., & Suresh, S. (2020). The impact of Covid-19 outbreak on United Kingdom infrastructure sector. *Smart and Sustainable Built Environment*, 10(4). doi: 10.1108/SASBE-05–2020–0068.

Kim, S., Chang, S., & Castro-Lacouture, D. (2020). Dynamic modelling for analysing impacts of skilled labor shortage on construction project management. *Journal of Management in Engineering*, 36, 04019035. https://doi.org/10.1061/(ASCE)ME.1943-5479.0000720.

Ling, F.Y.Y., Zhang, Z., & Yew, A.Y.R. (2022). Impact of COVID-19 pandemic on demand, output, and outcomes of construction projects in Singapore. *J. Manag. Eng.*, 38(2), 04021097(1–12). https://doi.org/10.1061/(ASCE)ME.1943–5479.0001020.

Ministry of Health Malaysia. (2020). *COVID-19: Social distancing guidelines for workplace, homes and individuals*. Available at http://covid-19.moh.gov.my/garis-panduan/garis-panduan-kkm/Annex_26_COVID_guide_for_Social_Distancing_24032020.pdf (Accessed 15 March 2022).

Ogunnusi, M., Omotayo, T., Hamma-Adama, M., Awuzie, B.O., & Egbelakin, T. (2021). Lessons learned from the impact of COVID-19 on the global construction industry. *Journal of Engineering, Design and Technology*, 20(1), 299–320. https://doi.org/10.1108/JEDT-05-2021-0286.

Raoufi, M., & Fayek, A.R. (2020). Identifying actions to control and mitigate the effects of the COVID-19 pandemic on construction organisations: Preliminary findings. *Public Works Manage. Policy*, 26(1), 1–9. https://doi.org/10.1177/1087724X20969164.

Simpeh, F., & Amoah, C. (2021). Assessment of measures instituted to curb the spread of COVID-19 on construction site. *International Journal of Construction Management*, 1–9.

The Sun. (2020). COVID-19 pandemic leaves lasting scar on Malaysian construction sector. Available at www.thesundaily.my/business/covid-19-pandemic-leaves-lasting-scar-on-malaysian-construction-sector-FL5782315 (Accessed 15 June 2022).

Tan, C.K.L., & Abdul-Samad, Z. (2022). A study of the impact of COVID-19 on construction workforce productivity in Malaysia. *International Journal of Productivity and Performance Management*. https://doi.org/10.1108/IJPPM-07-2021-0421.

Tan, S.Y., & Zainon, N. (2022). Impact of COVID-19 pandemic on the quantity surveying practices in Malaysia. *Engineering, Construction and Architectural Management*. https://doi.org/10.1108/ECAM-11–2021–0988.

Wang, Z., Liu, Z., & Liu, J. (2020). Risk identification and responses of tunnel construction management during the COVID-19 pandemic. *Advances in Civil Engineering*. Article ID: 6620539. https://doi.org/10.1155/2020/6620539.

WHO (World Health Organization). (2021). *WHO coronavirus (COVID-19) dashboard*. Available at https://covid19.who.int/ (Accessed 15 June 2022).

Zamani, S.H., Rahman, R.A., & Fauzi, M.A., & Yusof, L.M. (2021). Effect of COVID-19 on building construction projects: Impact and response mechanisms. Proceedings of the 4th National Conference on Wind & Earthquake Engineering, Putrajaya, Malaysia, 16–17 October 2020; *IOP Conference Series: Earth and Environmental Science Effect of COVID-19 on Building Construction Projects: Impact and Response Mechanisms* (Vol. 682, pp. 012049).

# 22 Facing the impacts of COVID-19 in construction

## The case of Chile

*Alfredo Serpell*

## Introduction

Starting in 2019, the world has been affected by the outbreak of a pandemic known as COVID-19. This pandemic has not only affected the health of people, but also the health of companies and organizations, including the construction industry (Ogunnusi et al., 2020). The COVID-19 crisis has produced different effects on world economies and the economic impacts have been significant, so many companies have had to find their way to understand, react, and learn lessons from this event (Reeves et al., 2020). Daily operational challenges due to social distancing, remote work requirements, absenteeism, as well as supply shortages and unplanned disruption to global supply chains, were part of these impacts (PWC, 2020).

The COVID-19 pandemic has significantly affected the construction sector, which, being an activity that is intensive in the use of labor and carried out directly on the ground, has had to face conditions that have restricted its operational capacity and continuity.

This chapter presents a description of the effects that the COVID-19 pandemic had on the Chilean construction industry in various aspects and how these effects have been addressed, both at the institutional level and at the level of each company, to protect the health and well-being of workers and maintain a productive activity.

For the Chilean construction industry, the impact of COVID-19 occurred at a time when the activity had already been strongly affected by a major social uprising that started on October 18, 2019, and which produced major economic and political impacts from which the construction industry was still affected. It had not recovered from this crisis by the time the pandemic reached Chile in early March 2020. Thus, the COVID-19 crisis came on top of this economic and political crisis.

Then, research was carried out about the construction industry situation during the pandemic. It was sought to collect information on the variables of interest corresponding to the following research questions:

1 What have been the main impacts of COVID-19 on the Chilean construction industry?
2 What actions were taken to address the impacts of COVID-19 and by who?

DOI: 10.1201/9781003278368-25

In addition, an analysis of the actions that were taken against the impacts of COVID-19 was carried out.

The chapter continues with a review of relevant concepts and then follows with a brief description of the research method. Subsequently, the main results obtained from the research are presented to continue with a discussion of these and an analysis of the implications for practice and research. Finally, the main conclusions of the chapter are presented.

## Perspectives

The construction sector, like other economic sectors in any country, has had to deal with a variety of global shocks that have produced different impacts on its performance over the years. For example, it is possible to remember the cases of the financial crisis of the years 2007–2008 and the crisis of the SARS virus, among others. In all these cases, lessons learned have been generated as follows: a) the importance of increasing the cash reserves of companies to face the rise of fund needs produced by this type of crisis to maintain the activity; b) to create governmental stimulus for economic growing; and c) to increase the public investment to keep the activity of construction sector and protect its employment. In the case of COVID-19, this pandemic has been changing since its inception and has caused social, cultural, and economic systems to adjust to this new reality (Rokooei et al., 2022).

### *Impacts of the COVID-19 pandemic*

It is necessary to point out that the economic effects of this type of event are very different from those of other types of crises, such as those of financial or fiscal origin, because due to the health restrictions (such as quarantines), there is not only a demand shock but also a supply shock due to an exogenous decrease in labor supply (Comisión Nacional de Productividad, 2020).

Since the construction industry has an important influence on the economy of any country, the impacts that affect it spread to many other sectors. Construction provides infrastructure that is critical for the development of countries and the economic activity of industries, providing housing for its inhabitants and generating many jobs. All these aspects are negatively affected when construction is affected severely. For example, in the global financial crisis of 2008, in Australia 22% of new housing contracts fell through (Rokooei et al., 2022).

Another effect refers to the legal implications of the impacts of COVID-19 on the normal progress of construction projects, producing losses to construction companies whose potential recovery varies according to the type of contracts and the country's legal practices. The pandemic has slowed down processes, causing interruptions and delays with projects even having to stop completely and restart later (Ogunnusi et al., 2020). These effects have been considered an occurrence of force majeure, which would normally allow an extension of time for delays due to the pandemic but not compensation for costs. However, these circumstances have been very complex to resolve, significantly affecting the Chilean construction companies involved in this type of situation.

### Health and safety impacts of COVID-19 in the construction industry

The COVID-19 pandemic has unleashed an unprecedented public health crisis coupled with an economic crisis unlike the world had seen in the past century (Bassoli and Probst, 2022). Occupational health and safety issues have become critical strategic concerns for organizations and industry sectors when making decisions about the management of business operations during the pandemic (Caligiuri et al., 2020).

Construction projects have been facing a unique challenge due to the pandemic; however, governments and organizations tried to minimize the risks of spreading the virus by issuing new requirements or guidelines on how to perform construction activities as the businesses started to reopen (Almohassen et al., 2023). For example, in the US, the federal guidelines place a focus on eight aspects for construction employers: (1) hazard assessment; (2) controlling and prevention; (3) promoting social distancing and face masks; (4) cleaning, disinfection, and hand hygiene; (5) managing sick workers; (6) return to work after worker exposure to COVID-19; (7) providing education, training, and communication; and (8) mental health and wellbeing considerations (CDC, 2020).

According to a report by the International Labor Organization, the increase in health risks associated with COVID-19 has exacerbated decent work deficits in the construction sector, which adds to occupational health and safety risks and the skills shortage of workers. Quarantines and mobility restrictions have affected those who must travel daily to the worksites. The workers that carry out their activity in remote works can run health risks on the way to and from if the means of transport used is very full of people and the opportune measures of risk control are not adopted. Apart from physical well-being, mental health is also a concern since higher levels of anxiety have been found among construction workers (ILO, 2021).

The quick spread of the pandemic has forced the development of adaptive capacity on the fly. Therefore, learning by doing, trial and error, and creativity have been clearly as necessary as predefined plans (Saurin, 2020).

Assaad and El-adaway (2021) propose that the short- and long-term impacts posed by the COVID-19 virus on the construction industry include (1) workforce-related issues, such as worker shortages because of infections and preventive quarantines and worker layoffs caused by project cancelations and delays; (2) project and workplace considerations, such as implementing new workplace practices and policies; (3) procurement and supply chain implications, such as the restrictions and closures in the international exchange markets; and (4) contractual, legal, and insurance aspects, such as issues regarding the applicability of the force majeure clause.

In terms of safety performance management and practices in construction, different studies provided different strategies and procedures to be used to boost the performance and mitigate the effects of the COVID-19 pandemic.

For example, Nnaji et al. (2022) report that fieldworkers believe that staggered breaks and lunches, remote work, project area isolation, remote worksite of pre-fabrication, and technologies for meetings were the most effective measures in increasing social distance and minimizing group gathering size to 10 persons. These approaches provide flexible worksites by only having essential field crews on sites, keeping unessential workers away from hazards, and establishing flexible work hours to limit the number of workers on-site at the same time.

COVID-19 has affected not only people's physical health, but also their mental health and wellbeing. Contractors have been observing their workers' mental health problems. Many workers feel stressed about their job stability, the need to work remotely, and/or the need to conduct field work amidst rising challenges to their health (Pamidimukkala and Kermanshachi, 2021).

### Actions against COVID-19

Many actions have been taken by governments and the construction industry to meet the challenges of COVID-19. According to Alsharef et al. (2021) in the US construction industry actions included: a) to adopt new safety measures, including the adoption of masks, the adoption of social distance, training on the risks of COVID-19 and the security measures to be adopted, and the temperature check together with the provision of sanitizers at the entrances to the workplaces; b) to manage other risks of the project through employees dedicated to analyzing government policies and the occurrence of delays and delays that were unavoidable; c) to reduce the impact of material delays and related challenges such as price increases; d) to review contracts in light of delays and price increases to assess expected impacts and provisions for their defense, such as full documentation recording events that have occurred; and e) to use government support programs to deal with cash flow problems.

According to PWC (2020), these measures can be divided into two main categories: stabilization measures and stimulation measures. The first would focus on preventing or halting the economic downturn and allowing key elements of the economy to continue to function. The second would be aimed at injecting capital and generating new demand in the economy or specific industries, such as construction.

## Method

The study presented has a descriptive scope, seeking to specify the important properties and characteristics of a specific phenomenon. The phenomenon under study concerns the occurrence of the COVID-19 pandemic and its impact on the construction industry.

This study has been based on the search and compilation of existing information from different local sources that covers from the beginning of 2020 to 2022. The following themes were used to carry out the search:

- COVID-19 in Chile.
- Impacts of COVID-19 on the construction industry in Chile.

- COVID-19 and construction in the world.
- Actions to address the impacts of the COVID-19 pandemic on construction in Chile.
- Evaluation of actions to face the COVID-19 impacts on the Chilean construction industry.

A thematic analysis was carried out by looking for specific entries in different sources, like professional journals, reports from Chilean construction organizations, government reports, news published in Chilean newspapers, and information found on the web. These sources are considered mostly reliable in the sense that they addressed the situation of the construction industry using data from this sector that was created by different studies. The information obtained was processed and structured, achieving an adequate classification for its analysis and use. The results are presented in the next section. Unfortunately, it was not possible to find information on the effectiveness of the actions to face the impacts of the pandemic on the Chilean construction industry at this time.

## Results and discussion

Like the rest of the world, construction in Chile was considerably affected by the arrival of COVID-19. The main results obtained from the study and analysis of the available information are presented here.

### *Economic impacts of the pandemic on the Chilean construction industry*

According to a descriptive analysis bulletin published by the Ministerio de Economía, Fomento y Turismo (2021) on the impacts of the pandemic on almost 900,000 companies in Chile, 62.4% of the companies registered a decrease in their sales between these years, with micro-enterprises being the most affected both in the proportion of companies that reduced their sales (63.1%) and in the magnitude of the decrease (-37.5%). In the case of construction (CO) and real estate (RE), the percentage variation by sector and size in a) sales; b) employment; and c) remuneration, as shown in Table 22.1.

The Comisión Nacional de Productividad (2020), in a similar study also based on the tax information of companies, presents aggregate statistics of variations in four indicators between the months of March and July 2020. Table 22.2 shows these results.

The Construction and Real Estate sectors have been strongly affected by the pandemic, being among the three most affected sectors at the national level, together with the Hotels and Restaurants and the Arts and Entertainment sectors. Regarding the decrease in purchases, the Real Estate sector sharply reduced its purchases, influenced by the reduction in demand and by the stoppage in construction. Regarding the variation of active companies, the analysis shows that the decrease occurred entirely in smaller companies. The number of small construction and real

*Table 22.1* Percentage change in sales, employment and wages by sector and company size. (Analysis Bulletin published by the Ministerio de Economía, Fomento y Turismo (2021)

| Sector | # | Sales (%) | | | | Employment (%) | | | | Wages (%) | | | |
|---|---|---|---|---|---|---|---|---|---|---|---|---|---|
| | | Micro | Small | Medium | Large | Micro | Small | Medium | Large | Micro | Small | Medium | Large |
| CO | 56,463 | −53.0 | −21.0 | −15.2 | −8.1 | −47.6 | −16.1 | −10.4 | −9.1 | −1.3 | 0.2 | 0.7 | 1.9 |
| RE | 20,432 | −57.8 | −44.9 | −41.0 | 3.2 | −19.9 | −3.5 | −3.4 | −5.0 | −5.2 | 1.3 | 1.8 | 5.5 |

Company size classified by Chilean IRS in annual sales at 07/15/2022 exchange rate:
Micro companies: from US$ 0.3 to 76,000
Small companies: from US$ 76,000 to 792,000
Medium companies: from US$ 792,000 to 3,167,000
Large companies: more than US$ 3,167,000

*Table 22.2* Aggregate variations in key indicators from March to July 2020.

| Sector | Variation in sales (%) | Variation in buying's (%) | Variation in the number of active companies (%) | Variation in employment (%) | Variation in number of employments |
| --- | --- | --- | --- | --- | --- |
| Construction | −39 | −38 | −21 | −20 | −115,000 |
| Real Estate | −25 | −40 | −14 | −12 | −4,900 |

estate companies that stopped selling reached 15,000 and 1,000 of medium-sized companies in all the sectors. In the case of construction and real estate, the variation of active companies between March and July of 2020 was minus 21% and minus 14% respectively.

Regarding employment, Figure 22.1 shows the evolution of employment in construction from 2007 to 2020.

For its part, ICR Chile (2020) indicates that the pandemic has exacerbated the negative impacts that the construction sector had been showing after the social revolt that occurred in October 2019. This same study indicates that regarding the supply of housing and civil works, a significant reduction in new projects is estimated. Figure 22.2 shows a general summary of the impacts of COVID-19.

According to a survey of 33 construction companies about specific impacts due to COVID-19, the following results were indicated (PMG, 2020): a) impacts on prevention or reaction plans to face the crisis and to maintain the operation of the company, like operational planning and adjustment, organizational restructuring, renegotiation and coordination with clients, and search of new financing sources, 96.1%; total or partial stoppage of projects 76.6%; impact on the sale/awarding of projects 76.6%; reduction and/or restructuring of personnel 71.4%; e) teleworking and remote coordination 71.4%; negotiation with suppliers or clients 55.8%; g) reduction or suspension of service contracts 40.3%; h) adjustments in individual remunerations 39.0%; i) working capital financing 39.0%; and j) reduced attendance 29.9%.

Another relevant economic impact on the Chilean construction sector due to the pandemic was the rise in the price of construction materials. In a news entry from the Senado de Chile (2021), it was reported that construction materials have experienced an increase of between 10 and 30% during the pandemic, affecting thousands of families who need to make improvements to their homes or who aspire to have their own house. In addition, it is added that the breakdown of stock of associated products adds to this uneasy situation for this productive sector.

This situation is also highlighted by the Instituto de la Construcción (2021), which reports that the sustained rise in the prices of construction materials and the breakdown of stock has caused a direct effect on the cost of the works and, therefore, on the final value of the projects. Given the low inventories, prices have had a sustained increase, reaching an average increase of 20 to 30% in materials

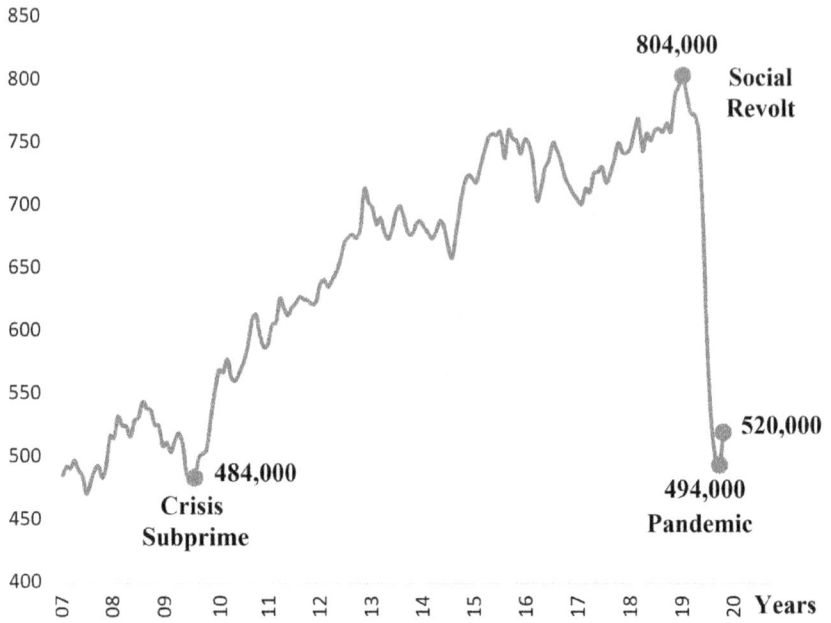

*Figure 22.1* Evolution of construction employment in Chile from year 2007 to year 2020.

*Source:* (adapted from Cámara Chilena de la Construcción (2020b)

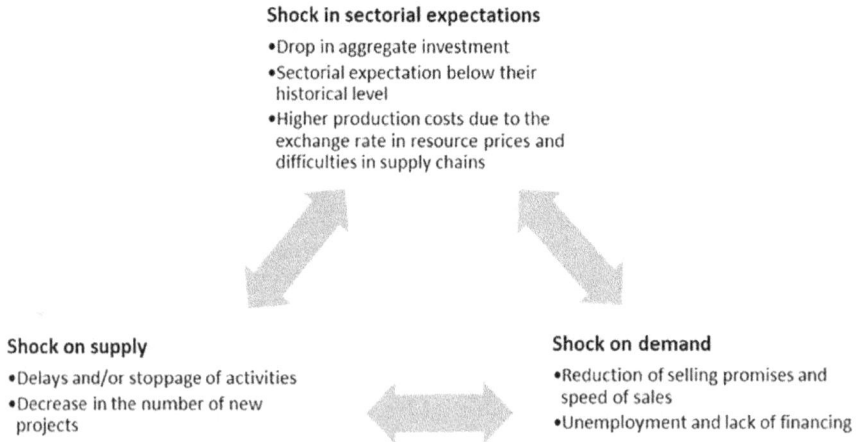

**Shock in sectorial expectations**

• Drop in aggregate investment
• Sectorial expectation below their historical level
• Higher production costs due to the exchange rate in resource prices and difficulties in supply chains

**Shock on supply**

• Delays and/or stoppage of activities
• Decrease in the number of new projects

**Shock on demand**

• Reduction of selling promises and speed of sales
• Unemployment and lack of financing

*Figure 22.2* Summary of impacts of COVID-19.

*Source:* (adapted from ICR Chile, 2020)

compared to 2019. Manufacturers of construction materials strongly reduced production due to health restrictions and quarantines in the country.

### Contractual impacts on construction activities

The COVID-19 pandemic has caused complexities in relation to the fulfillment of the contractual obligations assumed by the different parties to a construction contract. These complexities derive from different attitudes and interpretations regarding the consequences of the impacts of the pandemic on construction projects. In this regard, in Chile many clients demanded contractors to assume the costs implied by the pandemic, including those due to impacts such as described earlier: stoppage of projects, continuity of execution with low productivity, and unfavorable working conditions. There were also projects that did not stop and had to continue their execution under the pandemic conditions, particularly in the case of projects that were considered essential or critical.

The main problem in this area has been the lack of recognition by the clients of the economic impacts of the pandemic on the execution of projects, who have assigned all the economic consequences of these risks to contractors. This situation is considered by the latter as unfair and unbalanced, generating great concern and controversy in the construction sector. The main discussion has focused on the concept of "fortuitous event" or "force majeure", which must meet a series of requirements according to Chilean law: it must be unpredictable, irresistible, and external (outside of the will of the parties) and, if any of these three requirements is not met, the existence of a fortuitous event is ruled out (Tapia, 2020).

Therefore, the situation described has generated contractual conflicts between clients and contractors and economic losses for the latter in many cases. These conflicts and associated consequences that are still not solved will continue to be part of the discussion in the industry in the medium term.

### Actions to face the impacts of COVID-19

Different actions were implemented to face the impacts of COVID-19. The most relevant ones are described here:

#### Government protocol for construction

In 2020, the Chilean government established a management and prevention protocol for COVID-19 in the construction sector (Government of Chile, 2020). This was important because construction works were considered essential and allowed to continue working during the pandemic. This protocol established the preventive actions to be carried out in construction works and tasks to reduce the risk of contagion of COVID-19. This protocol was organized in the following sections: a) general actions for construction sites; b) actions for accessing the construction site; c) actions within the work; d) actions during lunch/snack time; e) actions to exit the work; f) actions for workers of greater vulnerability; and g) actions for workers during transportation.

It included mandatory prevention measures, like the use of a mask, physical distancing, hygiene measures, cleaning and disinfection, and the availability of sanitary information for the personnel. Additionally, it proposed self-care recommendations, such as always maintaining a distance of at least one meter between people, covering the nose and mouth with a forearm when coughing or sneezing, encouraging frequent hand-washing with soap and water or alcohol, salutations without physical contact and with distance, and so on.

It also included specific measures for the workplace, such as cleaning and disinfecting of dining rooms after use, reinforcing hygiene in bathrooms, and self-care measures for the personnel. Regarding entrances and exits of the sitework, it proposed the control of the access of people external to the company, including the taking of temperatures and a declaration of the state of health with the corresponding contact information. In the event of interaction with external companies, it should be ensured that preventive measures are complied with, cleaning and disinfecting and/or promoting it in the transport means for workers, and thorough hand-washing upon entry.

For workers, it promoted that each worker has their own tools or tools provided by the company and to clean those that must be shared, to control body temperature and visual check of the general state of health of all the people who enter the site, and, in case of somebody presenting with symptoms, to prohibit their entry to the site. It was also directed that face-to-face meetings should be avoided and to ensure that all actions were taken to avoid the contagion of personnel and avoiding crowds at the site.

### Protocol promoted by the Cámara Chilena de la Construcción (2020a)

This union organization, of great importance and influence in the sector, also generated a complementary protocol for its member companies, in line with the public policies developed by the Chilean government. It highlighted the importance of materializing these preventive measures and procedures in action protocols that are part of the company regulations, as well as the formulation of a Health and Safety Management System and a Work Site Committee. Additionally, this protocol proposed establishing specific order, cleaning and sanitization crews, and organizational measures such as flexible hours by establishing deferred hours for the entry and exit of workers.

### Response actions of construction and supplier companies

Companies were concerned with two central issues during the pandemic. The first was to keep the business operational and the second was how to deal with the measures taken by the authorities to control COVID-19 in a way that had the least impact on the business (PMG, 2020). According to this study, the actions that 33 construction companies carried out to face the COVID-19 contingency were as follows: a) actions aimed at maintaining continuity in the operation of works in 93.1% of cases; b) improving the planning and control of works by 72.4%; c) better coordination with suppliers in 55.2% of the cases; d) actions to ensure business continuity by 41.4%; and e) to maintain the continuity of the central office at 37.9%. When inquiring about the main issues that were pending resolution, most of the companies (90%) declared the continuity of the business, which leads to being able to execute works in a shorter period, adjust to a lower level of works, and prepare plans of operational efficiency and reduction of permanent expenses.

*Government measures to support construction*

The Chilean government implemented a large set of measures to deal with COVID-19 in different areas. Some of these measures were related to the construction industry, particularly in measures aimed at helping companies.

In 2020, guarantee funds were delivered for small and medium-sized entrepreneurs for a total of US$ 3,000 million, allowing to finance companies that had up to US$ 34 million in annual sales (at the exchange rate of March 15, 2020) to stimulate the economy and employment.

In the same year, the early return of income tax was established, benefiting almost 342,000 small and medium-sized companies. In 2021, a guarantee fund for small and medium-sized entrepreneurs was delivered to promote the reactivation and recovery of the economy, as well as to companies with annual sales of up to approximately US$41 million in this case (at the exchange rate of March 2021). Additionally, a bonus was established for small and medium-sized companies consisting of a contribution of around US$1,300 in addition to a set of tax measures for economic and employment reactivation (Dirección de Presupuestos de Chile, 2022).

Other measures were aimed at facilitating access to credit for small and medium-sized companies, as well as subsidies for hiring by companies in general. An ambitious plan of US$ 34,000 million was also created to promote both public and private investment to carry out public works of different types throughout the country in the first case, and concession works and land tenders for the development of private investment projects.

For its part, the Ministry of Housing and Urbanism established a complete contingency plan to guarantee the quality and continuity of the social housing construction works. One of the measures was to advance payment to construction companies to ensure the salary of workers as well as the necessary security measures to avoid contagion, to guarantee the development of the works in execution, protect the salary of workers, and protect health (MINVU, 2020).

It is evident that, considering the data presented, the COVID-19 pandemic and the health restrictions imposed by the authority on the operation of companies and the economy in general have caused significant damage to the construction sector, in addition to affecting the health of workers in the sector. Also, it is possible to appreciate the rapid, varied, and wide range of measures that were taken in the face of these challenges at the government, union, and business levels. Regarding the effectiveness of the measures taken, at this time there are no available studies in Chile that report on the assessment of the implementation of the measures described, which have apparently been postponed. Future revisions will help to review the criteria used in the selection of measures, as well as to analyze their merits.

## Implications for practice

The information presented in this chapter allows the identification of several implications of interest for practice. First, the analysis of the way construction dealt with the COVID-19 pandemic clearly shows the need to act incrementally as the characteristics of the pandemic were learned. A second implication has to do with the need to act in collaboration with the authorities to deal with this type of crisis, considering that the authority must act against conditions that affect the health of the entire population and not just one sector, like construction. A collaborative scheme makes it possible to keep in mind different important factors such as health, the economy, and social and labor aspects, and the consequences that are produced by their interaction.

In this regard, an unexpected consequence of the labor support provided by the Chilean government would have caused many workers to decide to live on government help and economic benefits and quit working, producing a significant reduction of the labor supply in construction according to the Chilean Construction Chamber. The new alternative sources of income, the withdrawal of pension funds, and the delays of financial obligations have altered the reserve salary of construction workers, i.e., the salary from which a person would be willing to work which, during the year 2020 and the beginning of 2021, has overcome the average salary in the construction activity by 21.3%. This situation indicated that the workers occupied in the sector registered a fall of 15% between January 2020 and January 2021, which means a decrease of 114,000 work positions (El Mercurio, 2021).

An important aspect that should be further studied regarding the COVID-19 crisis is the lessons learned on how to deal with it so that they can be used in future crises. The topic should be oriented to analyze how to increase the resilience of construction companies in the face of this type of crisis.

Some ideas that have been raised because of this experience are as follows (Cámara Chilena de la Construcción, 2020a):

- Promote the industrialization and standardization of construction components to work under controlled conditions and reduce the number of activities to be done on site, reducing in this way the number of people working at the site.
- Increase the use of technology to supervise workers, control flow situations and crowds, and help protect them.
- Disseminate good practices for handling the pandemic and apply new business models.
- Accelerate the digital transformation of the industry to facilitate teleworking for many of its activities. Also, increase process automation to reduce the number of interactions between people.

- Work collaboratively with suppliers to facilitate interaction with them and reduce the contacts between people.
- Another practical implication that is obtained from the contractual experiences is to have contracts with greater clarity regarding the consequences resulting from a pandemic like this so that it would be easier and quicker to resolve disputes due to this cause.

As for future research topics, one of the first is the study of the effectiveness of the measures taken to confront COVID-19, including an analysis of the usefulness of each measure. It is also proposed to investigate the decision-making process in companies in times of crisis in such a way that plans are established considering a systemic approach and accelerated implementation based on lessons learned during this and previous crises. Additionally, it is necessary to define which business model would be more appropriate to face future potential crises in an effective and resilient way by ensuring the ability to react quickly and maintain the operation of the company.

## Conclusions

This chapter reports on the impacts that the COVID-19 pandemic had on the Chilean construction industry, as well as the actions taken by the government, and by institutions and companies in the sector. An exhaustive review of the available information was attempted, with greater emphasis on the year 2020, which was when the greatest impacts occurred and where the sector had to react quickly to face this crisis. As can be seen from the literature review, many of the measures applied in Chile are similar to those applied in other countries.

Most data presented in this chapter refer to the economy, which caused strong economic and social impacts. Along with regretting the death of people due to the pandemic, the application of health protocols created very complex situations for the operational continuity of construction projects, causing the paralysis of a significant number of them. These stoppages had an impact on employment in the sector, on contractual relations between clients and contractors, and on sales in the sector, with a greater impact on smaller companies.

Although the pandemic is still with us, the construction industry in Chile has managed to recover its activity, maintaining the sanitary measures established in the existing protocols. One of the most complex aspects corresponds to the difficulties still present in the supply chains and the persistent increase in the costs of materials, which has led to a significant increase in the costs of construction and products in this sector.

The research carried out was based on published material available from various sources. Although an effort was made to address all the most important aspects for the objective of the investigation, it was not possible to find sufficient documentation about every aspect. However, the information provides a clear frame of reference for the situation of the Chilean construction industry in the face of the COVID-19 pandemic.

## References

Almohassen, A., Alkhaldi, M., & Essam, M. (2023). The effects of COVID-19 on safety practices in construction projects. *Ain Shams Engineering Journal*, 14(1), 101834. https://doi.org/10.1016/j.asej.2022.101834.

Alsharef, A., Banerjee, S., Uddin, S.M.J., Albert, A., & Jaselskis, E. (2021). Early impacts of the COVID-19 pandemic on the United States construction industry. *Int. J. Environ. Res. Public Health*, 18, 1559. https://doi.org/10.3390/ijerph18041559.

Assaad, R., & El-adaway, I.H. (2021). Guidelines for responding to COVID-19 pandemic: Best practices, impacts, and future research directions. *Journal of Management in Engineering*, 37, 06021001.

Bassoli, A., & Probst, T. (2022). COVID-19 moral disengagement and prevention behaviors: The impact of perceived workplace COVID-19 safety climate and employee job insecurity. *Safety Science*, 150, 105703. https://doi.org/10.1016/j.ssci.2022.105703.

Caligiuri, P., et al. (2020). International HRM insights for navigating the COVID-19 pandemic: Implications for future research and practice. *Journal of International Business Studies*, 51, 697–713.

Cámara Chilena de la Construcción (2020a). *El sector construcción frente a la crisis sanitaria, septiembre, Temuco, Chile (The construction sector facing the health crisis, September, Temuco, Chile)*. Available at www.ccc.cl/wp-content/uploads/2021/03/Barometro_informe_Experiencia-internacional-del-sector-de-la-construcci%C3%B3n-frente-a-la-crisis-sanitaria.pdf.

Cámara Chilena de la Construcción (2020b). *Informe MACh 55 Macroeconomía y construcción, diciembre (MACh 55 macroeconomics and construction report, December)*, p. 13.

Centres for Disease Control and Prevention (CDC). (2020). *Construction COVID-19 checklists for employers and employees* [Online]. Available at www.cdc.gov/coronavirus/2019-ncov/community/organizations/construction-worker-checklists.html.

Comisión Nacional de Productividad. (2020). *Efectos del COVID-19 en la actividad de las empresas en Chile (Effects of COVID-19 on the activity of companies in Chile)*. Santiago, Chile.

Dirección de Presupuestos de Chile. (2022). *COVID-19: evolución, efectos y políticas adoptadas en Chile y el mundo (COVID-19: Evolution, effects and policies adopted in Chile and the world)*. Available at www.dipres.gob.cl/598/articles-266625_doc_pdf.pdf.

El Mercurio. (2021). *Construcción revela escasez de trabajadores por efecto de ayudas económicas por pandemia (Construction reveals shortage of workers due to economic aid due to pandemic)*, 12 March, section B.

Gobierno de Chile. (2020). *Protocolo de manejo y prevención ante COVID-19 en sector construcción, Programa Paso a Paso, Chile (Management and prevention protocol against COVID-19 in the construction sector, Step by Step Program, Chile)*. Available at https://cdn.digital.gob.cl/public_files/Campa%C3%B1as/Corona-Virus/documentos/paso-a-paso/Protocolo-construccion.pdf.

ICR Chile. (2020). *Industria inmobiliaria y construcción (Real estate and construction industry)*. Available at https://icrchile.cl/noticia/ante-la-actual-contingencia-sanitaria-pr2261/.

Instituto de la Construcción. (2021). *Costos en la construcción se triplican y presionan un alza de hasta un 15% en el precio de la vivienda para los próximos meses (Construction costs triple and push up to a 15% rise in housing prices for the coming months)*. Available at www.iconstruccion.cl/2021/08/19/costos-en-la-construccion-se-triplican-y-presionan-un-alza-de-hasta-un-15-en-el-precio-de-la-vivienda-para-los-proximos-meses/.

International Labor Organization ILO. (2021). *The impact of COVID-19 in the construction sector, Informative sectorial note*. Available at www.ilo.org/sector/Resources/publications/WCM_800244/lang--es/index.htm.

Ministerio de Economía, Fomento y Turismo. (2021). *Boletín de análisis descriptivo del impacto de la pandemia sobre las empresas en Chile (Bulletin of descriptive analysis of the impact of the pandemic on companies in Chile)*. Santiago, Chile: Unidad de Estudios, División Política Comercial e Industrial.

MINVU. (2020). *Ministerio de Vivienda y Urbanismo anticipa pagos (Ministry of Housing and Urbanism anticipates payments)*. Available at www.minvu.cl/noticia/noticias/minvu-anticipa-pagos-para-asegurar-continuidad-de-obras-sueldos-y-seguridad-de-trabajadores/.

Nnaji, C., Jin, Z., & Karakhan, A. (2022). Safety and health management response to COVID-19 in the construction industry: A perspective of fieldworkers. *Process Safety and Environmental Protection*, 159, 477–488. https://doi.org/10.1016/j.psep.2022.01.002.

Ogunnusi, M., Hamma-Adama, M., Salman, H., & Kouider, T. (2020). COVID-19 pandemic: The effects and prospects in the construction industry. *International Journal of Real Estate Studies* [online], 14(Special Issue 2), 120–128. Available at www.utm.my/intrest/files/2020/11/2_Final_MS_CRES-Covid-025.pdf.

Pamidimukkala, A., & Kermanshachi, S. (2021). Impact of COVID-19 on field and office workforce in construction industry. *Project Leadership and Society*, 2, 100018. https://doi.org/10.1016/j.plas.2021.100018.

PMG. (2020). *Contingencia COVID-19 El modelo ganar: antecedentes y oportunidades en la construcción (COVID-19 contingency the win model: Background and opportunities in construction)*. Available at www.pmgchile.com/wp-content/uploads/2020/05/Modelo-GANAR-PMG-Constructoras.pdf.

PWC. (2020, mayo). *COVID-19: Impacto en infraestructura y construcción (Impact on infrastructure and construction)*. Available at www.pwc.com.uy/es/covid-19/pdfs-covid-19/covid19-impacto-infraestructura-construccion.pdf.

Reeves, M., Lang, N., & Carlsson-Szlezak, P. (2020, February 27). Lead your business through the Coronavirus crisis. *Harvard Business Review*.

Rokooei, S., Alvanchi, A., & Rahimi, M. (2022). Perception of COVID-19 impacts on the construction industry over time. *Cogent Engineering*, 9(1), 2044575. doi: 10.1080/23311916.2022.2044575.

Saurin, T.A. (2020, September). A complexity thinking account of the COVID-19 pandemic. *Saf Sci*, 134, 105087. https://doi.org/10.1016/j.ssci.2020.105087.

Senado de Chile. (2021). *Alza de materiales de la construcción: solicitan investigar razones y entregar información al SERNAC y la FNE (Rise in construction materials: Senators request to investigate reasons and deliver information to SERNAC and the FNE)*. Available at www.senado.cl/noticias/coronavirus/alza-de-materiales-de-la-construccion-solicitan-investigar-razones-y.

Tapia, M. (2020). *¿El COVID-19 es un caso fortuito? (Is COVID-19 a fortuitous event?)*. Available at www.derecho.uchile.cl/comunicaciones/columnas-de-opinion/el-covid-19-es-un-caso-fortuito---mauricio-tapia.

# 23 Factors that led to an increase of building collapses during the COVID-19 lockdown period in the Greater Kampala metropolitan area, Uganda

*Henry Alinaitwe and Richard Irumba*

## Introduction

The construction industry in Uganda has a poor safety record. Between 1996 and 1998, a total of 146 accidents were reported in the construction industry, 17 of which were fatal cases (Lubega et al., 2000). During the period of 2001 to 2005, the annual averages were 54 cases on building sites, 103 cases on construction sites including buildings and 384 cases for all industries, construction inclusive (Alinaitwe et al., 2007a, 2007b). Similarly, from 2006 to 2010, the construction industry in Uganda continued to witness fatal accidents, with a total of 49 fatalities reported in the Greater Kampala Metropolitan Area, GKMA (Irumba et al., 2010). Reportedly, the construction injury rate for Kampala City is 3797 per 100,000 workers, and the fatality rate is 84 per 100,000 workers (Irumba, 2014). Comparatively, the construction industry fatality rate for Kampala City is four times higher than the fatality rate for Sub-Saharan Africa, reported as 21 per 100,000 workers (CIDB, 2010).

The causes of construction accidents in the GKMA are not only numerous but also diverse given that they relate to both technical, management and policy cavities. Alinaitwe and Ekolu (2014) identified the five primary causes as poor materials and workmanship, design and construction errors, absence of professional supervision of site works, wrong implementation of construction methods and neglect of design approval procedures. In addition, Alinaitwe and Ekolu (2014) identified the secondary factors complicit to construction failure in the GKMA as attempts to severely minimize construction cost, neglect of inspection and monitoring by local authorities and influence peddling by proprietors. Following an industry-wide survey, Irumba (2014) ascertained that the three most prevalent causes of construction accidents in the GKMA are mechanical hazards (i.e. struck by machines, vehicles, hand tools, cutting edges etc.), being hit by falling objects and falls from height. Irumba (2014) demonstrates that site congestion and spatial factors (including tectonic forces associated with earthquakes and quarrying activities) also contribute to the occurrence of construction accidents in the GKMA.

Meanwhile, the spread of COVID-19 posed an unprecedented challenge with unpredictable economic consequences across the globe (McKibbin and Fernando,

DOI: 10.1201/9781003278368-26

2021). Uganda registered the first case of COVID-19 on 21st March 2020 and the first death due to COVID-19 on 23rd July 2020. The Government of Uganda (GOU) imposed the first lockdown due to COVID-19 on 20th March 2020. In order to minimize the spread of COVID-19, restrictions were imposed on many activities and movements. GOU categorized construction as an essential activity and therefore allowed construction projects to proceed. However, because of the suspension of public transport, the majority of workers and professionals could not visit the sites or do so regularly. GOU directed construction workers to stay in camps near the sites, but many developers could not afford that. There was also a shortage of construction materials on the market. These deficiencies, amongst other factors, resulted in collapse of buildings and at a rate higher than the usually reported cases in the country.

The purpose of this chapter is to report how COVID-19 contributed to the collapse of buildings under construction during the lockdown period in Uganda. This period extended from 20th March 2020 to 30th July 2021 (i.e., 16 months), when it was partially eased to allow opening of selected sectors and movements, but it maintained suspension of night curfews until 24th January 2022 (i.e., 22 months). Beyond the introduction, the chapter presents a literature review on quality and safety matters in construction, details the methodology adopted, presents and discusses results and finally highlights the conclusions and recommendations.

### Quality and safety in the construction process

The key performance indicators for construction projects include quality, cost and schedule while remaining within the work scope. Attention regarding performance in the industry has largely been placed on cost, schedule and scope with less emphasis on quality, to the detriment of the industry (Mbachu and Nkado, 2006). Quality failures in building construction are increasingly being noted, partly due to the prevailing environments (Kakitahi et al., 2015). The collapse of a building is evidence of total quality failure in the building process. The Ugandan construction industry has seen increased occurrences of quality failure and rework (Alinaitwe et al., 2007a). Quality is about meeting specifications and user and implied requirements (Kakitahi et al., 2015).

Kagioglou et al. (2000) developed an improved project process, the process protocol, which considers the whole lifecycle of a construction project whilst integrating its participants under a common framework. The lifecycle includes identification, appraisal, definition, approval, implementation and operation (Nigel, 2018). Failure of quality at each of the stages may manifest in the later stages and at the extreme event by collapse of the building. Hence, the collapse of a building is an example of extreme quality failure.

The occupational safety and health situation in the construction industry is still very much below expectations. Accidents and diseases still occur and are a cause for concern as the available statistics show that the percentage of accidents occurring in the workplace has alarmingly increased (Coble et al., 2000). A study carried out by

Alinaitwe et al. (2007b) found that the construction industry in Uganda is a major contributor of accidents, that the majority of accidents and fatalities are caused by being hit by objects including collapsing building elements and that accidents inflict on weighted average permanent incapacity of 37%for those who go through the ordeal.

A study of the Hong Kong construction industry concluded that mere legislation of safety requirements had been inadequate to protect the workers (Lo, 1997). It suggested that safety would be greatly improved by including its part in the existing quality management systems (Husrul et al., 2008). Husrul et al. (2008) contend that safety and quality are intertwined and that when safety is included in the quality standard, it would ensure that both are treated seriously.

In addition to the continuous improvement concept, Total Quality Management (TQM) concepts of teamwork and customer focus relate to safety. Quality management says "do it right first time"; TQM adds new emphasis of the idea that: doing it right" includes doing it safely. Thus, under TQM, safety is a quality issue (Husrul et al., 2008).

## Methodology

The most common research styles used in construction research include experimental, survey, action research, ethnographic research and case studies (Fellows and Liu, 2003). This chapter employed a case study methodology. A case study is an empirical inquiry that investigates a contemporary phenomenon within its real-life context, especially when the boundaries between phenomenon and context are not clearly evident (Yin, 2003). In a case study, a phenomenon is investigated within the context where variables are numerous and qualitatively different so that no single survey or data collection approach can be appropriately used to collect information about these variables.

Five case studies drawn from GKMA are presented here. The case studies are based on official accident investigation reports prepared by the National Building Review Board (NBRB), a policy body established under the Building Control Act (2013) to promote and ensure planned, decent and safe building structures that are developed in harmony with the environment, and incident reports by Kampala Capital City Authority (KCCA) a body established under the Kampala Capital City Act (2010) to govern and develop the capital city on behalf of central government. Summary details of case studies are presented here.

### Case study 1   Collapse of a building at Kitebi, Lubaga Division, Kampala City

The accident site is located in Kitebi along Wankulukuku road, Lubaga Division. The accident occurred during the night of 16th August 2021, resulting in the death of one person, a male adult 19 years old.

Based on records available at KCCA, on 10th February 2020, the developer was granted permission to construct Residential Apartments and a Boundary Wall on the subject land. The approved plans consisted of two proposed three-level apartment blocks. However, at the time of the accident, the building plan had been irregularly altered, introducing a third block of apartments occupying the space hitherto meant to be a parking area. Reportedly, this illegal third block of apartments is what collapsed on 16th August 2021.

On 25th March 2021, the Building Inspector for Lubaga identified the illegal construction activity and served the developer with a stop order notice to obtain a building permit for the structure or to demolish all the works which were done without a building permit. On 19th May 2021, KCCA reported this illegal construction activity (and many others) to the Executive Director National Building Review Board and the Executive Director National Physical Planning Board for a joint enforcement operation, which unfortunately was suspended because of the COVID-19 lockdown.

Records by the technical staff at KCCA show that the building block which collapsed lacked approved plans and was not being supervised by a qualified registered engineer. The speed of construction of the storeyed building was high, not allowing sufficient time for the building to set before being loaded. These lapses compromised the quality of the works, leading to the collapse of the building.

## Case study 2   Collapse of a building at Kisenyi, Central Division, Kampala City

The accident site is located in Kisenyi II Parish, Central Division. The accident occurred on 5th September 2021 at around 2:00 pm. Seven people died during the accident and five people were injured.

The building construction, which had reached the fourth level, did not have approved plans. The site was also not being supervised by a qualified Engineer. Reportedly, the supervising Engineer whom the developer communicated to KCCA following the collapse of the building died in 2020, one year before the accident occurred.

On 30th June 2021, the Physical Planner for Central Division issued a removal notice requiring the developer to halt the ongoing works and to provide approved plans, proof of inspection and a hoarding permit. Reportedly, construction work had commenced earlier than the date of serving the notice.

The Building Inspector was not inspecting works since he was away from duty because of COVID-19 staff rationing requirements. A follow-up enforcement notice was issued by the Physical Planner on 29th July 2021, requiring the developer to halt works and to provide a structural integrity report and a building permit within 27 days. Unfortunately, the building collapsed before the period of voluntary enforcement could expire.

At their 32nd sitting on 13th September 2021, the Building Committee of KCCA approved the demolition of the remaining three blocks, which evidently showed signs of failure and hence posed a grave risk to the public and neighboring structures. The developer was given three days to comply, effective 15th September 2021; if they failed to do so, KCCA would demolish the offending buildings at the cost of the developer. The developer did not comply and instead secured a court order barring KCCA from demolishing the building.

Based on analysis by KCCA, the concrete used during construction was weak, the water table was high, foundation soils were weak and the building foundation was weak. In combination, these lapses led to the collapse of the building.

## Case study 3   Collapse of a multi-storeyed Gate House at Kitubulu, Wakiso District

A multi-storeyed gate house located at Kitubulu, Wakiso District, GKMA collapsed on 20th April 2020. The gate house was a reinforced concrete structure comprising foundations, columns, beams and slabs. The architectural designs of the boundary wall and gate house had been approved by Katabi Town Council on 18th June 2018. Construction works are reported to have commenced immediately and while still casting concrete, the already cast bay of the slab collapsed, injuring some people.

An investigation conducted by NBRB established that the factors that contributed to the accident include a poorly designed/arranged temporary support system, poor structural design, inadequate supervision by professionals, especially due to restricted movements during the lockdown period, poor project management and failure of the local authority to stop construction due to the inadequacies. NBRB observed that the geometric specifications of the beams on site were smaller than what was shown on the drawings, which adversely affected the strength and robustness of the beams, especially those with wide spans. An interview with the architect revealed that the accident happened three weeks into the COVID-19 lockdown period and that the architect had not been able to visit the site during that period.

The engineer indicated that the roof design was changed from a structural steel truss system to a reinforced concrete canopy slab without approval. The contractor changed the work methodology by replacing the steel props with eucalyptus tree props/supports. Safety guidelines like hoarding off the site, provision of protective gear, warning vests or reflecting garments and proper management of equipment were ignored by the contractor. The last inspection by the engineer was on 28th March 2020 and by the time of the accident, the engineer was not supervising the site because of travel restrictions. The client affirmed that the altered designs were not approved by the local authority. NBRB established that the local authority lacked capacity to evaluate and approve building plans or to inspect a site of this magnitude.

In summary, NBRB concluded that the collapse was due to excessively weak support props which were not efficiently installed to cover the canopy height of six meters. The heavy weight of concrete caused differential settlement upon the weak soggy soil. Though there were minor injuries, the collapse dented the reputation of the construction industry and caused economic loss to the developer and Uganda.

## Case study 4   Collapse of a five-storeyed commercial building at Kansanga, Makindye Division, Kampala City

During the COVID-19 lockdown, a 5-storeyed commercial building located at Kiwempe, Kansanga, Makindye Division, Kampala City, which was under construction near the finished stage, collapsed on 9th May 2020 at 11:45pm, killing 13 workers who were sleeping in the incomplete building and injuring four others.

NBRB established that the factors contributing to the collapse of the building include:

a) The developer executed the building construction works in total disregard of the prevailing laws, and appointed unqualified people to carry out the roles of design, construction and supervision.
b) The construction was at a high speed with the 5-storeyeyed in-situ concrete building block having taken only three months to construct. In effect, the concrete did not gain sufficient strength before loading.
c) The use of inferior and poor-quality materials.
d) Lack of approved building plans including architectural and structural drawings.
e) Lack of geotechnical investigations.

f) Poor workmanship coupled with poor construction technology and not following procedures.

g) Failure of the city authority to adequately monitor and inspect building construction, which was exacerbated by the absence of key staff during the COVID-19 lockdown period.

NBRB noted that legislation and enforcement mechanisms to regulate the contractors to employ qualified personnel, adopt appropriate work methods and deploy the right materials are either missing or inadequate. In summary, the acts of omission and commission by the developer, site agents and the city authority contributed to the collapse of the building.

## Case study 5   Collapse of a four-storeyed apartment along Lubega Road, Makindye Division

During the COVID-19 lockdown period, a four-storeyed reinforced concrete building along Lubega Road, Makindye Division collapsed on the night of 11th September 2020 while still under construction. Construction was reported to have commenced around February 2020. The collapse led to economic losses, but there were no deaths or injury of persons.

NBRB established that the factors which contributed to the collapse of the building include:

i. The building had no approved architectural or structural designs, and even the available draft drawings were not correctly followed during construction.

ii. The critical columns and their footings were not able to carry the loads from the three suspended floors; the designs were appropriate for no more than two suspended floors.

iii. No geotechnical investigations were done; these were important in ascertaining the strength of the soils to support the building's foundations.

iv. There was overloading of the suspended floors by construction loads. For example, the sand that was hipped on the third floor for plastering the walls was the last nail in an already precarious situation. It is highly likely that the collapse of the building commenced from the weak position of the columns that were not braced but were carrying heavy loads from the sand hipped on the floors.

v. The quality control of materials and works was evidently inadequate. The laboratory tests conducted by the investigating team show that the concrete was less than the specified strength. Tests on the steel show that the steel bars had a mix of brittle, weak and ductile strong steel.

vi. Use of unqualified engineering personnel to execute the works. Falsification of professionals' records was noted, reportedly with the Architects Registration Board indicating that the alleged supervising architect ceased practicing in Uganda more than 10 years preceding the accident.

vii. Inadequate monitoring and inspection of the works by the skeleton staff of the city authority who were retained during the lockdown period.

NBRB noted concerns of corruption and professional negligence by staff of the city authority. The area physical planner and building inspector aided illegal construction and were reluctant to enforce the building regulations. In summary, a combination of technical, management and ethical lapses contributed to the collapse of the building.

The five case studies presented here depict trends in causal factors responsible for the collapse of buildings in the GKMA, some of which are factors inherent in the organization of the construction industry and others which are emerging trends due to COVID-19 restrictions. A detailed discussion of the findings is presented here.

**Results and discussion**

The COVID-19 pandemic has caused and is still causing havoc around the world. All sectors of the economy, including the construction sector, have been severely affected by COVID-19 (Simpeh and Amoah, 2021). In Uganda, the construction industry was left open during the lockdowns, though it was seriously constrained by restrictions imposed on transport and staff attendance rotas, amongst others.

Table 23.1 presents a summary of the causal factors for building collapses based on the case studies presented under the section on methodology. Included in Table 23.1 are statistics on the impact of accidents in the form of fatalities and injuries.

Based on the results presented in Table 23.1, the top five factors responsible for building collapses during the COVID-19 lockdown period include poor supervision of building works marked by absence or irregular site visits due to COVID restrictions on movements, poor monitoring of works by local authority, which was also related to COVID restrictions on movements, lack of approved building plans, poor construction methods and failure to carry out site investigations resulting in defective designs.

*Table 23.1* Building accidents causation factors in Greater Kampala Metropolitan Area.

| Case Study | Accident causal factors | | | | | | | | Impact | |
|---|---|---|---|---|---|---|---|---|---|---|
| | Lack of approved plans | Poor supervision | Poor monitoring by local authority | Poor constr. methods | Lack site investigations | Poor quality materials | Poor designs | Breach of safety protocols | Fatality | Injury |
| Case #1 | ✓ | ✓ | ✓ | ✓ | | | | | 01 | – |
| Case #2 | ✓ | ✓ | ✓ | ✓ | ✓ | | | | 07 | 05 |
| Case #3 | | ✓ | ✓ | | ✓ | | ✓ | ✓ | – | – |
| Case #4 | ✓ | ✓ | ✓ | ✓ | ✓ | ✓ | ✓ | | 13 | 4 |
| Case #5 | ✓ | ✓ | ✓ | ✓ | ✓ | ✓ | | | – | – |
| Totals/Freq. | 4 | 5 | 5 | 4 | 4 | 2 | 2 | 1 | 21 | 09 |
| Rank | 3 | 1 | 1 | 3 | 3 | 6 | 6 | 8 | 1 | 2 |

*Legend:* ✓ – presence of a causation factor encountered in the case.

## Poor project supervision

Poor project supervision manifested in two ways: irregular site inspection visits and deployment of unqualified personnel. Irregular site visits associated with COVID-19 restrictions on movement were evident, for example, in case 3 where the architect could not visit the site for three consecutive weeks following the declaration of the COVID-19 lockdown; similarly, the engineer did not visit site for about three weeks prior to the accident. Since there was a lockdown, the Government of Uganda directed all construction workers and supervisors to reside on sites, which the supervising professionals (i.e., architects, engineers, quantity surveyors etc.) could not do due to insufficient amenities on site. As a consequence, construction work proceeded without adequate supervision. Notably, when supervisors are not present on site, unsatisfactory work goes undetected and eventually results in building collapses (Irumba et al., 2010).

Beyond irregular site visits, there was evidence of using unqualified supervisors. For example, in case 4, the developer disregarded the prevailing laws and appointed unqualified people to carry out the roles of design, construction and supervision. Similarly, in case 5, unqualified people were deployed to execute works. As reported by Alinaitwe et al. (2009), many construction workers are trained on the job and many lack basic qualifications.

Cases of falsification of professional records, included an architect who ceased practicing more than 10 years before the collapse (see case 5) and a reportedly active engineer who in real terms died one year before the accident, were cited (see case 2). In essence, work on these sites progressed without supervision, compromising quality and hence contributed to occurrence of the accidents.

## Poor monitoring by local authority

Poor monitoring and inspection by local authorities was reported in all five case studies. While this is a historical problem resulting from lack of capacity and resource gaps, the problem was exacerbated by the 20–30% COVID-19 staff rationing requirement imposed by the Ministry of Public Service during the lockdown period. In case 2, the lack of capacity of the local authority to effectively scrutinize building plans prior to approval was noted. Whereas the architectural designs of the gate house and boundary wall were approved by the local authority, they were found defective by NBRB and reportedly the anomaly contributed to the occurrence of the accident. Matters of corruption, maladministration and professional negligence by staff of local authorities are ethical issues prevalent in Uganda (Irumba and Mwakali, 2007).

## Lack of approved plans

Evidently, cases 1 and 2 show that the clients flouted the planning approval procedures. There were no plans approved for the buildings that collapsed as provided for under the Physical Planning Act (2010) and the Building Control Act (2013). In case 3, construction was progressing without approved structural drawings. In case 4, there was a lack of approved building plans, including architectural and structural drawings. In case 5, the building had no approved architectural and structural designs, and even the available draft drawings were not correctly followed during construction. These findings are in line with what Alinaitwe and Ekolu (2014) observed. Notably, a number of clients are not keen on getting approval of their designs and therefore, some mistakes inherent in the designs are implemented which subsequently lead to building collapses.

### Poor construction methods

Poor construction methods are a common cause of building failure (Alinaitwe and Ekolu, 2014; Irumba et al., 2010). In case 3, the contractor changed the work methodology communicated by the supervising engineer by replacing the steel props with eucalyptus tree props/supports. As a result, the gate house slab collapsed while under construction because the weak support props could not hold the heavy weight of the concrete slab. In case 5, the suspended floors were overloaded with stockpiles of materials including sand hips, which contributed to the collapse of the building. Also in case 5, construction was at high speed and as a result the concrete did not gain sufficient strength before loading, contributing to building failure. Irumba et al. (2010) observe that the tendency to accelerate projects can lead to accidents. Notably, accelerated projects tend to experience high levels of unsatisfactory work compared to projects implemented following their planned schedule.

### Lack of site investigations

The Building Control Regulations (2020) state that developers/professional agents of multi-storeyed and public buildings must undertake investigations categorized as geotechnical, hydrological, environmental and social assessment and traffic impact assessment. This legal requirement is not being observed on many construction sites. For example, geotechnical investigations were not carried out for the multi-storeyed structures reported under cases 4 and 5, yet they were important to ascertain the strength of the soil to support the building foundation. The multi-storeyed gatehouse project under case 3 was being implemented in a fragile natural environment adjacent to Lake Victoria. This site is also characterized by soggy soil. However, there was no evidence to show that environmental and social assessment studies were done or that these studies informed the designs of the project. Reportedly, failure to carry out site investigations results in defective designs, which ultimately lead to building collapses.

### Other causal factors

Beyond these five factors which contributed to building collapses during the COVID-19 lockdown period, the other factors complicit in building collapses include poor designs, poor quality materials and breach of safety protocols. Poor design is a composite causal factor which can be linked to several other factors, including lack of site investigations, deployment of unqualified personnel and lack of capacity of the local authority to scrutinize and review building plans. Accidents related to handling of materials are common on construction sites (Perttula et al., 2003). The suitability and condition of materials is an important safety factor (Haslam et al., 2005). In case 4, use of poor-quality materials was cited as a causal factor for the building collapse and in case 5, the investigating team confirmed through laboratory tests that the construction materials did not meet the industry standards. On the other hand, safety protocols like hoarding off the site, provision of protective gear, warning vests or reflecting garments and proper management of equipment were ignored by the contractor in case 3. Failure to follow the required safety protocols increases the risk of occurrence of an accident and magnifies the impact when an accident actually occurs.

In terms of impact, more fatalities than injuries were recorded during the COVID-19 lockdown period. Reputation damage and economic loss are the other dimensions of the impact of building collapses during the COVID-19 lockdown period. When people die, their immediate families and relatives are affected, as a number of the workers have several dependents. Building collapse and fatalities lead to stagnation of economic and social development of communities and societies.

## Conclusions and recommendations

This chapter has analysed five cases of construction failure during the 16-month COVID-19 lockdown period in GKMA from March 2020 to July 2021. The analysis has been used to point out the causality of extreme building failure. Reportedly, the 16-month COVID-19 lockdown in Uganda was the longest lockdown period globally. The top five factors responsible for building collapses in GKMA during the COVID-19 lockdown period include poor supervision of building works, poor monitoring of works by local authorities, lack of approved building plans, poor construction methods and failure to carry out site investigations. The failure of or lack of efficiency in carrying out site supervision by professionals and monitoring/ inspection by local authorities was attributable to COVID-19 lockdown restrictions on movements and public service restrictions on staff quotas, respectively, greatly contributing to the occurrence of building collapses. In terms of impact, during the COVID-19 lockdown period, more fatalities were recorded than injuries in the GKMA. Reputation damage and economic loss are noted as the other dimensions of the impact of building collapses during the COVID-19 lockdown period. During future epidemics management, due attention should be paid to maintaining good site presence and work conditions for professional teams and local authority building staff, in order to mitigate building collapses.

## Acknowledgement

The authors would like to acknowledge Kampala Capital City Authority and the National Building Review Board for availing data and reports on which the chapter is based.

## References

Alinaitwe, H., & Ekolu, S. (2014). Structural failures in East Africa: A study of cases in Uganda. In S. Ekolu, M. Dundu, & X. Gao (eds.), *Construction materials and structures* (pp. 76–85). Johannesburg: IOS Press. ISBN: 978-1-61499-465-7.

Alinaitwe, H.M., Mwakali, J.A., & Hansson, B. (2007a). Factors affecting the productivity of building craftsmen: Studies of Uganda. *Journal of Civil Engineering and Management*, 13(3), 169-176.

Alinaitwe, H.M., Mwakali, J.A., & Hansson, B. (2007b). Analysis of accidents on building construction sites reported in Uganda during 2001–2005. In T.C. Haupt & R. Milford (eds.), *Proceedings of the international council for research and innovation in building and construction (CIB) world building congress on construction for development, 14–18th May 2007* (pp 1208–1221). Cape Town, South Africa: CIB Publication. ISBN: 1-920-01704-6.

Alinaitwe, H.M., Mwakali, J.A., & Hanson, B. (2009). Organizational effectiveness of Ugandan building firms as viewed by craftsmen. *Journal of Civil Engineering and Management*, 15(3), 281–288.

Building Control Act. (2013). *Government of Uganda*. Entebbe: Government Publishing House.

Building Control Regulations. (2020). *Government of Uganda*. Entebbe: Government Publishing House.

CIDB. (2010). *Report on construction health and safety in South Africa*. In J. Smallwood, T. Haupt, & W. Shakantu (eds.). Cape Town: Construction Industry Development Board of South Africa Publication, pp. 1–48.

Coble, R.; Hinze, J., & Haupt, T.C. (2000). *The management of construction safety and health*. Brookfield: CRC Press.

Fellows, R., & Liu, A. (2003). *Research methods for construction* (2nd ed.). Oxford: Blackwell Science.

Haslam, R.A., Hide, S.A., Gibb, A.G.F., Gyi, D.E., Pavitt, T., Atkinson, S., & Duff, A.R. (2005). Contributing factors in construction accidents. *Applied Ergonomics*, 36, 401–415.

Husrul, H., Hamminah, A., & Kamaruzaman, J. (2008). Management of safety for quality construction. *Journal of Sustainable Development*, 1(3), 41–48.

Irumba, R. (2014). Spatial analysis of construction accidents in Kampala, Uganda. *Safety Science*, 64(April), 109–120.

Irumba, R., & Mwakali, J. (2007). Ethics in construction: Examples from Uganda. In T.C. Haupt & R. Milford (eds.), *Proceedings of the international council for research and innovation in building and construction (CIB) world building congress on construction for development, 14–18th May 2007* (pp. 2094–2105). Cape Town: CIB Publication. ISBN: 1-920-01704-6.

Irumba, R., Wilhelmsson, M., & Kerali, A.G. (2010). Modelling the dynamics of safety on construction projects: An undiscovered rework perspective. In *Proceedings of the 18th international council for research and innovation in building and construction (CIB) world congress on building a better world, 10–13th May 2010* (pp. 227–240). Salford Quays, UK: CIB Publication 357. ISBN: 978-1-905732-91-3.

Kagioglou, M., Cooper, R., Aouad, G., & Sexton, M. (2000). Rethinking construction: The generic design and construction process protocol. *Engineering, Construction and Architectural Management*, 7(2), 141–153.

Kakitahi, J., Aliaitwe, H., Landin, A., & Mudaaki, S. (2015). A study of non-compliance with quality requirements in Uganda. *Management, Procurement and Law*, 168(1), 22–42.

Kampala Capital City Act. (2010). *The Kampala Capital City Act of 2010 as amended.* Kampala: Government of Uganda Publication.

Lo, A. (1997). A talk of safety experience. *A Hong Kong Journal of Safety Bulletin*, Occupational Safety and Health Association, 15(4), 6–7.

Lubega, H.A., Kiggundu, B.M., & Tindiwensi, D. (2000). An investigation of the causes of accidents in the construction industry in Uganda. In *Proceedings of the 2nd international conference on construction in developing countries: Challenges facing the construction industry in developing countries, 15–17 November 2000*, Gaborone, Botswana.

Mbachu, J., & Nkado, R. (2006). Conceptual framework for assessment of client needs and satisfaction in the building development process. *Construction Management and Economics*, 24(1), 31–44.

McKibbin, W., & Fernando, R. (2021). The global macroeconomic impacts of COVID-19: Seven scenarios. *Asian Economic Papers*, 20(2), 1–30. https://doi.org/10.1162.

Nigel, S. (2018). *Engineering management: Project cost estimating.* London: Thomas Telford.

Perttula, P., Merjama, J., Kiurula, M., & Laitinen, H. (2003). Accidents in materials handling at construction sites. *Construction Management and Economics*, 21, 729–736.

Physical Planning Act. (2010) *Government of Uganda*. Entebbe: Government Publishing House.

Simpeh, F., & Amoah, C. (2021). Assessment of measures instituted to curb the spread of COVID-19 on construction site. *International Journal of Construction Management*. doi: 10.1080/15623599.2021.187467.

Yin, R.K. (2003). *Applications of case study research* (2nd ed.). Thousand Oaks, CA: Sage.

# 24 A digital approach to health and safety management on-site

## A silver lining of the COVID-19 pandemic

*Nikdokht Ghadiminia and Salman Saeidlou*

## 1 Introduction

In the wake of the global pandemic brought by the COVID-19 virus, industries are now more inclined to invest in the digitalisation of their modus operandi. This trend is also evident throughout all businesses within the construction sector. Despite the historical lag of the construction industry in adopting digital solutions, the restrictions brought by the pandemic have had a substantial influence on those reluctant to change their traditional practices (Yang et al., 2021). This is mainly due to the sharp rise in the number of COVID infections amongst construction workers around the world. The figures at the start of the pandemic illustrated that the construction workers were 30% more at risk of testing positive compared to workers in other sectors (Olukolajo et al., 2022; Silao et al., 2021) This led to the introduction of health and safety measures to control the rapid increase of the positive COVID-19 cases amongst the construction workers. These measures were focused on monitoring symptoms on a daily basis, temperature checks of the site attendees, and procedures to contain the infections such as social distancing and sterilisation facilities (Sami Ur Rehman et al., 2022).

The health and safety measures to combat the wide spread of COVID-19 within the construction sector led to a sharp decline in the delivery output of the majority of construction stakeholders. The limited supply of materials, shortages of labour force, lack of investment in digital solutions, late payments and disputes, as well as the unprecedented local and global isolation of resources caused significant disruptions to the delivery of projects (Majumder and Biswas, 2021). The construction sector within the UK reported major delays in the delivery of projects, leading to financial loss, quality deprivation and client dissatisfaction (Li et al., 2022).

The pandemic has shed new light on the potential benefits associated with the use of the wide variety of digital tools and technologies now available. These include cyber-physical systems and devices, networks, robotic construction, virtual reality (VR) and augmented reality (AR), laser scanning, drones, building information modelling and many more (Majumder and Biswas, 2021; Sami Ur Rehman et al., 2022; Tan and Abdul-Samad, 2022).

Despite the advanced technologies and digital tools introduced to the construction industry, the potential of these facilities was impeded by the lack of

DOI: 10.1201/9781003278368-27

investments, digital incompetency of professionals and the reluctance to change business strategies. Now, the construction sector is proactively working to embrace the digital solutions available to ease the burden of the pandemic and improve project deliverables, health and safety of employees and client satisfaction (Lv et al., 2022; Yang et al., 2021).

Hence, the aim of this study was to explore the technologies and digital solutions used to diminish the adverse impacts of the pandemic on project deliveries, whilst increasing health and safety standards on site. This was achieved through the fulfilment of three main objectives as follows: 1. To investigate the limitations brought by the pandemic to construction sites, 2. To explore the digital tools and technologies introduced to overcome these limitations and 3. To investigate the feasibility of these digital solutions in tackling health and safety on-site.

The following sections will provide an overview of the pandemic-related challenges and the digital solutions deployed at the construction phase of projects during the pandemic.

## 2   Overview of H&S technologies in construction

Technology advancements in the construction sector were mainly focused on ameliorating project performance and optimising delivery output. Most commonly adopted technologies, BIM, digital twins, wearable equipment, Internet of Things devices (IoT), AR and VR tools and laser scanners were developed to tackle the challenges and limitations of traditional construction (Okorie and Musonda, 2020; Seagers et al., 2022). The combined use of technologies facilitates achievement of the optimum potential of each invention. However, these technologies were also found useful to minimise and thwart health and safety risks on site. Examples include the use of wearable equipment paired with artificial intelligence (AI) and information communication (ICT) technologies to monitor temperature of the work environments. Alternatively, AI technology can assist with supervising compliance with regulations regarding the use of personal protective equipment (PPE) on site. More recent technological advancements also facilitate the use of robots and automated tools to prevent human exposure to high-risk activities on site (Seagers et al., 2022).

In light of the global pandemic, business strategies were reshaped to accommodate new COVID-19-related health and safety measures whilst enabling maximum operability for the workers in offices and on site. There are a number of case studies demonstrating the use of various digital solutions and devices to tackle pandemic complications on construction sites (Seagers et al., 2022; Yang et al., 2021). They have mostly focused on the use of digital communication and data exchange platforms to enhance information exchange and real-time communication of team members and project stakeholders under the social distancing and lockdown measures. Building information modelling as one of the key enablers of seamless communication, information exchange, real-time data updates and project coordination, has shown great potential in facilitating easy communications during and post-pandemic (Lv et al., 2022). However, the on-site installations, productions and construction activities are more difficult to manage through digital platforms and cyber spaces. They require labour attendance on site to enable physical operations, installations and storage of materials and machineries. This has led to the invention of autonomous tools and technologies paired with IoT to deliver remote operations, management and monitoring of site activities (Dai et al., 2021).

Despite the availability of advanced technologies within the sector, there are many constraints associated with the deployment of these tools. The cost of procuring and operating robots and devices for semi-autonomous and autonomous manoeuvres and installations on site, and the expertise required to use digital platforms are the most common issues addressed by several existing studies. However, COVID-19 has demonstrated the significance of overcoming these challenges to ensure the benefits associated with a mature digitalisation can be extended to improve health and safety for construction workers on site. Henceforth, more studies are required to evidence the use of digital tools as part of the reformation of health and safety management on site, and to further investigate the potential solutions that may be offered by the regulatory bodies, policy makers, researchers and industry professionals.

### 2.1   Re-discovering digital health and safety management on the construction site

Since 2020, the COVID-19 pandemic has significantly affected all stakeholders in the architecture, engineering, construction and operations (AECO) industry. Statistics showed that the number of positive COVID-19 cases amongst construction employees, particularly those involved in on-site activities, had been relatively higher compared to other industry sectors in North America, Europe, and East Asia (Pamidimukkala and Kermanshachi, 2021). This raised the flag for the health and safety authorities to further investigate and control the health decline of the workers resulting from the pandemic. Due to the nature of on-site construction work, it is challenging to manage the common COVID-19 measures used across other sectors, such as disinfection and social distancing considerations (Nnaji et al., 2022). In the UK, an extended period of lockdown was enforced by the government for all sectors. This resulted in (Pamidimukkala and Kermanshachi, 2021) an adverse impact on the project deliveries, due to disrupted services, shortages of labour, isolated supply chains and limited availability of machinery and materials. The closure of on-site activities directly imposed schedule delays and financial loss for many ongoing projects, as well as a cut in payments and staff salaries and lowered profits. The wider impact of this negatively affected the UK economy, causing high rates of unemployment and a sharp fall in the national Gross Domestic Product (GDP) (Li et al., 2022).

Despite the adversities, the COVID-19 pandemic has spiked the deployment of strategies to maintain cleaner and safer working environments for the labour force on site. The Health and Safety Executive (HSE) provided detailed guidelines and best practices to effectively diminish the fast spread of the COVID-19 virus. These guidelines proactively encourage the use of digital tools to monitor the symptoms and facilitate optimum social distancing measures for site workers (Simpeh and Amoah, 2022; Umeokafor et al., 2022). The strategic changes to site management and the introduction of new policies have significantly raised the scale of demand and investment for the implementation of digital technologies and tools. This is backed up by the need to restore the pre-pandemic project performance levels that were compromised during the pandemic. Hence, the pandemic is believed to have unleashed new potentials for the available digital solutions, which were hindered in traditional working processes and procedures.

There are many studies on the use of technology to overcome on-site construction challenges. The main focus has always been on performance enhancement, rather than the health and safety of workers or crisis management. With the spread of COVID-19 on construction sites, organisations turned to these digital solutions to maintain productivity and operate in safer ways (Lv et al., 2022). This was highlighted through the increased understanding of the correlation between worker health and safety and project performance (Yang et al., 2021).

Some of the most popular digital solutions and tools, including building information modelling (BIM), common data environments (CDEs), digital communication platforms (e.g., Microsoft Teams) and augmented and virtual reality devices (AR/VR technologies), were re-considered in a new light, to ease much of the financial and health-related burden brought by the virus to the construction industry (Lv et al., 2022). The enhanced deployment of technologies resulted in improved efficiency of stakeholder communications through digital platforms, as well as maintaining productivity throughout the pandemic. However, this has not always been successful in all projects, due to the challenges of digitisation and digitalisation amongst many stakeholders. In particular, small and medium organisations are the hardest hit, due to their unreadiness to digitalise working processes and the lack of finance to invest in the technologies used by larger organisations (Li et al., 2022). Hence, it is important to revisit the application of digital tools and technologies during the pandemic and investigate the ways these digital solutions can reshape the management of health and safety on construction sites in the new post-COVID norm or in a similar crisis in future (Yang et al., 2021).

## 3.0 Methodology

In light of the challenges brought about by the COVID-19 crisis and its direct impact on all individuals, the need for a qualitative enquiry into the experiences of construction workers and the way in which they tackled the crisis using various technologies is signified. Qualitative studies enable us to capture new knowledge, beyond the traditional textbook assumptions of the digitalisation processes (Busetto et al., 2020). Through semi-structured interviews with 21 site workers, the true facets of digital communication and remote working using technology were revealed.

The semi-structured interviews enabled the interviewer to explore the upheavals of technology enablement of on-site operations, whilst capturing fresh knowledge about which existing digital tools and systems can be integrated with traditional building methods. Although various case studies could provide knowledge of the aftermath and delivery outcomes of technology-enabled projects, this study was more inclined to capture individual experiences of the workers in operating digital tools and communicating through digital platforms (Moser and Korstjens, 2018).

The selection of the 21 interviewees was based on a set criterion to ensure the validity and reliability of findings. The common recommendation for the sample size in qualitative enquiries that involve in-depth interviews is between 10–30. The respondents were invited from different SME construction firms, as they were evidently hit hardest by the pandemic. Interviewees with more than three years of site-related work experience were shortlisted to reflect on the particular challenges of health and safety management on site in the COVID-19 era, compared to pre-COVID times. Table 24.1 provides an overview of the interviewees' roles, years of experience and organisational size.

Interviews were conducted through video calls using Microsoft Teams and Zoom software to enable wider access to industry professionals from across the UK. The interview questions were designed to direct the discussion towards various existing digital tools and solutions. All interviews were voice recorded to enable accurate transcription. The transcriptions were later coded in NVIVO software to facilitate easier management of codes and sub-codes, resulting from an interpretive content

*Table 24.1* Interviewees Profile Overview

| Organisation | Company Size (No. Employees) | Role/Responsibility | Years of Experience |
|---|---|---|---|
| Builder | 76 | Construction Worker | 5 |
| General Contractor | 125 | Site Manager | 8 |
| Real Estate (renovations/ development) | 54 | Building Service Engineers | 6 |
| Renovations | 30 | Operatives | 5 |
| Construction Manager | 98 | Surveyor | 3 |
| Home Developer | 131 | Site Manager | 8 |
| Construction Contractor | 67 | Site Manager | 12 |
| Domestic sub-contractor | 16 | Site Engineer | 6 |
| Developer | 93 | Sie Supervisor | 9 |
| Construction Manager | 142 | Site manager | 8 |
| Construction Manager | 85 | Surveyor | 3 |
| Design and Build Contractor | 116 | Surveyor | 4 |
| Construction Management | 54 | Project Manager | 6 |
| Builder | 38 | Construction Worker | 8 |
| Builder | 35 | Installer | 7 |
| Home Builders | 83 | Site Supervisor | 7 |
| Renovations | 25 | Installer | 3 |
| Renovations | 27 | Engineer | 3 |
| Construction Manager | 36 | Site Engineer | 6 |
| Contractor | 15 | Construction Worker | 3 |
| Contractor | 45 | Site Supervisor | 5 |

analysis. Findings were summarised and sent to the respondents to ensure the data was not misinterpreted by the researchers. The interviews revealed the digital approaches used to manage health and safety on site during the pandemic, whilst also shedding light on the challenges and obstacles experienced by the employees.

## 4.0  Findings

The findings were codified and grouped into three main categories. The first category corresponded to information provided regarding the challenges faced by the organisations as a result of the pandemic and the measures that were put in place to manage the spread of COVID-19, such as lockdown, temporary closure of construction sites, self-isolation, sanitary and disinfectant measures and on-site symptom monitoring. The second category included existing digital technologies to manage health and safety on site, and their usage during the pandemic. The third category reported the interviewees' experience of technology implementation and application of digital solutions for on-site tasks, during and after the pandemic. The following sections demonstrate findings using quotations stated by the interviewees, as indicated by the letter R and the number of interviewee (Rn).

### 4.1  Category 1: pandemic challenges faced by the construction firms

The interviews illustrated the adverse impacts of COVID-19 on the on-time delivery of projects, resulting from limited on-site construction. The large number of construction workers who tested positive for the virus early in the pandemic resulted in fewer workers on site. A number of respondents also shed light on the difficulties in obtaining materials and machinery on time due to the global disruptions and isolation of the supply chain (R3, R11, R19). These challenges were mainly considered as the underlying cause of delays in hand-over or temporary halts of projects in the construction phase, which in turn added additional burdens on the budgetary allowances of the project.

As stated by all respondents, the pandemic also resulted in a sharp increase in costs related to site activities, including transportation costs, materials and machinery, labour and the newly introduced health and safety measures to tackle the virus on sites (R5, R7, R10, R19, R21). Respondents 6 and 7 also reported the termination of their contracts due to the clients' incapability to cover the expenses. However, most projects were subject to prolonged disruption until further funding was acquired by the client. In light of this, Respondents 4, 5, 17 pointed to the need for amendments in some of the contract clauses to address the crisis brought about by the pandemic and to manage the compensation rights and procedures.

Due to the many difficulties the construction stakeholders faced during the pandemic, many respondents reported a positive rush towards digitalisation by their organisations. Most respondents were knowledgeable of the digital technologies that can assist with the implementation of the new health and safety measures for construction sites; however, they were all concerned about the expenses associated with their procurement. Respondents 12 and 19 pointed to the challenges associated with acquiring new hardware and software to facilitate the online communication of the project team and ensuring optimum coordination of all project tasks. Many respondents also stated that the online communications were inefficient, and the contractors and subcontractors were struggling to invest in cloud solutions and the relevant technical training for their staff (R5, R9).

The following section presents the second category of findings on the technologies available to support health and safety management on site.

### 4.2 Category 2: digital enablers of enhancing health and safety on site during the pandemic

The interviews also focused on how respondents perceived the application of digital technologies in managing health and safety on site, particularly during the pandemic. Most responses corresponded to the professionals' theoretical knowledge of the potential of the existing technologies. Only a limited number of participants were personally involved with the use of advanced technologies to monitor and manage health and safety on site (i.e., R6, R10, R18, R19), mainly because of financial burdens and a lack of investment. However, there were a number of technologies which were repeatedly named by the respondents. The most popular digital solutions used by the organisations were the information communication technologies (ICTs) such as email, Microsoft Teams and Zoom to communicate with fellow project stakeholders (R3, R12, R20, R11, R17). Others pointed to the digital platforms that enabled the exchange, analysis and storage of projects' digital data, such as building information modelling (BIM) (R7, R11) and Primavera (R2, R19, R21), as well as other Autodesk software (R13, R19). Respondents 11 and 12 also stated that their organisations had invested in AI-based temperature monitoring devices and disinfectant facilities to limit contagion on sites. However, others (R2, R15) mentioned that the monitoring measures were not consistently applied on all sites. Table 24.2 lists the digital tools and technologies extracted from the interview transcriptions which were believed to have wide-ranging application in the management of health and safety during the pandemic.

The semi-structured interviews enabled in-depth discussions about personal interactions with the existing technologies in construction. Respondents reported a rise in technology adoption, in particular for communication and information exchange. Despite regulatory pressures from the government and policy makers, health and safety management had been inconsistently approached by the construction sector. Many respondents demonstrated fair awareness of the latest technological advancements in the sector, such as the integration of AI and robotics in construction sites. However, the awareness was mainly sourced from newsletters, word of mouth, websites, journals and conferences. Furthermore, the majority of respondents described the pandemic as a powerful driver of digital transformation for the construction industry; albeit the cultural, economic and managerial challenges are still ahead of most small and medium firms in the construction sector. The next section presents the third category of findings, outlining the challenges of

Table 24.2 Technologies for Health and Safety management on-site during COVID-19

| Technology | Applicability Domain | | H&S application on-site | | | Recognition Basis |
|---|---|---|---|---|---|---|
| | Office | Site | Pre-Pandemic | During Pandemic | Post-Pandemic | Experience/Theory |
| **AI Based thermal mass temperature screen devices** | X | X | Non reported | Widely used across different projects | Still in-use | Experience |
| **Virtual Inspection Management** | | X | Limited | Collaborative AI to perform virtual inspections using imagery data collection and minimize labour attendance on site | Under further development | Theory |
| **Microsoft Teams, Skype, Zoom, Google Meet** | X | | Limited | Support WFH and self-isolation rules | Continued | Experience |
| **Cloud Computing, Shared Drives, Primavera, Common Data Environment (CDE)** | X | | Varied use across different organisations | sharp rise in the use of digital platforms to share data | Continued and on the rise | Experience |
| **BIM/Autodesk** | X | | Varied maturity across different organisations | Not much change reported in the use of BIM for H&S management | Continued and on the rise | Experience |
| **Autonomous Operations (e.g.Tunnel Boring Machines)** | | X | Limited (Project/ Client dependent) | Limited (Project/Client dependent) | Limited (Project/ Client dependent) | Experience & Theory |
| **Drones** | | X | Limited (Project/ Client dependent) | Limited (Project/Client dependent) | Limited (Project/ Client dependent) | Theory |
| **Robotic Construction** | | X | None Reported | None Reported | None Reported | Theory |
| **AI Based PPE monitoring system** | | X | Limited (Project/ Client dependent) | Limited (Project/Client dependent) | Limited (Project/ Client dependent) | Theory & Limited Experience |

implementing technology in the management of health and safety on construction sites, based on responses provided by the interviewees.

### 4.3    Category 3: feasibility of technology implementation and application of digital solutions on-site

The pandemic has brought disastrous impacts to all industry sectors, including the construction industry. Projects at the construction phase require a well-functioning supply chain including wide-ranging sectors, such as electrics and electronics, logistics and transportation and manufacturing. The financial adversaries of the local and global economy certainly hit all organisations in the construction sector, particularly the small and medium organisations, with limited financial backup. The majority of interviewees raised concerns about the financial losses during the pandemic. Respondents 12 and 19 shed light on the significant fall in investments for new projects. Some reported the early halt of projects mid-construction, due to insufficient funds (R18). Interviewees pointed out that the measures to monitor and manage the infection rates were too costly to be implemented consistently across all construction sites (R6, R12, R16). Respondents 9 and 17 signified a lack of motivation on the client side to spend more on the deployment of new technologies for their projects.

It was further reported that the use of digital solutions, such as the AI-enabled monitoring technologies, virtual site inspections, drones and robots were not practically viable for their projects. Respondents 10 and 21 also stated that the digital temperature screening devices were not always accurate. The lack of a reliable internet connection was reported as a key barrier to the use of advanced technologies on site (R6, R19). Participants had different views on the implementation and use of BIM for the management of health and safety on site (R12, R14, R20). Most participants were certain that BIM can potentially optimise the prediction and mitigation of health and safety hazards on site; however, not many of them expressed full readiness for using the technology to its full potential. Interviewees described a sudden pressure to self-train on the use of information communication solutions and digital platforms, without sufficient support from their employers. A number of participants further stated that the online training was insufficient to prepare them for the day-to-day tasks.

Many respondents claimed that more work needs to be done to seamlessly integrate digital solutions with on-site operations and activities (R13, R17, R18, R21). Many of the interviewees pointed to the need for a cultural shift, where construction workers and stakeholders involved in the supply-chain are well trained to use technologies and tools for both site operations and real-time communication of project information with other project members. In light of this, respondent 11 stated the following: "We need to develop readiness and establish reliable baselines to achieve the full potentials of digitalisation for projects; only then the clients will understand the value of investment in advanced technologies and digital tools in projects."

The results of this study highlighted that the unprecedented arrival of the pandemic in the UK and the immediate adversities forced the construction industry to shift towards new working methods without having the essential underpinnings for this fast-paced change. It was also found that the impact of workers' health and safety on project performance has positively influenced health and safety measures on site. Findings also demonstrated that the social distancing measures put in place by the UK government, including working from home measures and self-isolation rules, may have pushed an immediate digitisation rather than the digitalisation of working strategies. Interviews illustrated that many organisations did not have the necessary infrastructure to accommodate the shift towards digital ways of working.

## 5.0 Conclusions

Despite the promising advancement of technology for the construction sector, the study demonstrates the uncertainty of both clients and construction stakeholders in the feasibility of the application and deployment of these digital tools on site. Amid the challenges brought by the pandemic to the on-site construction work, the construction industry has been pushed towards a speedy implementation of digital practices, with limited organisational readiness across the sector. Findings from the in-depth interviews with on-site construction professionals showed limited knowledge and experience of the application of digital solutions in health and safety management on-site. Findings also emphasised the impediments of digital working methods on-site and their potential advantages in improving the efficiency of project deliveries, in similar pandemic conditions or the new normal.

Thus, the present findings add value to the existing knowledge about the challenges of digital transformation amongst small and medium construction firms during the pandemic. The lessons learnt from the management of health and safety during the crisis are key assets to post-pandemic organisational strategies and project management plans. Future research should also look into the successful projects where digital solutions were seamlessly used to achieve optimum on-site health and safety. It would be of value to focus on real-world case studies to identify the missing links between the anticipated potentials of these technologies and the real benefits derived from a mature digitalisation of health and safety management on site. This would encourage both clients and industry professionals to consider a wider adoption of technology for their future projects and would also ensure an easier transformation within the sector, as more clients will acknowledge the benefits and more investments will support the organisational digital transformation.

## References

Busetto, L., Wick, W., & Gumbinger, C. (2020). How to use and assess qualitative research methods. *Neurological Research and Practice 2020 2:1*, BioMed Central, 2(1), 1–10.

Dai, F., Olorunfemi, A., Peng, W., Cao, D., & Luo, X. (2021). Can mixed reality enhance safety communication on construction sites? An industry perspective. *Safety Science*, Elsevier, 133, 105009.

Li, Z., Jin, Y., Li, W., Meng, Q., & Hu, X. (2022). Impacts of COVID-19 on construction project management: A life cycle perspective. *Engineering, Construction and Architectural Management*, Emerald Group Holdings Ltd. https://doi.org/10.1108/ECAM-10-2021-0873/FULL/HTML.

Lv, Z., Chen, D., & Lv, H. (2022). Smart city construction and management by digital twins and BIM big data in COVID-19 scenario. *ACM Transactions on Multimedia Computing, Communications, and Applications*. Association for Computing Machinery (ACM). https://doi.org/10.1145/3529395.

Majumder, S., & Biswas, D. (2021). COVID-19 impacts construction industry: Now, then and future. *Lecture Notes on Data Engineering and Communications Technologies*, Springer Science and Business Media Deutschland GmbH, 60, 115–125.

Moser, A., & Korstjens, I. (2018). Series: Practical guidance to qualitative research. Part 3: Sampling, data collection and analysis. *European Journal of General Practice*, Taylor and Francis Ltd., 24(1), 9–18.

Nnaji, C., Jin, Z., & Karakhan, A. (2022). Safety and health management response to COVID-19 in the construction industry: A perspective of fieldworkers. *Process Safety and Environmental Protection*, Elsevier, 159, 477.

Okorie, V.N., & Musonda, I. (2020). An investigation on supervisor's ability and competency to conduct construction site health and safety induction training in Nigeria. *International Journal of Construction Management*, Taylor and Francis Ltd., 20(5), 357–366.

Olukolajo, M.A., Oyetunji, A.K., & Oluleye, I.B. (2022). Covid-19 protocols: Assessing construction site workers compliance. *Journal of Engineering, Design and Technology*, Emerald Group Holdings Ltd., 20(1), 115–131.

Pamidimukkala, A., & Kermanshachi, S. (2021). Impact of Covid-19 on field and office workforce in construction industry. *Project Leadership and Society*, Elsevier, 2, 100018.

Sami Ur Rehman, M., Shafiq, M.T., & Afzal, M. (2022). Impact of COVID-19 on project performance in the UAE construction industry. *Journal of Engineering, Design and Technology*, Emerald Group Holdings Ltd., 20(1), 245–266.

Seagers, J., Liu, Y., & Jebelli, H. (2022). Smart robotic system to fight the spread of COVID-19 at construction sites. In *Construction Research Congress 2022: Health and safety, workforce, and education: Selected papers from Construction Research Congress 2022* (Vol. 4-D, pp. 452–461). American Society of Civil Engineers (ASCE).

Silao, J.F., Guerrero, R.L., Pantalunan, C., Renomeron, C., & Jr., S.L. (2021). Pandemic risk management in construction projects. *International Journal of Recent Technology and Engineering (IJRTE)*, Blue Eyes Intelligence Engineering and Sciences Engineering and Sciences Publication – BEIESP, 10(2), 1–4.

Simpeh, F., & Amoah, C. (2022). COVID-19 guidelines incorporated in the health and safety management policies of construction firms. *Journal of Engineering, Design and Technology*, Emerald Group Holdings Ltd., 20(1), 6–23.

Tan, C.K.L., & Abdul-Samad, Z. (2022). A study of the impact of COVID-19 on construction workforce productivity in Malaysia. *International Journal of Productivity and Performance Management*, Emerald Group Holdings Ltd. https://doi.org/10.1108/IJPPM-07-2021-0421/FULL/24924/IJABM/2017.11/V5.ISS2/53.67.

Umeokafor, N., Evangelinos, K., & Windapo, A. (2022). Strategies for improving complex construction health and safety regulatory environments. *International Journal of Construction Management*, Taylor and Francis Ltd., 22(7), 1333–1344.

Yang, Y., Chan, A.P.C., Shan, M., Gao, R., Bao, F., Lyu, S., Zhang, Q., et al. (2021). Opportunities and challenges for construction health and safety technologies under the COVID-19 pandemic in Chinese construction projects. *International Journal of Environmental Research and Public Health*, Multidisciplinary Digital Publishing Institute (MDPI), 18(24), 13038.

# 25 Digitalisation differently

## An inclusive digital twin model for climate risk management in major projects in the post-COVID era

*Andrea Yunyan Jia, Fidelis Emuze and John Smallwood*

## Introduction

The COVID-19 pandemic has accelerated the Fourth Industrial Revolution (4IR) (WEF, 2022). In the construction sector, the accelerated digital transformation has dual impacts on the SHW of the PiC. It brings about efficiency and centralisation, yet reduces opportunities for workers' participation in system-level decisions. Centralisation leads to exclusion; exclusion loses information and results in the system being unresponsive to the reality of context. To de-centralise, it needs to keep the system open. This chapter contributes a critical review on the state of the 4IR technologies in managing weather information in significant projects, through which an inclusive digital twin (DT) model is envisioned to enable worker engagement, individual-level risk mitigation, more innovative project planning, and cross-project learning.

Osunsanmi et al. (2018) cluster 4IR technologies applied in construction into three categories, including an intelligent construction site, which includes prefabrication/modularisation, Internet of things (IoT), automation, Internet of services, product lifecycle management, human-computer interaction, additive manufacturing, radio-frequency identification (RFID), robotics, cyber-physical systems (CPS), and embedded systems; *simulation tools*, which includes Building Information Modelling (BIM), virtual reality (VR), and augmented reality (AR); and visualisation tools, which covers mobile computing, social media, big data, and cloud computing. Aghimien et al. (2019) classify 4IR technologies in construction into ten categories: IoT, cloud computing, big data, automation and robotics, BIM, additive manufacturing, simulation-based tools (such as VR, AR, and mixed reality), unmanned aerial vehicles (drones), and sensors/laser scanners. Other 4IR technologies applied in other parts of the world include georeferencing technologies such as global positioning systems (GPS), geospatial analytical tools such as geographic information systems (GIS), and data collection tools such as thermal imagery, wearables, and embedded sensors. These technologies come together to support a core concept in digital transformation: the DT. Hence, the study focuses on a multi-level DT concept for improving construction SHW, explicitly managing the heat stress risk related to the climate.

The natural environment is both a resource and a hazard in construction projects. PiCs' exposure to climatic risks is patterned by the works, products, rules,

DOI: 10.1201/9781003278368-28

and routines of the project process. In this sense, construction projects mediate between the local climate and the people working within it to produce a health and safety (H&S) outcome for the people working on the construction sites as their workplace. Hazards from the natural environment include ultraviolet exposure, air pollution, and vector-borne disease (Chigara and Smallwood, 2016). One of these risks is heat stress on the construction site from the local weather. The delivery of significant construction projects mainly involves organising a large workforce, which makes risk management a more substantial task (Narayanan and Huemann, 2021, Locatelli et al., 2021).

To become weather-responsive, construction projects must develop climate intelligence to manage weather information. Weather impacts the project through both extreme events and daily conditions. Severe weather conditions such as heavy rain, flooding, lightning, and typhoons bring direct safety risks to the PiC. Daily weather conditions such as heat render an accident-prone context for other construction activities. On construction sites, climatic heat is a systemic hazard to workers' H&S and a factor responsible for low productivity (Rowlinson, 1997, Dunne et al., 2013, Rowlinson et al., 2014). Apart from its direct consequence on heat stroke incidents on site and its long-term health consequences (Tawatsupa et al., 2012), heat stress is a catalyst for many other incidents that can impair workers' mental performance in hazardous work environments like construction sites (NECA, 2004, Mazlomi et al., 2017, Byrne et al., 2020). Suicide, an increasing mental health problem among construction workers, is conceptually linked to seasonality and weather conditions (Alashwal and Moustafa, 2022). The conceptual idea suggests that the potential for suicide may follow a seasonality pattern with a link between suicide rate and temperate (heat) conditions. Such observations show that weather issues affect the PiC, and efforts must not be spared in unpacking the solutions.

This chapter proposes a multi-level inclusive process DT model and reviews its enabling technologies for effective weather information management in significant projects. The following research questions guided the reported study:

• What characteristics of weather information interface with digital transformation in construction?
• What are the enabling technologies for data capturing, processing and risk management for a digital twin of the project process in response to real-time weather information?
• What are the characteristics of a digital twin model for managing climatic risks in major project delivery in the post-COVID era?

In the subsequent sections, this chapter will showcase how H&S issues will be addressed in the post-COVID-19 era, where technologies influence prevention, detection, and mitigation efforts in construction. From administrative practices to technologies, scholars have demonstrated how the COVID-19 pandemic impacts construction business and project aspects (Emuze, 2022). Improved planning and sequencing of work will secure sites (Jones et al., 2022), apart from the use of technologies such as DT and the internet of things (IoT) for telemonitoring (Mahmood and Rafaa, 2022). The chapter highlights the role of DT in the next section.

## Digital twins for SHW in construction

DT is "a digital representation of a physical asset, process or system" (CDBB, 2022). DT is created by a CPS as a virtual copy of the physical production system (Sawhney et al., 2020). A DT generally involves three key elements: the physical and digital parts, and the link. The digital part is more than a mere description of its physical twin but is in a dynamic relationship with its physical twin, driven by data. This involves data storage, model, analytics, and insights to support decision-making. Through machine learning and artificial intelligence, the digital part can formulate intervention for the physical aspect. For example, through data visualisation and analytics, DT can suggest options for decision-making or predictions (Sacks et al., 2020). In practice, DTs have been developed to serve different purposes and functions at different scopes, scales, and levels of detail.

Sacks et al. (2020) proposed a model of DT information systems that enables a data-driven approach for project planning and control. The DT model is centred on a plan-do-check-act cycle. They suggest five levels of feedback and control loops for handling different aspects of project delivery: (1) real-time monitoring and feedback for physical products and processes; (2) real-time monitoring and daily feedback on the supply of construction resources; (3) daily monitoring and daily to weekly feedback on product and process performance; (4) weekly to monthly analysis and feedback for systematic planning; and (5) project archive information for learning and long-term planning. They suggest "potential interactions between project digital twins of systems in the surrounding environments" as an area for future research. Sacks et al. (2020)'s multi-level DT model is adopted in this research as a conceptual framework to guide a literature review on the characteristics of weather information in construction projects and supporting technologies for handling it.

## Methodology

The research is a longitudinal study taking an abductive approach (Fellows and Liu, 2008). A longitudinal study in this research means understanding a phenomenon through observation over a prolonged period of time in different contexts. This approach allows deeper insights to be developed from the iteration between empirical observation and theoretical conceptualisation. The investigation was initiated based on empirical observations of on-site practice of work health and safety (WHS) management. First, the author did ethnographic fieldwork on construction projects from 2012 to 2017. Gaps in H&S risk management and utilisation of technologies were observed and meditated over time, from which cross-case commonalities were drawn. These observations and patterns were a snapshot of the state of regular practice before the COVID-19 pandemic, in 2011, 2012, and 2015, respectively. Based on the literature research, the initial insights and potentials were initially framed with Sacks et al. (2020)'s DT concept. Starting from this general framework, we thoroughly reviewed relevant research, and emerging technologies were expedited. The review envisions a DT model for weather information management in major projects and effective mitigation of H&S risks on the PiC site.

## Results and discussion

In this section, we first illustrate three cases from observation which set the base condition of on-site practice and its gaps before COVID-19. We then analyse the types of information needed for climate risk management in major projects. This is followed by a comprehensive review of the technologies and their potential to bridge the gaps. We then present a multi-level DT model for an inclusive digitalisation strategy.

### *On-site observations: state of the SHW practice before COVID-19*

#### *Case 1: digitization of H&S reporting*

Case 1 was observed in a residential building construction site in Queensland, Australia, in 2015. A site manager was inundated with loads of paperwork for reporting and documenting hazards and risks. In trying to delegate the task while saving cost, he developed an app that enables direct input of information on hazards, risks, and incidents into the iPad, which is uploaded to a central database. In this way, the project digitised H&S documentation.

#### *Case 2: three levels of risk assessment*

Case 2 was observed in a liquidated natural gas (LNG) facilities construction megaproject in Darwin, Australia, in 2015–17. During the project, a three-tier risk assessment procedure was implemented. These included a safe work method statement (SWMS) upon starting every new task, a job hazard analysis (JHA) being done every three months, and a personal risk assessment (PRA) that each worker needed to fill in three times a day. The SWMS and JHA were conducted by safety advisors or supervisors. The observed gap is that the PRAs were not followed up with immediate risk mitigation measures. The filled forms were used for project documentation only. The potential is to digitalise the PRA and utilise it as a tool to mobilise personal-level risk mitigation. The digitalisation of the PRA will also enable centralised data collection of the risks in association with their temporal and environmental conditions as a base for artificial intelligence to work on to generate smart (real-time and interactive) and personal alerts.

#### *Case 3: dynamic risk assessment*

Case 3 was observed in an underground railway project in Hong Kong in 2012. A dynamic risk assessment (DRA) exercise was conducted during a leadership walk around the site by an H&S management team led by the Construction Manager

(CM). Risks were effectively identified and noted. However, the identified risks were not resolved. The identified risks were not mitigated immediately for two reasons. First, the CM was overwhelmed by the day's production tasks and unprepared for the extra time and resources to handle H&S issues. Second, the intervention would request a holistic assessment of the interdependencies between the risk and its environment. The removal of one risk may generate new risks through the alteration of the environment. Here the gap and potential for digitalisation is in the automation of systemic risk assessment which will enable dynamic risk mitigation.

In summary, the three observed cases provide an empirical account for the gaps and technological potentials in the SHW management system before digitalisation. An essential task in SHW practice is reporting hazards and incidents and mitigating risks. Traditionally, this is done manually in paperwork. Most of it was done for documentation, yet mitigation action is often lost in reporting and is either ineffective or untimely. Digital transformation of risk reporting has dramatically improved the efficiency of SHW management. Yet it has not been mobilised to enable effective risk mitigation.

### Types of information needed for managing heat risks in major projects

The thermal environment is a context and condition for all on-site construction activities. Specific characteristics characterise the information on the thermal state on-site: First, it is workplace-specific, varying with spatial attributes within a construction site. Second, it is constructed between the thermal environment and work activities. Third, it is personal, based on physiological and health conditions. Finally, it is temporal, changing with project lifecycle stages and varying with the time of the day. The types of information needed for managing the personal heat stress of a construction worker are summarised in Table 25.1.

Climate patterns and project practice define weather information relative to major projects at the project level. In construction project management, weather-related factors such as heat stress are significant causes of project delay, but not all are legitimate reasons for granting project extensions (Assaf and Al-Hejji, 2006; Jung et al., 2016). Thorpe and Karan (2008, p. 816) note that most general conditions of project contracts only recognise adverse weather as a foreseeable factor that is legitimated for granting an extension of project duration, while average weather is not. Relative to this concern, Tian and de Wilde (2011) suggest differentiating between foreseeable and unforeseeable weather in climate projection modelling. It is also a necessity by the legal requirement to discriminate abnormal weather from abnormal weather conditions (Nguyen et al., 2010). Heat stress embedded in average weather thus causes a hazard to workers while the solution is not allowed. This is a gap to be addressed by 4IR technologies. The goal is a digital model with the capability of productivity forecast to facilitate setting realistic expectations for productivity and project schedules accordingly, which will help more scientific management of heat stress among the workers.

*Table 25.1* Types of information needed for managing personal heat stress on site.

| Parameter | Scale of variance | | Heat load contribution |
|---|---|---|---|
| | Time scale | Location/scale | |
| Temperature | Hour-Minute | Worksite-specific | Environmental heat |
| Humidity | Hour-Minute | Worksite-specific | Environmental heat |
| Solar radiant heat | Hour-Minute | Worksite-specific | Environmental heat |
| Wind speed | Minute | Worksite-specific | Heat dissipation |
| Workload | Hour-Minute | Task-Person | Metabolic heat |
| Work pace | Hour-Minute | Team-Person | Metabolic heat |
| Continuous work time | Hour-Minute | Project-Team | Metabolic heat |
| Fatigue | Day-Night | Person | Vulnerability to heat risk |
| Age/Gender | – | Person | Body's thermal regulation; personal risk propensity |
| Body mass | – | Person | Body surface area; metabolic heat |
| Body temperature | – | Person | Base temperature to a safe threshold |
| Health conditions | – | Person | Metabolic heat; vulnerability |
| Hydration status | Hour-minute | Person-Team | Body core temperature |
| Clothing | Daily | Person-Project | Heat dissipation capacity |

Ballesteros-Pérez et al. (2017) developed a methodology for estimating the impact of weather on the productivity of building projects, which varies with location and season, as does project duration. Using meteorological data to calculate and compare 15 scenarios of a building project in 15 regions of Spain, they demonstrated that in terms of the context of climate in Spain, projects starting in summer have the shortest durations in comparison to those starting in winter or autumn; projects located in regions of good weather have a shorter duration than those of bad weather. Nguyen et al. (2010) classify construction activities (e.g., excavation, foundation, and roofing) by three attributes: weather sensitivity, duration of the work activity, and the probability of the impacting weather condition, to estimate project schedule delay.

Weather conditions need to be forecasted to estimate productivity and project duration. Ballesteros-Pérez et al. (2018) developed a methodology of using national historical weather data to produce a set of weather delay maps for different climate zones in the UK. Using a sine curve, the methodology can predict productivity loss from daily weather variables and project delay. They suggested three steps to develop a weather-aware schedule for construction projects: (1) identifying weather-sensitive activities among the tasks, (2) estimating the needed time for each weather-sensitive activity, and (3) calculating the sum of time and the schedule extension needed. They found half-year projects are the most weather-sensitive types, while longer-term projects can offset this variability through the passing of seasons. However, the starting season of the project can make a difference of 5.7% to 38.3% in the duration of the extension. On this basis, they suggest considering the project starting date and seasonal patterns of regional climate in project scheduling. Furthermore, weather conditions vary vertically in the delivery of high-rise building projects. Such information is not available in the public meteorological system. Jung et al. (2016) developed a simulation model to profile vertical variance of the weather, including variances in solar radiation, maximum temperature, minimum temperature, average wind speed, average dew point temperature, and precipitation, for a finer forecast of project delay in high-rise building construction.

Regarding adopting 4IR technologies, Aghimien et al. (2019) identified the two most used 4IR technologies in South Africa: IoT and cloud computing. Smuts (2022) found that design and construction practitioners in South Africa anticipated the benefit of VR (including desktop-based VR, immersive VR, 3D Game-based VR, BIM-enabled VR, and AR) in terms of facilitating H&S training, specifically in providing immersive and realistic situations of workplace hazards to develop workers' capability in hazard identification and risk mitigation on site. However, despite the anticipation, they found none of the VR technologies were used in the practice of H&S training. These studies indicate a rapid increase in 4IR awareness among construction practitioners, but their actual adoption lags.

**Digital tools for personal heat risk management**

MeteoSwiss has set up an operating system for the prediction of heat stress and early warning linked to the monthly weather forecast by the European Centre for Medium-Range Weather Forecasts (ECMWF), based on data from weather stations throughout Europe (Noti et al., 2017). Rajagopalan et al. (2018) developed a mobile app to capture environmental heat data with a range of sensors, e.g., sensor-laden drones, Energy Buses, weather stations, stationery Temp-RH sensors, portable Temp-RH sensors, and portable infrared cameras, through citizen participation. The participating citizens help harvest the data from these sensors with their mobile app through Bluetooth low energy (BLE) technology via Wi-Fi and 4G cellular system. The mobile app could predict the thermal comfort level and suggest a simple heat stress mitigation tool. This protocol is potentially applicable to the work context of the construction site.

At the individual level, the United States (US) government developed a mobile app, a Heat Safety Tool (NIOSH, 2021), for personal use. The app provides real-time Heat Index information and hourly forecasts through automatic retrieval from the National Meteorological Service, anchored by Apple's location service. The app assesses the heat risk and provides related knowledge linked with first-aid methods, acclimatisation protocol, training, emergency plan, hydration protocol, and reminders for early signs and rest periods, etc. Project managers are using the app to justify time variations for completing their duties.

**Georeferencing and BIM-GIS integration**

To georeference BIM models, BuildingSMART Australasian developed a framework for integrating BIM and GIS by embedding BIM into its environmental context based on a set of laws, practices, and web protocols. Integrating BIM and GIS provides georeferenced BIM models of the built project, which will facilitate emergency responses during disaster situations such as fire, storm, flood, or earthquake (buildingSMART, 2012). Deng et al. (2019) developed a protocol to integrate 4D BIM and GIS for supplier selection and supply chain management. A BIM-GIS integrated model anchored information on transportation distance and material unit price. During a construction project undertaken in The Hague, Ohor et al. (2018) developed a system that allows adding georeferencing information to Revit 2018, which enabled the designers to relate the design information to the geographical knowledge of the environment and the site. Ponjavic and Karabegovic (2019) developed a location intelligence system that integrates BIM and GIS using a WebGIS solution based on OpenGeo architecture. The system was used for asset management of an airport, enabling smartphone access to the infrastructure database for inspection. The system can visualise the dynamic information of staff location, aircraft location, wildlife hazard (such as birds) assessment, and features that inform emergency decisions. They suggest a digital archive system for the relevant information for maintenance, upgrading, and further development of the airport. Such a system provides a prototype for managing the dynamic process of a significant construction project. They suggest using the Web Service Bus as part of Enterprise Architecture to facilitate integration.

**Enabling technologies for worker engagement**

Agent-based modelling provides an enabling technology for more active engagement of the PiCs. It enables responses to emergent situations by developing agents of specific behavioural characteristics. For example, Hattab and Hamzeh (2018) combine agent-based modelling with social network analysis to examine how the adoption of BIM has changed the design workflow. Trivedi and Rao (2018) used it to analyse scenarios of human panic behaviours to evaluate emergency evacuation strategies and identify possible bottlenecks and deficiencies indicated by evacuation time and agents' physical discomfort. Matthews et al. (2015) present a case of the RC frame (formwork, reinforcement concrete) in a commercial office development project in Perth's New City Link project using cloud-based BIM to manage the progress of the RC structure construction process. They re-engineered the project's paper-based process to align it with the information structure needed by the cloud-based BIM. They also designed a real-time object-oriented bi-directional system to capture on-site information and synchronise it with a federated BIM model. The modelling process acted as a system integrator during which the tasks aligned with the schedule, and the Quality Assurance procedures with the completed studies reporting made the data searchable. In this process, the site engineers and forepersons played an essential role in capturing and reporting real-time progress data with an iPad to the project planner, through the cloud-based BIM, for regular project schedule updates.

**Envisioning a process digital twin**

With the review of the state and potential of technologies, a multi-level process digital twin (PDT) model is envisioned to enable the project to respond to the changing weather information for the health benefit of the PiCs. PDTs are currently adopted in the manufacturing industry with the support of three advanced technologies, including cognitive services and advanced analytics; bot framework visual and speech recognition; and artificial intelligence, which feeds new insights to the supply chain (Microsoft, 2017). Data must be centralised to inform strategic decisions and localised for effective risk mitigation. The PDT needs to have the following four key characteristics:

- *Inclusive* – allow a lower level of information to be fed back upward, and the system is adapted accordingly to fit the SHW of the people at the bottom.
- *Informative* – people at all system levels must be informed of the thermal environment conditions at different times and in workplaces.
- *Responsive* – the PDT can respond to the identified risks and systemic adaptation on mitigation of the risks, and
- *Predictive* – the PDT can make customised daily heat stress forecast for preventive measures.

The multi-level PDT model is illustrated in Figure 25.1. Local actors are engaged and empowered for personal risk mitigation with a mobile digital tool at the individual level. A mobile app is needed to input and analyse the parameters of the specific workspace and the workers' health information. These data should be available to the individual worker only to ensure privacy while providing personalised user information for a heat risk assessment at a specific workplace. The anonymised data is then pooled for project schedule updates and planning. Beyond a project is the portfolio of projects of the client or the consultant's firm. The data pool enables inter-project learning and firm-level decisions on tendering and estimation. The team level and the site level PDT are between the individual and the project levels, which are periodically updated for more efficient coordination and daily work arrangement. The PDT has the same objective as a typical H&S report. An H&S report raises the awareness of PiC from the general worker to the craftsperson and the manager, to show the status of the use of SOPs (safe operating procedures) in work practices.

COVID-19 has transformed the worksite in construction. Scholars such as Alrashed et al. (2022) contend that DT can facilitate remote working during pandemic outbreaks by reducing the burden on physical services and infrastructure. Such observations resonate with the implications of PDT for COVID-19 in this chapter. PDT implies the ability to analyse data and study the impact on various body organs. For example, PDT can assist contractors and relevant PiC in the frontline to prepare for unforeseen health crises resulting from extreme or changing weather conditions.

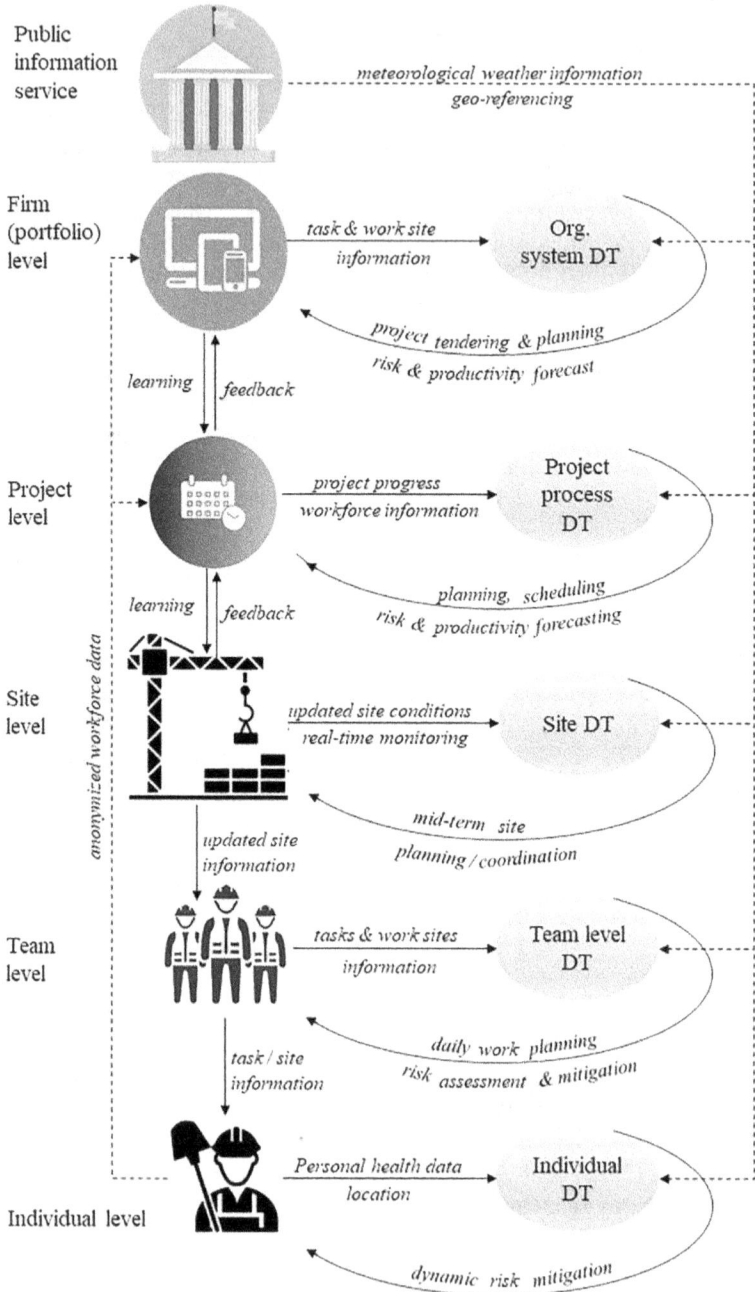

*Figure 25.1* A multi-level process digital twin framework for managing weather information in major projects.

*Source:* The authors

# Conclusion

This chapter presents a brief review of the state of the technology for weather information management on major construction projects. Through a review of existing technologies, the chapter envisions an inclusive model of a process digital twin that facilitates practical assessment and mitigation of SHW risks for the PiC. The use of PDT in the post-COVID-19 era can help to reduce the impact of changes in the worksite, especially with the analysis of real-time data that will handle health challenges. PDT is also open to engaging workers to participate in and contribute to the weather information management process. The information exclusively owned by individual workers is their personal health information and their local knowledge of the spatial environmental characteristics of the workplace and the task, which is of value to inter-project level and industry-level planning. A participatory georeferenced multi-level PDT model is envisioned to mitigate the heat stress risk locally while collecting anonymised data on the complex conditions of construction sites for future project planning. A central database is needed at an inter-project level to store and corroborate such information, which should be submitted to a national database for future estimation of project cost and duration in tendering. The challenge with system design is registering the complex spatial characteristics in the workplaces on construction sites, and how to put feasible and low-cost sensors to capture and transmit the needed data, including radiant heat and air velocity. This study contributes to a solution-oriented bottom-up approach to weather information management in major construction projects.

# Acknowledgement

The first author would like to acknowledge the University of Hong Kong, Curtin University Australia, National University of Singapore, and the University of Melbourne for their financial support when she worked with these institutions as Postdoctoral Fellow, Research Fellow, and Senior Lecturer over the past decade, during which the conceptualisation of the model was conceived and matured.

# References

Aghimien, D., Matabane, K., Aigbavboa, C., & Oke, A. (2019). Industry 4.0 diffusion in the South African construction industry: Construction professionals' perspective. In Haupt, T. & Akinlolu, M. (eds.), *Proceedings of the 13th Built Environment Conference, 2–3 September 2019*. Durban, South Africa: Association of Schools of Construction of South Africa.

Alashwal, A., & Moustafa, A.A. (2022). Weather and suicide of construction workers in Australia. *Proceedings of World Building Congress: Building our future, 27–30 June 2022*. Melbourne: RMIT.

Alrashed, S., Min-Allah, N., Ali, I., et al. (2022). COVID-19 outbreak and the role of digital twin. *Multimedia Tools and Applications*, 81, 26857–26871. https://doi.org/10.1007/s11042-021-11664-8.

Assaf, S.A., & Al-Hejji, S. (2006). Causes of delay in large construction projects. *International Journal of Project Management*, 24, 349–357.

Ballesteros-Pérez, P., Rojas-Céspedes, Y.A., Hughes, W., Kabiri, S., Pellicer, E., Mora-Melià, D., & Campo-Hitschfeld, M.L.D. (2017). Weather-wise: A weather-aware planning tool for improving construction productivity and dealing with claims. *Automation in Construction*, 84, 81–95.

Ballesteros-Pérez, P., Smith, S.T., Lloyd-Papworth, J.G., & Cooke, P. (2018). Incorporating the effect of weather in construction scheduling and management with sine wave curves: Application in the United Kingdom. *Construction Management and Economics*, 36, 666–682.

Buildingsmart. (2012). *National building information modelling initiative volume 1: Strategy, buildingSMART Australiasia.* Available at https://buildingsmart.org.au/wp-content/uploads/2014/03/NationalBIMIniativeReport_6June2012.pdf (Accessed 24 March 2019).

Byrne, J., Ludington-Hoe, S.M., & Voss, J.G. (2020). Occupational heat stress, thermal comfort, and cognitive performance in the OR: An integrative review. *AORN Journal*, 111, 536–545.

CDBB. (2022). *Gemini paper: What are connected digital twins?* Cambridge, United Kingdom: University of Cambridge, Centre for Digital Built Britain.

Chigara, B., & Smallwood, J. (2016). The impact of environmental thermal changes on construction health and safety in Zimbabwe. In E.M. Mwanaumo, I. Musonda, F. Muleya, M. Muya, J.N. Agumba, & C.S. Okoro (eds.), *Proceedings of the DII-2016 Conference on infrastructure development and investment strategies for Africa: Achieving solutions for renewable energy and sustainable development, 31 August–2 September 2016, Livingstone, Zambia.* Johannesburg: The Development and Investment in Infrastructure (DII) Conference Series.

Deng, Y., Gan, V.J.L., Das, M., Cheng, J.C.P., & Anumba, C. (2019). Integrating 4D BIM and GIS for construction supply chain management. *Journal of Construction Engineering and Management*, 145.

Dunne, J.P., Stouffer, R.J., & John, J.G. (2013). Reductions in labour capacity from heat stress under climate warming. *Nature Climate Change*, 3, 563–566.

Emuze, F. (2022). Guest editorial. *Journal of Engineering, Design and Technology*, 20(1), 1–5.

Fellows, R., & Liu, A. (2008). *Research methods for construction* (3rd ed.). Oxford: Wiley-Blackwell.

Hattab, M.A., & Hamzeh, F. (2018). Simulating the dynamics of social agents and information flows in BIM-based design. *Automation in Construction*, 92, 1–22.

Jones, W., Gibb, A.G.F., & Chow, V. (2022). Adapting to COVID-19 on construction sites: What are the lessons for long-term improvements in safety and worker effectiveness? *Journal of Engineering, Design and Technology*, 20(1), 66–85.

Jung, M., Park, M., Lee, H.-S., & Kim, H. (2016). Weather-delay simulation model based on vertical weather profile for high-rise building construction. *Journal of Construction Engineering and Management*, 142(6), 4016007. https://doi.org/10.1061/(ASCE)CO.1943-7862.0001109.

Locatelli, G., Greco, M., Invernizzi, D.C., Grimaldi, M., & Malizia, S. (2021). What about the people? Micro-foundations of open innovation in megaprojects. *International Journal of Project Management*, 39, 115–127.

Mahmood, A.F., & Rafaa, M.M. (2022). Designing a collection of two IoT-Systems for real time health telemonitoring. *Journal of Engineering, Design and Technology*, 20(1), 86–98.

Matthews, J., Love, P.E.D., Heinemann, S., Chandler, R., Rumsey, C., & Olatunj, O. (2015). Real time progress management: Re-engineering processes for cloud-based BIM in construction. *Automation in Construction*, 58(October 2015), 38–47.

Mazlomi, A., Golbabaei, F., Dehghan, S.F., Abbasinia, M., Khani, S.M., Ansari, M., & Hosseini, M. (2017). The influence of occupational heat exposure on cognitive performance and blood level of stress hormones: A field study report. *International Journal of Occupational Safety and Ergonomics*, 23, 431–439.

Microsoft. (2017). *The process digital twin: A step towards operational excellence*. Redmond, Washington, United States of America: Microsoft Corporation.

Narayanan, V.K., & Huemann, M. (2021). Engaging the organizational field: The case of project practices in a construction firm to contribute to an emerging economy. *International Journal of Project Management*, 39, 449–462.

NECA. (2004). *The effect of temperature on productivity*. Washington, DC: National Electrical Contractors Association.

Nguyen, L.D., Kneppers, J., de Soto, B.G., & Ibbs, W. (2010). Analysis of adverse weather for excusable delays. *Journal of Construction Engineering and Management*, 136(12), 1258–1267. https://doi.org/10.1061/(ASCE)CO.1943-7862.0000242.

NIOSH. (2021). *OSHA-NIOSH heat safety tool app*. Cincinnati, Ohio, United States of America: National Institute of Occupational Safety and Health.

Noti, P.-A., Spirig, C., Casanueva, A., Bhend, J., & Liniger, M. (2017). *Operational setup and skill analysis of a seb-seasonal forecasting system for detecting heat stress*. Zurich, Switzerland: Federal Office of Meteorology and Climatology MeteoSwiss.

Ohor, K.A., Diakité, A., Krijnen, T., Ledoux, H., & Stoter, J. (2018). Processing BIM and GIS models in practice: Experiences and recommendations from a GeoBIM project in the Netherlands. *ISPRS International Journal of Geo-Information*, 7.

Osunsanmi, T.O., Aigbavboa, C., & Oke, A. (2018). Construction 4.0: The future of the construction industry in South Africa. *International Journal of Civil and Environmental Engineering*, 12, 206–212.

Ponjavic, M., & Karabegovic, A. (2019). Location intelligence systems and data integration for airport capacities planning. *Computers*, 8.

Rajagopalan, P., Andamon, M. M., Paolini, R., & Santamouris, M. (2018). Developing experimental protocol for collecting large scale urban microclimate data through community participation. In P. Rajagopalan & M.M. Andamon (eds.), *Engaging architectural science: Meeting the challenges of higher density: 52nd international conference of the architectural science association 2018* (pp. 561–568). Melbourne, Australia: The Architectural Science Association and RMIT University.

Rowlinson, S. (1997). *Hong Kong construction site safety management*. Hong Kong: Sweet & Maxwell Limited.

Rowlinson, S., Jia, A.Y., Li, B., & Ju, C.C. (2014). Management of climatic heat stress risk in construction: A review of practices, methodologies, and future research. *Accident Analysis and Prevention*, 66, 187–198.

Sacks, R., Brilakis, I., Pikas, E., Xie, H.S., & Girolami, M. (2020). Construction with digital twin information systems. Data-Centric Engineering, 1, 1–26.

Sawhney, A., Riley, M., Irizarry, J., & Pérez, C.T. (2020). A proposed framework for Construction 4.0 based on a review of literature. *ASC 2020 (EPiC Series in Built Environment Vol. 1)*, 1, 301–309.

Smuts, D. (2022). *The use of virtual reality technology in health and safety training solution for construction sites*. BSc Hon dissertation, Port Elizabeth, South Africa, Faculty of Engineering, the Built Environment, and Technology, Nelson Mandela University.

Tawatsupa, B., Lim, L.L.-Y., Kjellstrom, T., Seubsman, S.-A., & Sleigh, A. (2012). Association between occupational heat stress and kidney disease among 37,816 workers in the Thai Cohort Study (TCS). *Journal of Epidemiology*, 22, 251–260.

Thorpe, D., & Karan, E.P. (2008). Method for calculating schedule delay considering weather conditions. In A. Dainty (ed.), *Procs 24th annual ARCOM conference, 1–3 September 2008* (pp. 809–818). Reading, United Kingdom: Association of Researchers in Construction Management.

Tian, W., & de Wilde, P. (2011). Uncertainty and sensitivity analysis of building performance using probabilistic climate projections: A UK case study. *Automation in Construction*, 20, 1096–1109.

Trivedi, A., & Rao, S. (2018). Agent-based modelling of emergency evacuations considering human panic behaviour. *IEEE Transactions on Computational Social Systems*, 5, 277–289.

WEF. (2022). *Regional action group for Africa: Attracting investment and accelerating fourth industrial revolution adoption in Africa.* White Paper, World Economic Forum.

# Index

For Product Safety Concerns and Information please contact our EU
representative  GPSR@taylorandfrancis.com
Taylor & Francis Verlag GmbH, Kaufingerstraße 24, 80331 München, Germany

www.ingramcontent.com/pod-product-compliance
Lightning Source LLC
Chambersburg PA
CBHW052117230326
41598CB00080B/3797

9 7 8 1 0 3 2 2 4 3 9 1 7